Child and Adolescent Psychiatry for the General Psychiatrist

Guest Editors

MALIA McCARTHY, MD
ROBERT L. HENDREN, DO

PSYCHIATRIC CLINICS OF NORTH AMERICA

www.psych.theclinics.com

March 2009 • Volume 32 • Number 1

SAUNDERS an imprint of ELSEVIER, Inc.

W.B. SAUNDERS COMPANY
A Division of Elsevier Inc.

1600 John F. Kennedy Boulevard ● Suite 1800 ● Philadelphia, PA 19103-2899

http://www.theclinics.com

PSYCHIATRIC CLINICS OF NORTH AMERICA Volume 32, Number 1
March 2009 ISSN 0193-953X, ISBN-13: 978-1-4377-0534-8, ISBN-10: 1-4377-0534-0
Editor: Sarah E. Barth
Developmental Editor: Donald Mumford

Psychiatric Clinics of North America (ISSN 0193-953X) is published quarterly by Elsevier Inc., 360 Park Avenue South, New York, NY 10010-1710. Months of issue are March, June, September, and December. Business and Editorial Offices: 1600 John F. Kennedy Blvd., Suite 1800, Philadelphia, PA 19103-2899. Periodicals postage paid at New York, NY and additional mailing offices. Subscription prices are $230.00 per year (US individuals), $398.00 per year (US institutions), $116.00 per year (US students/residents), $275.00 per year (Canadian individuals), $495.00 per year (Canadian Institutions), $342.00 per year (foreign individuals), $495.00 per year (foreign institutions), and $171.00 per year (international & Canadian students/residents). Foreign air speed delivery is included in all *Clinics'* subscription prices. All prices are subject to change without notice. **POSTMASTER:** Send address changes to *Psychiatric Clinics of North America*, Elsevier Periodicals Customer Service, 11830 Westline Industrial Drive, St. Louis, MO 63146. Customer Service: 1-800-654-2452 (US). From outside the United States, call 1-314-453-7041. Fax: 1-314-453-5170. E-mail: JournalsCustomer Service-usa@elsevier.com (for print support) and JournalsOnlineSupport-usa@elsevier.com (for online support).

Reprints. For copies of 100 or more, of articles in this publication, please contact the Commercial Reprints Department, Elsevier Inc., 360 Park Avenue South, New York, New York 10010-1710. Tel.: (212) 633-3813, Fax: (212) 462-1935, E-mail: reprints@elsevier.com.

Psychiatric Clinics of North America is covered in *MEDLINE/PubMed (Index Medicus)*, *Current Contents/Social and Behavioral Sciences*, *Social Science Citation Index*, *Embase/Excerpta Medica*, and PsycINFO.

Printed and bound by CPI Group (UK) Ltd, Croydon, CR0 4YY
Transferred to Digital Print 2011

Contributors

GUEST EDITORS

MALIA McCARTHY, MD
Associate Clinical Professor, Child and Adolescent Psychiatry Training Director,
Department of Psychiatry and Behavioral Sciences; and The M.I.N.D. Institute, University
of California, Davis Medical Center, Sacramento, California

ROBERT L. HENDREN, DO
Professor and Chief, Child and Adolescent Psychiatry, Department of Psychiatry and
Behavioral Sciences; and Executive Director, The M.I.N.D. Institute, University
of California, Davis Medical Center, Sacramento, California

AUTHORS

JIMMARK ABENOJAR, MD
Child and Adolescent Psychiatry Resident, Department of Psychiatry and Behavioral
Sciences, University of California, Davis, School of Medicine, Sacramento, California

THOMAS F. ANDERS, MD
Distinguished Professor (Emeritus), Department of Psychiatry and Behavioral Sciences,
University of California, Davis, School of Medicine, Sacramento, California

AMY BARKER, MD
Division of Child and Adolescent Psychiatry, Department of Psychiatry, Creighton
University/University of Nebraska Medical Center, Omaha, Nebraska

GAIL A. BERNSTEIN, MD
Endowed Professor in Child and Adolescent Anxiety Disorders; and Head, Program in
Child and Adolescent Anxiety and Mood Disorders, Division of Child & Adolescent
Psychiatry, University of Minnesota Medical School, Minneapolis, Minnesota

KIAH BERTOGLIO, BS
Department of Psychiatry and Behavioral Sciences and The M.I.N.D. Institute, University
of California, Davis Medical Center, Sacramento, California

ROBINDER K. BHANGOO, MD
Assistant Clinical Professor, Department of Psychiatry and Behavioral Sciences,
University of California, Davis, Sacramento, California

CAMERON S. CARTER, MD
Professor, Department of Psychiatry and Behavioral Sciences, University of California,
Davis, Sacramento, California

LOVINA CHAHAL, MD
Resident, Department of Psychiatry and Behavioral Sciences, Stanford University School
of Medicine, Stanford, California

SUFEN CHIU, MD, PhD
Assistant Clinical Professor, Department of Psychiatry and Behavioral Sciences, University of California, Davis, Sacramento, California

LINDSEY CORR, MD
Division of Child and Adolescent Psychiatry, Department of Psychiatry, Creighton University/University of Nebraska Medical Center, Omaha, Nebraska

CARL FEINSTEIN, MD
Professor, Department of Psychiatry and Behavioral Sciences; and Director, Division of Child and Adolescent Psychiatry, Lucile Packard Children's Hospital, Stanford University School of Medicine, Stanford, California

ROBERT FINDLING, MD
Director, Child and Adolescent Psychiatry, University Hospitals Case Medical Center, Case Western Reserve University School of Medicine, Cleveland, Ohio

SARAH A. FOTTI, MD
Assistant Professor of Psychiatry, Department of Psychiatry, PsycHealth Centre, University of Manitoba, Winnipeg, Manitoba, Canada

ROBERT L. HENDREN, DO
Professor and Chief, Child and Adolescent Psychiatry, Department of Psychiatry and Behavioral Sciences; and Executive Director, The M.I.N.D. Institute, University of California, Davis Medical Center, Sacramento, California

DAVID HESSL, PhD
Associate Professor of Clinical Psychiatry, Department of Psychiatry and Behavioral Sciences, The M.I.N.D. Institute, University of California, Davis, Sacramento, California

ROBERT HORST, MD
Assistant Clinical Professor, Department of Psychiatry, University of California at Davis; Medical Director, Sacramento County Child and Adolescent Psychiatry Services (CAPS), Sacramento, California

LAURENCE Y. KATZ, MD
Associate Professor of Psychiatry, Department of Psychiatry, PsycHealth Centre, University of Manitoba, Winnipeg, Manitoba, Canada

PENELOPE KNAPP, MD
Professor Emeritus, Psychiatry & Pediatrics, Department of Psychiatry and Behavioral Sciences, University of California, Davis, The M.I.N.D. Institute, Sacramento, California

CHRISTOPHER J. KRATOCHVIL, MD
Professor of Psychiatry and Pediatrics, Division of Child and Adolescent Psychiatry, Department of Psychiatry, University of Nebraska Medical Center, Omaha, Nebraska

VISHAL MADAAN, MD
Division of Child and Adolescent Psychiatry, Department of Psychiatry, Creighton University/University of Nebraska Medical Center, Omaha, Nebraska

ANN M. MASTERGEORGE, PhD
Assistant Adjunct Professor/Researcher, Human Development and Family Studies, University of California, Davis, The M.I.N.D. Institute, Davis Medical Center, Sacramento, California

MALIA McCARTHY, MD
Associate Clinical Professor, Child and Adolescent Psychiatry Training Director, Department of Psychiatry and Behavioral Sciences, University of California, Davis, School of Medicine; and The M.I.N.D. Institute, University of California, Davis Medical Center, Sacramento, California

MOLLY McVOY, MD
Fellow, Child and Adolescent Psychiatry, University Hospitals Case Medical Center, Cleveland, Ohio

W. PETER METZ, MD
Clinical Professor of Psychiatry, Division of Child and Adolescent Psychiatry, University of Massachusetts Medical Center, Worcester, Massachusetts

SUSAN MILAM-MILLER, MD
Volunteer Clinical Faculty, University of California Davis School of Medicine, Davis; Staff Psychiatrist, Sonoma County Mental Health; and Private Practice, Santa Rosa, California

EMILY OLSEN, BS
Imaging Research Center, University of California, Davis, Sacramento, California

LARA POSTL, MD
Resident in Psychiatry, Faculty of Medicine, PsycHealth Centre, University of Manitoba, Winnipeg, Manitoba, Canada

DAVID S. RUE, MD
Clinical Professor of Psychiatry, Department of Psychiatry and Behavioral Sciences, University of California Davis School of Medicine; and Medical Director, Child and Adolescent Services, Sutter Center for Psychiatry, Sutter Medical Center, Sacramento, California

MARJORIE SOLOMON, PhD
Assistant Professor of Clinical Psychiatry, Department of Psychiatry and Behavioral Sciences, Imaging Research Center, The M.I.N.D. Institute, University of California, Davis, Sacramento, California

BRIGETTE S. VAUGHAN, MSN, APRN
Division of Child and Adolescent Psychiatry, Department of Psychiatry, University of Nebraska Medical Center, Omaha, Nebraska

ANDREA M. VICTOR, PhD
Assistant Professor, Division of Child & Adolescent Psychiatry, University of Minnesota Medical School, Minneapolis, Minnesota

ASHLEY WHEELER, MD
Division of Child and Adolescent Psychiatry, Department of Psychiatry, Creighton University/University of Nebraska Medical Center, Omaha, Nebraska

NANCY C. WINTERS, MD
Associate Professor of Psychiatry, Division of Public Psychiatry, Oregon Health & Science University, Portland, Oregon

YUHUAN XIE, MD
Resident Physician, Division of Child and Adolescent Psychiatry, Department of Psychiatry and Behavioral Sciences, University of California Davis School of Medicine, Sacramento, California

Contents

Preface   xiii

Malia McCarthy and Robert L. Hendren

DISORDERS

New Developments in Autism   1

Kiah Bertoglio and Robert L. Hendren

The substantial increase in the prevalence of autism necessitates that practicing physicians become more familiar with the presentation of symptoms to improve early diagnoses and interventions, thus improving the prognosis for affected children. Autism is a complex neurodevelopmental disorder with a triad of core impairments in social interactions, repetitive behaviors, and communication. Clinically, autism appears as a spectrum, with many variations in the severity of defining behaviors and associated symptoms among children. Although the etiology of autism is unknown, it is thought to involve a genetic susceptibility that may be triggered by environmental factors. Because of the high variability in behaviors, biologic findings, and response to treatment, many specialists are assuming a theory of many different autisms, each of which may have a somewhat different etiology and response to treatment. Although there is no known cure for autism, many treatments are available to improve core and associated symptoms.

Psychiatric Phenotypes Associated with Neurogenetic Disorders   15

Carl Feinstein and Lovina Chahal

Advances in understanding the human genome and clinical application have led to identification of genetically based disorders that have distinctive behavioral phenotypes and risk for serious psychiatric disorders. Some patients have unrecognized genetic disorders presenting as psychiatric symptoms. Practitioners must be knowledgeable about the association between symptoms and underlying genetic bases. Treatment of neurogenetic disorders includes providing information about causes and prognoses. Patients are served best if they remain long term with a multidisciplinary team of providers who recognize the realities of a lifetime course, the high risk for symptom recurrence, and the need for providing information and support to families and coordinating medical and psychiatric care.

**Review of Pediatric Attention Deficit/Hyperactivity Disorder for the General
Psychiatrist**   39

Christopher J. Kratochvil, Brigette S. Vaughan, Amy Barker, Lindsey Corr,
Ashley Wheeler, and Vishal Madaan

Attention deficit/hyperactivity disorder (ADHD) is a common and impairing psychiatric condition, affecting significant numbers of children and adolescents. General psychiatrists serve, both by choice and out of necessity, in the assessment and treatment of children and adolescents who have ADHD and in the education of patients and their families. For many clinicians, however, there are numerous unanswered questions regarding the diagnosis and therapeutic interventions for ADHD. This article provides general psychiatrists with a practical overview and update on the assessment, diagnosis, and treatment of pediatric ADHD. Background information, recent relevant research, current evidence-based practice guidelines, and tips for clinical practice are reviewed in this article. The information is presented in a question-answer format.

Anxiety Disorders and Posttraumatic Stress Disorder Update   57

Andrea M. Victor and Gail A. Bernstein

Anxiety disorders are one of the most common categories of psychopathology in children and adolescents. This article provides an overview of several anxiety disorders that are diagnosed often during childhood and adolescence, including separation anxiety disorder, generalized anxiety disorder, social phobia, obsessive-compulsive disorder, and posttraumatic stress disorder. Although anxiety disorders commonly show similar clinical characteristics during childhood and adulthood, this article highlights some of the differences that may present across the life span.

Diagnostic Issues in Childhood Bipolar Disorder   71

Robert Horst

The field of psychiatry has largely discounted the existence of bipolar disorder (BD) in children and viewed adolescent-onset BD as uncommon until recently. Evidence demonstrating that a significant number of adults with BD report symptom onset before age 19 has led to an explosion in the recognition of childhood BD over the past decade. Because children and adolescents, including preschoolers, are being diagnosed with BD in rapidly increasing numbers, the criteria for mania are being adjusted in children and adolescents to accommodate various presentations of emotional dysregulation into the paradigm of BD. Still, it has yet to be seen whether these presentations will develop in adulthood into what we have traditionally considered to be BD. This blurring of the diagnostic lines has led to significant controversy in the field of child and adolescent psychiatry. This article introduces current thinking about this controversial diagnosis through two case examples.

Very Early Interventions in Psychotic Disorders   81

Robinder K. Bhangoo and Cameron S. Carter

It is well accepted that most serious psychiatric conditions begin in adolescence and are characterized by initial symptoms that predate the full manifestation of illness. This early period often consists of nonspecific symptoms, making accurate detection difficult. Classification as "prodromal" is only possible retrospectively, after a patient has developed positive psychotic symptoms. To monitor these patients prospectively, we must identify and follow patients who are at risk for psychosis, understanding that this group may also include false positives who do not go on to develop psychotic illness. Improving detection of at-risk individuals gives us an opportunity to intervene earlier in the course of the disorder, creating a window of opportunity to improve outcome and decrease overall burden of illness.

TREATMENT

Cognitive-Behavioral Therapy and Dialectical Behavior Therapy; Adaptations Required to Treat Adolescents

95

Laurence Y. Katz, Sarah A. Fotti, and Lara Postl

Conducting psychotherapy with adolescents is qualitatively different from psychotherapy with adults. Cognitive-behavioral therapy and dialectical behavior therapy are two types of psychotherapy commonly used in the treatment of adolescents. A brief review of the current state of research on these treatments is provided with a focus on anxiety disorders and depressive disorders. This article also describes adaptations of these treatments that will help the general psychiatrist to effectively conduct these treatments with adolescents in their practice.

Child and Adolescent Psychopharmacology Update

111

Molly McVoy and Robert Findling

Understanding pediatric psychopharmacology often is an important part of the practice of a general psychiatrist, as a substantial number of children and adolescents are affected by a major psychiatric illness. A general psychiatrist should consider some key issues before he or she begins prescribing psychotropic medications to children and adolescents. Some agents that are effective in adults may not be effective in youths, and similarly, medications that are well tolerated in adults may be associated with accentuated or additional risks when prescribed to young people. This article is an effort to summarize the recent advances in medication therapy of the pediatric population and bring the general psychiatrist up to date on the evidence-based psychopharmacologic treatment of children and adolescents.

SERVICE DELIVERY

The Wraparound Approach in Systems of Care

135

Nancy C. Winters and W. Peter Metz

Child and adolescent psychiatrists and general psychiatrists who serve children and adolescents with complex mental health needs, generally find themselves interfacing with multiple child-serving systems, including mental health, child welfare, juvenile justice, developmental disabilities, addictions services, and primary health care. In these systems of care, psychiatrists will likely encounter the term "wraparound," which describes a key intervention ushered in with the system-of-care model of service delivery. This article describes the wraparound approach, which has been at the forefront of mental health service delivery for children and youth with serious emotional disturbance since the mid-1980s. Wraparound is an empirically supported, family-driven, strengths-based planning approach that provides individualized care using an array of formal services and natural supports.

Disparities in Treating Culturally Diverse Children and Adolescents   153

David S. Rue and Yuhuan Xie

This article considers disparities in the psychiatric care of racial and ethnic children and adolescents, with respect to their under-utilization and under-treatment, especially with psychotropic medications. Culturally adapted psychotherapeutic approaches are discussed, as well as the notion of a culturally competent clinician who strives to apply his or her clinical skills while constantly making adjustments to the beliefs, habits, and circumstances of culturally diverse children and their parents, one patient at a time.

The Psychiatrist as Consultant: Working Within Schools, the Courts, and Primary Care to Promote Children's Mental Health   165

Susan Milam-Miller

This article presents a broad description of psychiatric consultation to schools to introduce concepts relevant in all child and adolescent psychiatric consultation outside of the hospital setting. A model of the consultation process is presented, which includes: (1) the consultant's entry into the system that is requesting consultation, (2) the process of defining the question posed, (3) identification of the focus of consultation and the consultant's role, and (4) measuring outcomes. Cases from psychiatric consultation to schools, juvenile justice, and primary care illustrate the various roles that a consultant may fill in providing consultative services for children and adolescents. Current trends in psychiatric consultation are described, including a shift away from indirect consultation and toward a collaborative role.

CONCEPTUAL ISSUES

Clinical Implications of Current Findings in Neurodevelopment   177

Penelope Knapp and Ann M. Mastergeorge

Research in the last decade has advanced our knowledge about biological factors underlying neurodevelopmental processes in childhood. Genetic research has gone beyond mapping the human genome to identifying epigenetic factors and explicating gene-environment interactions. Biological markers of vulnerability to specific disorders have been identified. The functions of and interactions between neuroanatomic regions have been illuminated by new imaging and other noninvasive techniques, such as EEG, event-related potentials, and functional magnetic resonance imaging, that allow us to link earliest signs of disorders to neurological changes. This article provides an overview of current findings in neurodevelopment, and discusses diagnostic factors, prevention and intervention, and clinical implications.

Towards a Neurodevelopmental Model of Clinical Case Formulation   199

Marjorie Solomon, David Hessl, Sufen Chiu, Emily Olsen, and Robert L. Hendren

Rapid advances in molecular genetics and neuroimaging over the last 10 to 20 years have been a catalyst for research in neurobiology, developmental psychopathology, and translational neuroscience. Methods of study in psychiatry, previously described as "slow maturing," now are becoming sufficiently sophisticated to more effectively investigate the biology of higher mental processes. Despite these technologic advances, the recognition that psychiatric disorders are disorders of neurodevelopment, and the importance of case formulation to clinical practice, a neurodevelopmental model of case formulation has not yet been articulated. The goals of this article, which is organized as a clinical case conference, are to begin to articulate a neurodevelopmental model of case formulation, to illustrate its value, and finally to explore how clinical psychiatric practice might evolve in the future if this model were employed.

Child and Adolescent Psychiatry for the Future: Challenges and Opportunities   213

Malia McCarthy, Jimmark Abenojar, and Thomas F. Anders

In this article, the authors focus on three particularly salient sets of issues that face the field of child and adolescent psychiatry as a sub-specialty of general psychiatry today—those related to workforce, public perception, and professional identity. In an article directed at the general psychiatrist, the authors present possibilities for refocusing the activities of the child and adolescent psychiatrist to emphasize consultative and collaborative roles. The authors embrace working in systems of care with communities and families as partners. Finally, they discuss the training implications of such shifts in professional identity, and the need to maintain the centrality of a scientifically-based developmental biopsychosocial formulation.

Index   227

FORTHCOMING ISSUES

June 2009
Ethics
Laura W. Roberts, MD, MA and
Jinger G. Hoop, MD, MFA, *Guest Editors*

September 2009
Anxiety
Uli Wittchen, MD and
Andrew T. Gloster, PhD, *Guest Editors*

December 2009
Schizophrenia Comorbidities
Michael Hwang, MD and
Henry Nasrallah, MD, *Guest Editors*

RECENT ISSUES

December 2008
Sexually Compulsive Behavior:
Hypersexuality
Mark F. Schwartz, ScD and
Fred S. Berlin, MD, PhD, *Guest Editors*

September 2008
Recent Research in Personality Disorders
Joel Paris, MD, *Guest Editor*

June 2008
Suicidal Behavior: A Developmental
Perspective
Maria A. Oquendo, MD and
J. John Mann, MD, *Guest Editors*

RELATED INTEREST

Child and Adolescent Psychiatry Clinics of North America, January 2009
(Vol. 18, No. 1)
Eating Disorders and Obesity
Beate Herpertz-Dahlmann, MD and Johannes Hebebrand, MD, *Guest Editors*
(see table of contents in the back of this issue)

Child and Adolescent Psychiatry Clinics of North America, April 2009 (Vol. 18, No. 2)
Bipolar Disorder
Jeffrey I. Hunt, MD and Daniel P. Dickstein, MD, *Guest Editors*

THE CLINICS ARE NOW AVAILABLE ONLINE!

Access your subscription at:
www.theclinics.com

Preface

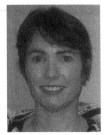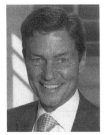

Malia McCarthy, MD   Robert L. Hendren, DO
Guest Editors

Because of a shortage and maldistribution of child and adolescent psychiatrists, general psychiatrists increasingly are being asked to evaluate and treat children and adolescents who are suspected of having or who have mental disorders. Improved recognition of the onset of many mental disorders early in their trajectory, increasing initiation of pharmacologic treatment at younger ages, interest from parents and teachers in getting the "best performance" from children who have behavioral, emotional, and cognitive difficulties, and the availability of newer pharmacologic agents with potentially fewer or less severe side effects are some of the reasons commonly given for this increased demand.

In spite of excellent efforts to increase the number of child and adolescent psychiatrists and to find better ways to share expertise with underserved areas, the supply has not kept pace with demand. This issue of the *Psychiatric Clinics of North America* is intended to deliver the latest information about some of the most common child and adolescent mental health issues that might involve a general psychiatrist. We hope this compilation of articles will be a useful reference in the offices of practitioners who have a background knowledge in general psychiatry but would like a quick review of the latest thinking and practice of child and adolescent psychiatry that is relevant to the general psychiatrist working in underserved areas.

The first section of this issue addresses topics organized as disorders. The articles are sequenced in the approximate developmental order in which these disorders might present in children. Autism spectrum disorders have increased dramatically in prevalence in recent years. "New Developments in Autism"

Psychiatr Clin N Am 32 (2009) xiii–xv
doi:10.1016/j.psc.2008.12.002   **psych.theclinics.com**

discusses some of the controversial issues pertaining to the pathophysiology of autism and provides a balanced discussion of interventions, including alternative treatments. "Psychiatric Issues in Genetic Syndromes" describes the current state of knowledge pertaining to genetically based disorders with distinctive behavioral phenotypes. "Review of Pediatric Attention Deficit/Hyperactivity Disorder for the General Psychiatrist" is an especially readable review of the most clinically relevant information pertaining to pediatric attention-deficit hyperactivity disorder. "Anxiety Disorders and Posttraumatic Stress Disorder Update," written by psychiatrists from a subspecialty child anxiety disorders clinic, provides an up-to-date review of the topic, highlighting differences across the lifespan. Because anxiety disorders often persist into adulthood, this article provides a useful perspective even for psychiatrists who do not treat children. Finally, perhaps one of the questions most frequently asked by general psychiatrists is "What is childhood bipolar disorder?" "Diagnostic Issues in Childhood Bipolar Disorder" addresses this controversial topic, while "Very Early Interventions in Psychotic Disorders" describes the emerging data regarding prodromal psychotic patients and associated interventions. Clearly, the implications for understanding these early processes are immense.

The next section, titled "Treatment," involved difficult decisions on our part, because the range of psychiatric interventions for children and adolescents is vast, and our page allotment is limited. Ultimately, we decided to focus on the interventions that we believe general psychiatrists in clinical practice treating children are most likely to use. "Cognitive-Behavior Therapy and Dialectical Behavior Therapy: Adaptations Required to Treat Adolescents" addresses exactly what its title describes. "Child and Adolescent Psychopharmacology Update" is as comprehensive and current a review as one is likely to find on this topic.

Section three, "Service Delivery," provides a context for the provision of child psychiatric care and emphasizes some of the unique aspects of treating children and adolescents. "The Wraparound Approach in Systems of Care" describes this widely used and potentially highly effective approach to treating children who have psychiatric disorders in community settings. "Disparities in Treating Culturally Diverse Children and Adolescents" addresses the underutilization and undertreatment of children from non-majority cultures. "The Psychiatrist as Consultant: Working within Schools, the Courts, and Primary Care to Promote Children's Mental Health" illustrates this increasingly relevant role for child psychiatrists.

The final section, "Conceptual Issues," begins with "Towards a Neurodevelopmental Model of Clinical Case Formulation." Case formulation is central to child psychiatric treatment, and many approaches are described in the literature. This article proposes another approach that we may find ourselves using increasingly in the future as our knowledge of the roles of and interactions between genes, environment, brain development, pathophysiology, neuropsychology, and behavior, as they pertain to child psychiatric disorders, grows. "Clinical Implications of Current Findings in Neurodevelopment" describes some of the latest such findings. Finally, "Child and Adolescent Psychiatry for the Future: Challenges and Opportunities" addresses current challenges to providing psychiatric treatment to children and adolescents, especially as related to workforce issues, public perception, and professional identity, and proposes future directions, with an emphasis on the role of the general psychiatrist.

We hope that this issue proves useful to you. We would like to thank Sarah Barth at Elsevier Publishing for her excellent guidance and support throughout this project.

We direct an ongoing workshop based on this issue at the annual meeting of the American Psychiatric Association and will appreciate knowing what is helpful to you and what is missing.

Malia McCarthy, MD
Department of Psychiatry and Behavioral Sciences
University of California, Davis
Medical Investigation of Neurodevelopmental Disorders (M.I.N.D.) Institute
2825 50th Street
Sacramento, CA 95817, USA

Robert L. Hendren, DO
Department of Psychiatry and Behavioral Sciences
University of California, Davis
Medical Investigation of Neurodevelopmental Disorders (M.I.N.D.) Institute
2825 50th Street
Sacramento, CA 95817, USA

E-mail addresses:
mmccarthy@ucdavis.edu (M. McCarthy)
rlhendren@ucdavis.edu (R.L. Hendren)

New Developments in Autism

Kiah Bertoglio, BS[a], Robert L. Hendren, DO[a],*

KEYWORDS

• Autism • Diagnosis • Psychopharmacology • Etiology
• Treatment • Epidemiology

The dramatic increase in the prevalence of autism within the past decade has been accompanied by an abundance of new research and treatment strategies. Although there is still no known cause or cure, the substantial progression of knowledge about the disorder in such a short period has left many professionals without adequate training on how to recognize and deal with the many cases suddenly presenting in their practice. This article is designed to provide basic information on the disorder to help equip the practicing physician with tools needed to identify early signs of autism, work with families of affected individuals, and implement optimal treatments.

Autism is characterized by a spectrum of abnormal behaviors that include marked impairment in reciprocal social interaction; communication difficulties; and restricted, repetitive, and stereotyped patterns of interests and activities.[1] Although the prognosis for children with autism is variable, most children with an early diagnosis of autism are not completely independent as adults[2] and the disorder generally has lifelong effects on a child's ability to be social, to care for himself or herself, and to participate in the community.[3] Autism often has a devastating impact on the affected child and his or her family members, who may experience associated anxiety, stress, mental illness, and lost productivity.[4] There is no effective means of prevention, no fully effective treatment, and no cure. Improved early diagnosis and a growing body of research are leading to the development of promising treatments and improved outcomes for affected individuals, however.

The increase in the prevalence of autism from 1 in 2500 in the 1980s to 1 in 150 in the past decade has raised great concern.[5,6] Substantial controversy exists as to whether this is attributable to the more frequent emergence of the disorder from an increase in potential triggers, such as environmental toxins, or is simply the result of evolving

This work was partly supported by grant 3031 from Autism Speaks, grant 1R21MH080026-01A1 from the National Institutes of Health, grants CN138179 and CN138180 from Bristol Meyer Squib, Inc., and grant NPL-2008-4-AUTUS-004 from Neuropharm, LTD.
Department of Psychiatry and Behavioral Sciences and The M.I.N.D. Institute, University of California, Davis Medical Center, 2825 50th Street, Sacramento, CA 95817, USA
* Corresponding author.
E-mail address: rlhendren@ucdavis.edu (R.L. Hendren).

diagnostic practices and a heightened attention to the disorder that have led to more sensitive diagnostic measures and more frequent diagnoses.[7]

Demographic findings on the disorder have been slim and varied. Autism is four times more likely to emerge in boys compared with girls, although the reasons for this are not fully understood.[8] Although most studies have not identified differences in race among affected individuals,[9] some have revealed variations. Most studies report a higher incidence of autism among immigrants when compared with natives.[10] Additionally, a recent study identified lower rates of autism in Latino populations when compared with non-Latino populations, with comparably similar rates in other ethnicities. The same study also identified lower rates of autism in populations with lower socioeconomic status.[11] It is unclear whether this represents a true difference in prevalence or whether it reflects fewer diagnoses being made in underserved and less educated populations, however. No well-established studies have consistently identified differences in the rates of autism across ethnicities or demographic backgrounds. Therefore, most professionals maintain a belief that the occurrence of autism is not influenced by economic, social, racial, or ethnic background.[12]

DIAGNOSIS
Characteristic Features of Autism

In the *Diagnostic and Statistical Manual of Mental Disorders, Fourth Edition* (DSM-IV), autism is classified as one of the five pervasive developmental disorders (PDDs) and is characterized by impairments in the three domains of social interaction, communication, and repetitive behaviors.[1] Autism is often referred to as autism spectrum disorder (ASD), because the severity and manifestation of these symptoms vary widely, ranging from modest social ailments to severe developmental and behavioral challenges.[13]

Impaired social interactions may include but are not limited to poor eye contact, difficulty in understanding and relaying appropriate social gestures, trouble in interpreting facial expressions, lack of joint attention, and limited or inappropriate facial expressions. Poorly developed empathy and lack of reciprocity are also characteristic traits of the disorder. Many children with autism express the desire to have friends but do not know how to initiate or maintain relationships, and often do not have a clear understanding of what friendship involves.[14–16]

Nonverbal and verbal communication is often impaired in autism. The development of language is delayed in most affected children. Thirty percent of children with autism experience regression, usually before 36 months of age, wherein they frequently lose any previously acquired language.[17] Although many are able to reacquire verbal skills, some never develop language. Individuals with autism who do exhibit adequate speech usually have difficulty in initiating and sustaining conversations outside of their focused interests. Their speech is often repetitive and rote, echoing phrases from surrounding individuals, movies, video games, or books. Children with autism also typically have difficulty in understanding and integrating abstract concepts, focusing their discord on concrete ideas. Nonverbal communication is also impaired in autism, because these children typically use inadequate or inappropriate gestures, which may include failing to point or to shake their head for "yes" or "no".[18]

In addition to impaired social interaction and communication, children on the spectrum display repetitive behaviors or stereotyped patterns of interests. This may include a wide range of behaviors involving excessive circumscribed preoccupations, inflexible mannerisms, and preoccupation with parts of the whole. For example, children who have autism may have their interest overly focused on parts of toys as opposed to the toy as a whole or may be interested in objects of a more unusual nature, such as pipes, fans, or vents. These children may have a strong desire to read the same book incessantly or to watch the same movie. Some of these behaviors, called self-stimulatory behaviors or "stimming," may arise from the child's unusual sensory integration, which may be satisfied by behaviors, such as spinning, flapping arms, or repetitive blinking.[18]

Differentiating Autism from Other Pervasive Developmental Disorders

In the DSM-IV, autistic disorder, Asperger's disorder, and PDD not otherwise specified (PDD-NOS) are the most commonly diagnosed disorders, and perhaps the most difficult to differentiate within the PDD category. When the symptoms of autism are present without significant language or cognitive delay, a diagnosis of Asperger's disorder is often assigned. The diagnostic assignment of autism is also often appropriate, however, because language delay is usually present but not required for a diagnosis of autism, although impairment is.[19,20] Such extensive overlapping criteria between the disorders have created substantial debate as to whether Asperger's disorder is on the continuum of ASD as an equivalent to high-functioning autism (HFA)[20] or whether it represents a separate disorder.[21] Individuals with Asperger's disorder and those with HFA may be obsessed with certain topics; may have learning disabilities in reading, writing, and mathematics; may have an unusually accurate memory for certain information and facts; may exhibit peculiar referencing during conversations; and may be hypersensitive to loud sounds, lights, and odors. Studies conducted by Szatmari and colleagues[22] and Fine and colleagues[23] suggest that children who have HFA have more frequent echolalia, pronoun reversal, and difficulty with conversation and intonation compared with children who have Asperger's disorder. Contradictory studies have found no difference in the frequency of these symptoms between the two disorders, however.[24] Conversely, a diagnosis of PDD-NOS is often assigned to children who exhibit subthreshold symptoms, when repetitive behaviors are not present, or when language develops late. Rett's syndrome and childhood disintegrative disorder, the other two diagnoses within the PDD category, are much less common and are associated with characteristic neurologic regression, making them more easily differentiated from ASDs.

Diagnostic Tools

An autism diagnosis is best made by an experienced clinician using the DSM-IV. A reliable diagnosis may also require the addition of the Autism Diagnostic Observation Schedule (ADOS), an interactive assessment with the child using one of four modules, which is selected based on the amount of language the child has developed.[25] The Autism Diagnostic Interview, Revised (ADI-R) is the other main diagnostic tool, consisting of an extensive interview with the caregiver that focuses on details of the child's development between the ages of 3 and 4 years.[26] Diagnosis is most accurately confirmed when both tests are used, providing an extensive parent-reported history of the child along with a clinician's objective evaluation through a standardized test.

Although the ADOS and the ADI-R are the most reliable assessments to diagnose autism, they require extensive training, certification, and time to administer and were designed to be used for research studies. Other assessments that may be used include the Social Communication Questionnaire (SCQ), Childhood Autism Rating Scale (CARS), Autism Behavior Checklist (ABC), Checklist for Autism in Toddlers (CHAT), Modified Checklist for Autism in Toddlers (M-CHAT), and Pervasive Developmental Disorder Screening Test (PDDST). Although these assessments do not provide definitive diagnoses, they may serve as valuable screening tools that may help a clinician to determine whether a referral for more extensive evaluation is indicated.

Early Identification

Although periods of developmental delay may be observed in typically developing children, they are often among the earliest presenting symptoms in children who have ASDs. Primary care practitioners (PCPs) are often the first professionals to whom parents turn when they are concerned about their child's development. It is therefore important that PCPs be sensitive to early diagnostic signs and that they be familiar with referral resources for diagnostic confirmation and behavioral, speech, and pharmacologic treatment so as to provide affected children with the earliest possible intervention.

Characteristic emerging symptoms of autism may be identified in children only a few months old. Autism may be reliably diagnosed around the age of 2 years. The hallmark symptom for evaluation is delayed or abnormal development of speech. Many other characteristic symptoms, including absent or impaired joint attention, affect sharing, eye contact, interest in other children, simple pretend play, and responding to name, may present before obvious disturbances in language development, however. Social referencing, the process of understanding others through observation and changing one's behaviors accordingly, is also limited in autism. These behaviors reliably distinguish children with early-onset autism from those with other developmental disorders.[27,28] Therefore, the first indication of these behaviors warrants close monitoring, and the maintenance and progression of these symptoms necessitate diagnostic evaluation.[27,28] Indications for an immediate evaluation include no babbling or gesturing by 12 months of age, no single word by 16 months of age, no two-word phrases by 24 months of age, and any loss of language or social skills at any age.[29] Other red-flag concerns include sensory issues, such as being hyperreactive or hyporeactive, in addition to problems with sleep, feeding, and coordination.[28]

Before assigning a diagnosis of autism, other causes of developmental disturbances ought to be ruled out. If pica is present, lead poisoning should be assessed, which can present symptoms similar to those of autism. Genetic disorders that need to be ruled out include fragile X syndrome, neurofibromatosis, tuberous sclerosis, velocardiofacial syndrome, 15 q duplications, and Angelman's syndrome. Audiologic and visual examinations also need to be conducted, because hearing loss may account for the presentation of some emerging autistic behaviors.[30]

PATHOPHYSIOLOGY
Genetic Susceptibility to an Environmental Trigger

Autism is thought to involve a complex interaction between multiple and variable susceptibility genes,[31] epigenetic effects,[32] and environmental factors.[33] Many believe that autism results when a genetically susceptible child is exposed to an environmental trigger. Research into the pathophysiology of autism suggests multiple potential mechanisms, further supporting the likelihood of different groups of autisms. Although no consistent biomarkers have been identified, results from these studies suggest a role of inflammation, abnormal immunity, and neuronal disconnect in at least some types of autism.

A genetic basis for autism is well accepted among most researchers in the field. There is an increased risk for autism among siblings, with a 4% to 10% risk for subsequent offspring developing the disorder.[1] Identical twins share a 36% to 96% likelihood of having ASD compared with fraternal twins, who have up to a 30% risk for sharing the disorder.[34] In addition, one study reported that men 40 years of age or older are almost six times more likely to father a child who has autism than men younger than 30 years of age.[35] Although a specific gene for autism has not been identified, several potential genetic factors have been linked to autism, suggesting that susceptibility to the disorder may involve a combination of various genes. Specific genes implicated in ASD include genes at the loci 2q, 7q31 to 7q36, 15q11 to 15q13, and 16p13.[34,36,37] One recent study showed a strong association of the mesenchymal-epithelial transition factor (MET) receptor gene at the locus 7q31 with ASD, suggesting an immune gut-brain connection.[38] These studies and others provide compelling evidence for a genetic contribution to the development of autism.

The nature of the environmental trigger, proposed to be the next step in the development of autism, is more controversial. Documented environmental factors associated with autism include prenatal or early postnatal exposure to viral infections, valproic acid (Depakote), or thalidomide (Thalomid).[39] There is substantial controversy regarding the potential role of mercury, lead, and other heavy metals, in addition to vaccines and chemicals, in the etiology of autism. Although some studies have found high levels of heavy metals, such as mercury, in children with autism, it is unclear whether or not they are etiologically related to the disorder. A potential mechanism of heavy metal influence is the induction of oxidative stress.[40] Similarly, the role of vaccines in the disorder is heavily debated, with many parents reporting regression in their child immediately after vaccination. No causative link has been found between vaccines and autism,[7] and it is vastly important for children to continue to be immunized to prevent the emergence of other diseases. Some studies have shown a higher incidence of autism with increased exposure to mercury from Thimerosal-containing vaccines, however, warranting the continued removal of Thimerosal from vaccines.[41] A safe suggestion for parents hesitant to vaccinate their child may be to spread out their vaccines over a period of several months instead of administering all vaccines during one visit, especially if immune deficiencies are suspected.

Research to date has identified immune, oxidative stress, neurotransmitter, and epileptiform abnormalities in many affected individuals, although consistent biomarkers for these potential pathogeneses have not been identified.[34] Although there is evidence for depressed immunity in some affected individuals, as supported by their frequent infections and other findings, such as low lymphocyte numbers, substantial research has also shown an overactive immune system in many individuals who have the disorder. High levels of leukocytes, autoantibodies, and inflammatory cytokines support a hyperimmunity and an overall inflammatory process that may be influential in the development of ASD. An inflammatory process might also explain the common gastrointestinal symptoms and frequent allergies seen in many affected children.[42] Although approximately 30% of children who have autism have seizures, as many as 65% have abnormal electroencephalographic activity, suggesting potential dysfunctional neuronal connectivity.[43,44] This is further supported by findings of high levels of glutamate in children who have autism, creating an environment known to cause excitoxicity.[45] All these abnormalities can be antagonized by, and contribute to, oxidative stress. This finding has been noted in many children with autism who have been identified as having high levels of reactive oxidative species, such as nitric oxide, xanthine oxidase, and thiobarbituric acid reactive substances,[46,47] and low levels of antioxidants, such as glutathione (GSH)[48] and superoxide dismutase.[49]

Although brain abnormalities in autism are complex and not consistently identified,[50] studies have discovered an intriguing pattern of brain growth. This research indicates that infants with autism have the same or slightly smaller sized brains than typically developing children,[51] which then rapidly enlarge until the age 4 years, after which growth slows during subsequent stages of development.[52–54] By adolescence, most children with autism have a similar overall brain size as typically developing children but with varying abnormalities, which often include enlarged white matter and decreased Purkinje cells.[55,56] This pattern exemplifies one finding that is consistent with the theories of inflammation, oxidative stress, and underconnectivity. Nevertheless, it is difficult to ascertain whether these abnormalities are primary mechanisms in the pathogenesis of autism or whether they are secondary to the disorder.

Many Different Autisms?

The spectrum of symptoms and their severity, variety of associated symptoms, inconsistent physiologic findings, and varying response to treatment strongly support the presence of subgroups within the disorder, each of which may have a somewhat different etiology and response to treatment. An excellent example of this is fragile X syndrome, a genetic mutation that accounts for approximately 2% of autism cases through a unique etiology. Children with fragile X syndrome possess clinical features that are distinct from those of other autisms (see the article by Solomon elsewhere in this issue).[57]

Although we do not yet know the causes of the other "autisms," many clinicians cluster cases into groups based on commonly associated symptoms. Thirty percent of children with autism exhibit regression.[58] An additional 30% of children have seizures, and up to 65% display abnormal electroencephalograms.[43,44] Mental retardation is found in 70% of children with autism, according to the DSM-IV Text Revision (TR), whereas few affected children possess savant skills.[59] Frequent infections, allergies, and chronic gastrointestinal symptoms are also often associated with the disorder.[60–62]

Commonly associated behaviors include inattention, aggression, impulsivity, hyperactivity, excessive compulsions, affective instability, and, occasionally, psychosis. Studies report widely varying comorbidities of autism with attention deficit hyperactivity disorder (ADHD), obsessive compulsive disorder, Tourette's disorder, bipolar disorder, and schizophrenia, however.[63] Additionally, many children exhibit subthreshold symptoms of these disorders, which makes it difficult to discern whether or not these symptoms are simply variations in the autism spectrum or represent full comorbid diagnoses. Regardless of whether the children are diagnosed with a full comorbidity, treatment needs to be targeted to address their symptoms.

TREATMENT

The abundant anecdotal reports of promise with early intervention are increasingly supported by studies demonstrating substantial cortical plasticity during early development[64] and positive outcomes from many early educational and behavioral intervention programs.[65] Therefore, routine screening and diagnostic evaluation of children exhibiting early signs of the disorder, along with more studies focused on early identification, are crucial in the path toward a better prognosis. Better outcome is associated with higher IQ, language ability and the ability to perform cognitive shifts.[66] Although core features of autism may not dramatically change, behavioral and medical intervention often substantially improves adaptive skills, showing most promise when implemented in conjunction with each other.

Behavioral Interventions

Applied behavior analysis (ABA), an in-home or school one-on-one behavioral intervention program, is one of the most studied treatments for autism and is often effective in helping the child to develop adaptive functioning skills.[65] Such behavioral programs may include up to 40 hours per week of intervention, with younger children usually assigned more treatment hours. The Denver Model is a promising expansion of ABA and other more child-centered approaches, which integrate developmental, behavioral, and relationship-based interventions.[67] Other approaches are often used during in-home programs, including Treatment and Education of Autistic and Related Communication Handicapped Children (TEACCH), which targets characteristic traits of autism, such as impaired visuospatial skills, need for structure, and strengths in visual over verbal communication,[68] and pivotal response training, which involves using child-centered reinforcers and motivational factors to teach communication, self-help, academic, social, and recreational skills.[69] Parent training is often also incorporated to provide consistency with the implemented program and to help parents learn how to meet the needs of their child most effectively.

Occupational therapy (OT) can also be extremely beneficial by addressing the child's unique sensory integration needs and by providing learning skills to obtain sensory input for more effective self-regulation independently and appropriately. Regular sessions with a speech therapist or the use of assistive technologies, such as pictures and computers, also often helps to address the language delays experienced by most affected children.

Pharmacologic Treatments

Although pharmacologic treatments do not target the core symptoms of autism, many medications are available to ameliorate associated symptoms, which often prove to be the most disturbing in the lives of affected children and their families. When considering pharmacologic treatment, it is important to identify the potential target symptom and its likelihood of response. Some medications used to address these symptoms are briefly discussed here but are also thoroughly elaborated on elsewhere.[70]

Aggression, self-injurious behavior, and irritability are the only associated symptoms of autism that have a pharmacologic treatment approved by the US Food and Drug Administration with the atypical antipsychotic risperidone. Clinical findings also support the use of risperidone for rigidity and transitions, in addition to cognitive disorganization. Children who do not respond to risperidone, or who experience side effects from the medication, may benefit from another medication in this class, such as aripiprazole (Abilify) or quetiapine (Seroquel), which have also been found to be effective in treating these symptoms. Weight gain and sedation are the most common side effects of the atypical antipsychotics, although akasthia and extrapyramidal symptoms do rarely occur.[71]

Repetitive and compulsive behaviors, in addition to cognitive rigidity and anxiety associated with autism, are often improved by selective serotonin reuptake inhibitors (SSRIs), such as fluoxetine. Starting at low doses with slow upward titration often dramatically reduces common side effects, such as activation and decreased appetite.[72] For example, when prescribing fluoxetine for a child with autism, beginning with a dose of 2 mg/d and titrating up by 2 to 4 mg every week may reduce potential side effects and also often identifies a lower optimal dose than might typically be considered. Irritability stemming from extreme cognitive rigidity and self-injurious behavior rooted in compulsions may also be improved by SSRIs, although they are not as frequently prescribed for this use.

ADHD symptoms of distractible inattention, hyperactivity, and impulsivity may be treated with stimulants, including amphetamines and methylphenidate. Frequent side effects include irritability, increased stereotypies, insomnia, and aggression.[73] If stimulants are ineffective or induce unacceptable or unmanageable adverse effects, α-agonists, such as guanfacine and clonidine, may also be used. Side effects include sedation and hypotension.[74,75] The norepinephrine reuptake inhibitor Strattera is often an effective alternative that may help with inattention and hyperactivity. The most common side effects of Strattera are fatigue and nausea.[76]

Symptoms of mood dysregulation and affective instability may be improved by mood stabilizers, such as divalproex sodium. A retrospective pilot study of 14 patients with ASDs, including autism, Asperger's disorder, and PDD-NOS, demonstrated improvement in mood instability, impulsivity, and aggression after treatment with divalproex sodium for an average of 10 months.[77] Seventy-one percent of patients who completed a trial of divalproex sodium were rated as having a sustained response to treatment.[77] A more recent double-blind placebo-controlled study comparing divalproex sodium with placebo found significant improvement in repetitive behaviors as measured by the Children's Yale-Brown Obsessive Compulsive Scale (CY-BOCS) scale with 13 patients in an 8-week trial.[78] Therefore, divalproex sodium is a potentially promising treatment for mood dysregulation and repetitive behaviors in patients who have ASD. Because as many as 68% of children with autism have been found to exhibit epileptic abnormalities, which some studies have shown to be normalized by divalproex sodium, the efficacy of divalproex sodium for treating autism is thought by some to be, in part, attributable to its antiepileptic properties.[44] Along with most of these medications, however, larger double-blind controlled studies need to be performed to draw any steadfast conclusions about their efficacy in treating autism and their mechanisms of action in ameliorating these symptoms.

Biomedical Treatments

Biomedical treatments, also called complementary and alternative medical (CAM) treatments, are commonly used by individuals with autism. Recent surveys reveal the prevalence of CAM use in children with autism to be between 30% and 95%. Although this variability is likely related to the substantial differences in survey design and the populations studied,[79–81] these studies clearly demonstrate the common use of CAM treatments among individuals with autism. Numerous anecdotal reports from parents and clinicians have indicated CAM benefits ranging from slight improvement to claims of cure.

A group of physicians, referred to as Defeat Autism Now (DAN) doctors, strongly believe in CAM treatments (so-called because they are scientifically unproved), and many have reportedly developed systems to treat subgroups of autism effectively by targeting their biologic dysfunction. Examples of CAM treatments include hyperbaric oxygen therapy[82] and omega-3 fatty acids[83] to target an inflammatory process, methyl B_{12}[48] and GSH to target oxidative stress, and chelation to target heavy metal toxicity.[84] Other popular nutritional CAM approaches include the gluten- and casein-free (GF/CF) diet,[85] based on the theory that some children on the spectrum develop gut inflammation. Some hypothesize that this may involve compromised permeability of the intestinal mucosa, which may allow digestive products to enter the blood, a condition referred to as "leaky gut".[86] Many parents report substantial benefits from the GF/CF diet and describe substantially exacerbated autistic symptoms on the child's reintroduction to milk products or wheat. Other innovative treatments include using pharmaceutic drugs to target potential mechanisms. Examples include peroxisome proliferator-activated receptors gamma (PPARg) agonists, which are approved to treat diabetes and to target inflammation in autism,[87] and the Alzheimer's disease drug memantine to treat the core symptoms of autism by potentially minimizing excitotoxicity.[88]

Despite the vast number of individuals using CAM treatments and the frequently reported benefits to children with autism, few studies have been conducted to evaluate their efficacy scientifically. Additionally, many of the CAM treatments come at a cost to affected families, requiring varying investments of time, energy, and money. CAM treatments with a plausible mechanism of action and a surplus of positive anecdotal reports need to be subjected to double-blind studies to determine their efficacy in treating the symptoms of autism objectively. Furthermore, because there are many autisms, each of which may respond differently to treatments, these studies need to be approached by identifying a subgroup of responders with corresponding improved biomarkers. This is in contrast to putting a broad group of subjects with autism in a treatment study, which is unlikely to show significance, assuming that many autisms exist. Therefore, it is essential that good double-blind studies are conducted and analyzed in a manner that does not wash out an effective treatment for a subgroup of autism.

Because of the large number of families using CAM treatments, it is important that the practitioner be aware of the various treatments. Some families seem to be pressured to commit to strictly CAM treatments or to strictly pharmacologic treatments, depending on whether they see a traditional doctor or a DAN doctor. When working with families interested in CAM treatments, however, it is important to provide them with accurate information about the likelihood of response and potential side effects of CAM and traditional treatments. For example, families ought to be informed that these alternative treatments are available, used by many children with autism, and maintain positive anecdotal reports but are not proved effective by any well-done published studies. So that they can ultimately make the best informed decision for their child, families ought to be educated about the placebo effect that may contribute to the positive anecdotal reports in autism, and they need to be aware of the benefits and potential side effects that they might expect from any treatment.

Strategy for Implementing Treatments

The complexity of the disorder frequently requires complex treatment strategies, which may include the integration of many treatments that may need to be altered throughout the child's development. Principles to guide such treatment include the following: (1) identify and monitor target symptoms, (2) maximize each medication dose before adding or discontinuing an agent, (3) change and adjust only one drug at a time, (4) monitor medication side effects carefully, and (5) discontinue the drug of least benefit. Pharmacologic treatment of individuals who have autism should always be part of a comprehensive treatment program that includes behavioral, psychosocial, speech, and language therapy in addition to treatment of medical comorbidities. Maintaining strong rapport and treatment partnerships with patients and families is essential if one is to be able to guide decision making, monitor side effects, and provide guidance and referral to educational and support groups effectively.

WORKING WITH FAMILIES

Once you have confirmed a diagnosis of autism, you ought to begin to work with the child's family members to provide them with the support and resources that lead to the optimal outcome for the child and family. They ought to be advised that although there is not a cure for autism, many behavioral and pharmacologic treatments are available with the potential to improve their child's adaptive functioning and quality of life vastly. As a physician, you may also want to inform parents of some of the controversies surrounding the diagnosis of autism, ranging from extremes from groups claiming that autism should not be treated to other extremes suggesting a devastating prognosis for all affected individuals. Instead, parents ought to be encouraged that their child may have unique and special qualities resulting from the disorder, but they also need to be prepared for the challenges they are going to face.

Many services are available to children with autism, although locating and obtaining them often require dedication and persistence. On diagnosis, an individual family service plan for preschool children and an individualized education plan for school-aged children are required by law.[89] Many services are often covered by the local regional center, including in-home behavioral therapy, OT, and speech therapy. A parent-based advocate society for children who have autism, called Families for Early Intervention and Treatment (FEAT), offers excellent support and resources for families to help them obtain services and overcome the everyday challenges of caring for a child with autism, such as finding a dentist who is able to accommodate their child's behaviors. The Autism Society of America[90] and Autism Speaks[91] also provide a large amount of Web-based information and resources.

ACKNOWLEDGMENTS

The authors thank Debra Matsumoto for her assistance in reviewing and preparing this manuscript for submission.

REFERENCES

1. American Psychiatric Association. Diagnostic and statistical manual of mental disorders. 4th edition. Arlington (VA): American Psychiatric Association; 2000. p. 84.
2. Lord C, Spence S. Autism spectrum disorders: phenotype and diagnosis. In: Moldin SO, Rubenstein JLR, editors. Understanding autism: from basic neuroscience to treatment. Boca Raton (FL): CRC Press; 2006. p. 1–24.
3. Lord C, McGee J, editors. Educating children with autism. Washington, DC: National Academy Press; 2001.
4. Ganz ML. The costs of autism. In: Moldin SO, Rubenstein JLR, editors. Understanding autism: from basic neuroscience to treatment. Boca Raton (FL): CRC Press; 2006. p. 475–502.
5. Bertrand J, Mars A, Boyle C, et al. Prevalence of autism in a United States population: the Brick Township, New Jersey, investigation. Pediatrics 2001;108(5): 1155–61.
6. Steinhausen HC, Gobel D, Breinlinger M, et al. A community survey of infantile autism. J Am Acad Child Psychiatry 1986;25(2):186–9.
7. Taylor B. Vaccines and the changing epidemiology of autism. Child Care Health Dev 2006;32(5):511–9.
8. Yeargin-Allsopp M, Rice C, Karapurkar T, et al. Prevalence of autism in a US metropolitan area. JAMA 2003;289(1):49–55.
9. Fombonne E, Simmons H, Ford T, et al. Prevalence of pervasive developmental disorders in the British nationwide survey of child mental health. J Am Acad Child Adolesc Psychiatry 2001;40(7):820–7.
10. Dyches TT, Wilder LK, Sudweeks RR, et al. Multicultural issues in autism. J Autism Dev Disord 2004;34(2):211–22.
11. Liptak GS, Benzoni LB, Mruzek DW, et al. Disparities in diagnosis and access to health services for children with autism: data from the National Survey of Children's Health. J Dev Behav Pediatr 2008;29(3):152–60.
12. What is autism? Advocate: the newsletter of the Autism Society of America. 2000; 33(3).
13. Pediatrics AAo. The pediatrician's role in the diagnosis and management of autistic spectrum disorder in children. Pediatrics 2001;107:1221–6.
14. Mundy P. Annotation: the neural basis of social impairments in autism: the role of the dorsal medial-frontal cortex and anterior cingulate system. J Child Psychol Psychiatry 2003;44(6):793–809.

15. Rogers SJ, Hepburn SL, Stackhouse T, et al. Imitation performance in toddlers with autism and those with other developmental disorders. J Child Psychol Psychiatry 2003;44(5):763–81.
16. Tuchman R. Autism. Neurol Clin 2003;21(4):915–32, viii.
17. Rogers SJ. Developmental regression in autism spectrum disorders. Ment Retard Dev Disabil Res Rev 2004;10(2):139–43.
18. Karande S. Autism: a review for family physicians. Indian J Med Sci 2006;60(5): 205–15.
19. Eisenmajer R, Prior M, Leekam S, et al. Comparison of clinical symptoms in autism and Asperger's disorder. J Am Acad Child Adolesc Psychiatry 1996; 35(11):1523–31.
20. Miller JN, Ozonoff S. The external validity of Asperger disorder: lack of evidence from the domain of neuropsychology. J Abnorm Psychol 2000;109(2):227–38.
21. Klin A, Volkmar FR. Asperger syndrome: diagnosis and external validity. Child Adolesc Psychiatr Clin N Am 2003;12(1):1–13, v.
22. Szatmari P, Bremner R, Nagy J. Asperger's syndrome: a review of clinical features. Can J Psychiatry 1989;34(6):554–60.
23. Fine J, Bartolucci G, Szatmari P, et al. Cohesive discourse in pervasive developmental disorders. J Autism Dev Disord 1994;24(3):315–29.
24. Macintosh KE, Dissanayake C. Annotation: the similarities and differences between autistic disorder and Asperger's disorder: a review of the empirical evidence. J Child Psychol Psychiatry 2004;45(3):421–34.
25. Lord C, Rutter M, Goode S, et al. Autism diagnostic observation schedule: a standardized observation of communicative and social behavior. J Autism Dev Disord 1989;19(2):185–212.
26. Lord C, Rutter M, Le Couteur A. Autism Diagnostic Interview-Revised: a revised version of a diagnostic interview for caregivers of individuals with possible pervasive developmental disorders. J Autism Dev Disord 1994;24(5):659–85.
27. Baird G, Charman T, Baron-Cohen S, et al. A screening instrument for autism at 18 months of age: a 6-year follow-up study. J Am Acad Child Adolesc Psychiatry 2000;39(6):694–702.
28. Palomo R, Belinchon M, Ozonoff S. Autism and family home movies: a comprehensive review. J Dev Behav Pediatr 2006;27(2 Suppl):S59–68.
29. Filipek PA, Accardo PJ, Ashwal S, et al. Practice parameter: screening and diagnosis of autism: report of the Quality Standards Subcommittee of the American Academy of Neurology and the Child Neurology Society. Neurology 2000;55(4): 468–79.
30. Hansen R. Contributions of pediatrics. In: Ozonoff S, Rogers SJ, Hendren RL, editors. Autism spectrum disorders: a research review for practitioners. Washington, DC: American Psychiatric Publishing, Inc.; 2003. p. 87–109.
31. Keller F, Persico AM. The neurobiological context of autism. Mol Neurobiol 2003; 28(1):1–22.
32. Beaudet AL. Is medical genetics neglecting epigenetics? Genet Med 2002;4(5): 399–402.
33. London EA. The environment as an etiologic factor in autism: a new direction for research. Environ Health Perspect 2000;108(Suppl 3):401–4.
34. Freitag CM, Kleser C, von Gontard A. Imitation and language abilities in adolescents with Autism Spectrum Disorder without language delay. Eur Child Adolesc Psychiatry 2006;15(5):282–91.
35. Reichenberg A, Gross R, Weiser M, et al. Advancing paternal age and autism. Arch Gen Psychiatry 2006;63(9):1026–32.

36. Philippe A, Martinez M, Guilloud-Bataille M, et al. Genome-wide scan for autism susceptibility genes. Paris Autism Research International Sibpair Study. Hum Mol Genet 1999;8(5):805–12.
37. Muhle R, Trentacoste SV, Rapin I. The genetics of autism. Pediatrics 2004;113(5): e472–86.
38. Campbell DB, Sutcliffe JS, Ebert PJ, et al. A genetic variant that disrupts MET transcription is associated with autism. Proc Natl Acad Sci U S A 2006; 103(45):16834–9.
39. Miyazaki K, Narita N, Narita M. Maternal administration of thalidomide or valproic acid causes abnormal serotonergic neurons in the offspring: implication for pathogenesis of autism. Int J Dev Neurosci 2005;23(2–3):287–97.
40. Mutter J, Naumann J, Schneider R, et al. Mercury and autism: accelerating evidence? Neuro Endocrinol Lett 2005;26(5):439–46.
41. Young HA, Geier DA, Geier MR. Thimerosal exposure in infants and neurodevelopmental disorders: an assessment of computerized medical records in the Vaccine Safety Datalink. J Neurol Sci 2008;271(1–2):110–8.
42. Ashwood P, Wills S, Van de Water J. The immune response in autism: a new frontier for autism research. J Leukoc Biol 2006;80(1):1–15.
43. Tharp BR. Epileptic encephalopathies and their relationship to developmental disorders: do spikes cause autism? Ment Retard Dev Disabil Res Rev 2004; 10(2):132–4.
44. Chez MG, Chang M, Krasne V, et al. Frequency of epileptiform EEG abnormalities in a sequential screening of autistic patients with no known clinical epilepsy from 1996 to 2005. Epilepsy Behav 2006;8(1):267–71.
45. Aldred S, Moore KM, Fitzgerald M, et al. Plasma amino acid levels in children with autism and their families. J Autism Dev Disord 2003;33(1):93–7.
46. Zoroglu SS, Armutcu F, Ozen S, et al. Increased oxidative stress and altered activities of erythrocyte free radical scavenging enzymes in autism. Eur Arch Psychiatry Clin Neurosci 2004;254(3):143–7.
47. Sogut S, Zoroglu SS, Ozyurt H, et al. Changes in nitric oxide levels and antioxidant enzyme activities may have a role in the pathophysiological mechanisms involved in autism. Clin Chim Acta 2003;331(1–2):111–7.
48. James SJ, Cutler P, Melnyk S, et al. Metabolic biomarkers of increased oxidative stress and impaired methylation capacity in children with autism. Am J Clin Nutr 2004;80(6):1611–7.
49. Yorbik O, Sayal A, Akay C, et al. Investigation of antioxidant enzymes in children with autistic disorder. Prostaglandins Leukot Essent Fatty Acids 2002;67(5): 341–3.
50. Bauman ML, Kemper TL. Neuroanatomic observations of the brain in autism: a review and future directions. Int J Dev Neurosci 2005;23(2–3):183–7.
51. Courchesne E. Abnormal early brain development in autism. Mol Psychiatry 2002;7(Suppl 2):S21–3.
52. Courchesne E, Karns CM, Davis HR, et al. Unusual brain growth patterns in early life in patients with autistic disorder: an MRI study. Neurology 2001; 57(2):245–54.
53. Sparks BF, Friedman SD, Shaw DW, et al. Brain structural abnormalities in young children with autism spectrum disorder. Neurology 2002;59(2):184–92.
54. Redcay E, Courchesne E. When is the brain enlarged in autism? A meta-analysis of all brain size reports. Biol Psychiatry 2005;58(1):1–9.
55. Herbert MR. Large brains in autism: the challenge of pervasive abnormality. Neuroscientist 2005;11(5):417–40.

56. Kern JK. Purkinje cell vulnerability and autism: a possible etiological connection. Brain Dev 2003;25(6):377–82.
57. Kielinen M, Rantala H, Timonen E, et al. Associated medical disorders and disabilities in children with autistic disorder: a population-based study. Autism 2004;8(1):49–60.
58. Werner E, Dawson G. Validation of the phenomenon of autistic regression using home videotapes. Arch Gen Psychiatry 2005;62(8):889–95.
59. Mottron L, Dawson M, Soulieres I, et al. Enhanced perceptual functioning in autism: an update, and eight principles of autistic perception. J Autism Dev Disord 2006;36(1):27–43.
60. Cohly HH, Panja A. Immunological findings in autism. Int Rev Neurobiol 2005;71: 317–41.
61. Ashwood P, Van de Water J. A review of autism and the immune response. Clin Dev Immunol 2004;11(2):165–74.
62. Erickson CA, Stigler KA, Corkins MR, et al. Gastrointestinal factors in autistic disorder: a critical review. J Autism Dev Disord 2005;35(6):713–27.
63. Munesue T, Ono Y, Mutoh K, et al. High prevalence of bipolar disorder comorbidity in adolescents and young adults with high-functioning autism spectrum disorder: a preliminary study of 44 outpatients. J Affect Disord 2008;11(2): 170–5.
64. Huttenlocher PR. Synapse elimination and plasticity in developing human cerebral cortex. Am J Ment Defic 1984;88(5):488–96.
65. Lovaas OI. Behavioral treatment and normal educational and intellectual functioning in young autistic children. J Consult Clin Psychol 1987;55(1):3–9.
66. Seltzer MM, Shattuck P, Abbeduto L, et al. Trajectory of development in adolescents and adults with autism. Ment Retard Dev Disabil Res Rev 2004;10(4):234–47.
67. Rogers SJ, Hayden D, Hepburn S, et al. Teaching young nonverbal children with autism useful speech: a pilot study of the Denver Model and PROMPT interventions. J Autism Dev Disord 2006;36(8):1007–24.
68. Mesibov GB. Commentary: facilitated communication: a warning for pediatric psychologists. J Pediatr Psychol 1995;20(1):127–30.
69. Koegel P, Sullivan G, Burnam A, et al. Utilization of mental health and substance abuse services among homeless adults in Los Angeles. Med Care 1999;37(3): 306–17.
70. Findling RL. Pharmacologic treatment of behavioral symptoms in autism and pervasive developmental disorders. J Clin Psychiatry 2005;66(Suppl 10):26–31.
71. Barnard L, Young AH, Pearson J, et al. A systematic review of the use of atypical antipsychotics in autism. J Psychopharmacol 2002;16(1):93–101.
72. Hollander E, Phillips A, Chaplin W, et al. A placebo controlled crossover trial of liquid fluoxetine on repetitive behaviors in childhood and adolescent autism. Neuropsychopharmacology 2005;30(3):582–9.
73. Findling RL, Steiner H, Weller EB. Use of antipsychotics in children and adolescents. J Clin Psychiatry 2005;66(Suppl 7):29–40.
74. Scahill L, McCracken J, McDougle CJ, et al. Methodological issues in designing a multisite trial of risperidone in children and adolescents with autism. J Child Adolesc Psychopharmacol 2001;11(4):377–88.
75. Wolraich ML, Wibbelsman CJ, Brown TE, et al. Attention-deficit/hyperactivity disorder among adolescents: a review of the diagnosis, treatment, and clinical implications. Pediatrics 2005;115(6):1734–46.
76. Hazell P. Does the treatment of mental disorders in childhood lead to a healthier adulthood? Curr Opin Psychiatry 2007;20(4):315–8.

77. Hollander E, Dolgoff-Kaspar R, Cartwright C, et al. An open trial of divalproex sodium in autism spectrum disorders. J Clin Psychiatry 2001;62(7):530–4.
78. Hollander E, Soorya L, Wasserman S, et al. Divalproex sodium vs. placebo in the treatment of repetitive behaviours in autism spectrum disorder. Int J Neuropsychopharmacol 2006;9(2):209–13.
79. Goin-Kochel RP, Mackintosh VH, Myers BJ. How many doctors does it take to make an autism spectrum diagnosis? Autism 2006;10(5):439–51.
80. Green VA, Pituch KA, Itchon J, et al. Internet survey of treatments used by parents of children with autism. Res Dev Disabil 2006;27(1):70–84.
81. Wong HH, Smith RG. Patterns of complementary and alternative medical therapy use in children diagnosed with autism spectrum disorders. J Autism Dev Disord 2006;36(7):901–9.
82. Rossignol DA, Rossignol LW, James SJ, et al. The effects of hyperbaric oxygen therapy on oxidative stress, inflammation, and symptoms in children with autism: an open-label pilot study. BMC Pediatr 2007;7:36.
83. Amminger GP, Berger GE, Schafer MR, et al. Omega-3 fatty acids supplementation in children with autism: a double-blind randomized, placebo-controlled pilot study. Biol Psychiatry 2007;61(4):551–3.
84. Levy SE, Hyman SL. Novel treatments for autistic spectrum disorders. Ment Retard Dev Disabil Res Rev 2005;11(2):131–42.
85. Millward C, Ferriter M, Calver S, et al. Gluten- and casein-free diets for autistic spectrum disorder. Cochrane Database Syst Rev 2008;(2):CD003498.
86. White JF. Intestinal pathophysiology in autism. Exp Biol Med (Maywood) 2003; 228(6):639–49.
87. Boris M, Kaiser CC, Goldblatt A, et al. Effect of pioglitazone treatment on behavioral symptoms in autistic children. J Neuroinflammation 2007;4:3.
88. Chez MG, Burton Q, Dowling T, et al. Memantine as adjunctive therapy in children diagnosed with autistic spectrum disorders: an observation of initial clinical response and maintenance tolerability. J Child Neurol 2007;22(5):574–9.
89. Filipek PA, Steinberg-Epstein R, Book TM. Intervention for autistic spectrum disorders. NeuroRx 2006;3(2):207–16.
90. Available at: www.Autism-Society.org. Accessed September 13, 2008.
91. Available at: www.AutismSpeaks.org. Accessed September 13, 2008.

Psychiatric Phenotypes Associated with Neurogenetic Disorders

Carl Feinstein, MD[a,b,*], Lovina Chahal, MD[a]

KEYWORDS

- Neurogenetics • Psychiatric disorders
- Velocardiofacial syndrome • Fragile X syndrome
- Down syndrome • Prader-Willi syndrome • Turner's syndrome
- Klinefelter's syndrome • Sex chromosome aneuploidy

OVERVIEW

Psychiatry has long sought to determine specific genetic risk for or causal factors in mental illness and to better understand the interaction between genetic and environmental factors that underlie psychiatric disorder. The general method has been to use a variety of increasingly powerful genetic and genomic screening tools to detect risk genes associated with the disorder being studied. This approach has proved difficult and slow, because current diagnostic categories consist of behaviorally defined clusters of symptoms and lack biologic validation or clear biologic markers that could guide researchers toward underlying genetic or genomic mechanisms. In addition, heterogeneity in quality, quantity, and type of symptoms within the currently defined psychiatric disorders continues to pose great challenges to studying genetic influences of any but the strongest effect.

In contrast, the burgeoning discipline of behavioral neurogenetics begins with known gene abnormalities or variations that can be determined and validated by reliable biologic tests and studies the effects of those specific genetic factors in individuals or groups of individuals who are homogeneous for the genetic variation being studied. The effect of the genetic variation then can be studied developmentally with reference to gene, protein, brain structure and function, cognition, and a wide range of behaviors and symptoms.[1,2]

---

[a] Department of Psychiatry and Behavioral Sciences, Stanford University School of Medicine, 401 Quarry Road, Stanford, CA 94305, USA
[b] Division of Child and Adolescent Psychiatry, Lucile Packard Children's Hospital, Stanford University School of Medicine, 401 Quarry Road, Stanford, CA 94305-5719, USA
* Corresponding author. Division of Child and Adolescent Psychiatry, Lucile Packard Children's Hospital, Stanford University School of Medicine, 401 Quarry Road, Stanford, CA 94305-5719.
E-mail address: carlf@stanford.edu (C. Feinstein).

Psychiatr Clin N Am 32 (2009) 15–37
doi:10.1016/j.psc.2008.12.001
0193-953X/08/$ – see front matter © 2009 Elsevier Inc. All rights reserved.

psych.theclinics.com

A vast and informative array of behavioral neurogenetic findings is being elucidated with the use of animal models.[3,4] This new information, often involving complex processes, such as social, communicative, and mating behaviors, has been gained partly by studying naturally occurring or bred variant strains or closely related species of many animals from drosophila to bees, fish, voles, mice and other rodents, songbirds, and primates.[4] Variations in behaviors are correlated with genomic data. Increasingly, however, experimental animal models have been used for the study of traits, such as sociability, stereotypic behavior, and behaviors related to anxious inhibition versus impulsivity by using gene knockout and insertion techniques.[4,5]

For clinical psychiatrists, however, there are several significant genetically based neurodevelopmental disorders that also may be viewed as a type of human model for specific behaviors or psychiatric disorders. These are conditions in which known gene mutations, chromosomal deletions, or copy number variations are associated with highly distinctive behavioral phenotypes.[6] Such behavioral phenotypes may be associated with specific psychiatric disorders in addition to cognitive and behavioral profiles that are unique to each genetically based disorder. In these situations, the specific chromosomal or gene-based neurodevelopmental disorder can be viewed as a homogeneous model (sharing a common genetic, biologically validated genetic basis) for studying the underlying pathophysiologic processes that might underlie specific behavioral traits or psychiatric disorders.

This review summarizes findings for some of the most prevalent genetic neurodevelopmental disorders, emphasizing the psychiatric aspects of their behavioral phenotypes. These include velocardiofacial syndrome (VCFS), fragile X syndrome (FXS), Down syndrome (DS), Prader-Willi syndrome (PWS), and the sex chromosome aneuploidies. These genetic neurodevelopmental disorders challenge psychiatrists, psychologists, and clinical neuroscientists partly because patients who have these conditions may present to clinicians with a clear psychiatric disorder but, unlike all other psychiatric conditions, they have a known biologic cause that can be validated by a laboratory test. In that sense they stimulate thinking about the nature of gene-brain-behavior relationships. They also present a challenge because if clinicians fail to recognize or test for the underlying genetic disorder, patients and families are deprived of a deeply meaningful and useful explanation for their condition and prognosis and all chances for genetic counseling are lost.

VELOCARDIOFACIAL SYNDROME

VCFS, also widely known as the 22q11.2 deletion syndrome, is the most common known microdeletion syndrome in humans.[7] In addition to the many congenital medical problems that result from VCFS, it has highly significant behavioral effects in childhood and in adulthood, including acting as the single most common known genetic risk factor for schizophrenia.[7,8] Most cases of VCFS are sporadic and derive from de novo mutations in one parent's germ cells; however, between 6% and 28% are inherited from a parent who has VCFS as an autosomal dominant trait.[9] When this occurs, the parent who has VCFS who has a child who has VCFS is likely to manifest few or only mild medical traits and cognitive deficits and may never have been diagnosed.[9]

VCFS first was described by Kirkpatrick and DiGeorge, with the diagnosis based primarily on a congenitally absent thymus in 1968.[10] In 1978, a more comprehensive account of the syndrome that included the "velo" (palate), "cardio," and "facial" (facial dysmorphism), along with learning disabilities and multiple associated medical and cognitive disabilities, was published by Shprintzen and colleagues.[11] VCFS results in a numerous and wide array of congenital medical defects that are variably present, the most common of which are cardiac/major truncal vessel malformations, palate defects, hypoparathyroidism with hypocalcemia, thymic hypoplasia, characteristic facial dimorphism, urinary system abnormalities and a range of hematologic problems.[7,12,13] Laboratory diagnosis has been based on cytogenetic fluorescence in situ hybridization (FISH) testing since approximately 1993.[7] The microdeletion most commonly is a homozygous 1.2–3 Mb microdeletion, always involving the COMT gene, on chromosome 22q11.2.[14]

Because population-based laboratory screening by FISH is prohibitively expensive, prevalence data are based on referral to genetics clinics, triggered in the vast majority of cases by congenital cardiac and aortic malformation or palate anomalies presenting in infancy. This minimum prevalence was found in a recent study (2003) to be approximately 1 in 5950 births.[15] Congenital anomalies of these types (that commonly trigger a genetics consultation in infancy), however, occur in only approximately 75% of individuals who have the deletion.[16] Therefore, the deletion is undetected in infancy in a substantial number of individuals. The most commonly cited prevalence estimate for VCFS is 1 per 4000.[12]

Because of the recent use of FISH testing and the not infrequent occurrence of individuals who have the deletion and who may not have pronounced cardiac or palate defects, there are occult and undetected cases of individuals who have VCFS in the general population. These may present to psychiatrists with serious psychiatric conditions, such as schizophrenia and mood disorders; the VCFS diagnosis secondary to a low index of suspicion may be missed.[17]

Childhood cognitive disabilities are a prominent feature of VCFS and can lead to the appropriate FISH testing and VCFS diagnosis in cases where the mild nature of the congenital abnormalities do not trigger a comprehensive genetic evaluation. Most toddler and preschool children who have VCFS are impaired by mild gross motor delays and severe language delays. Measures of intelligence in VCFS children in this age range tend toward the borderline to mild intellectual disability range.[17–20]

The cognitive profile in school-aged children, adolescents, and adults continues to include group mean IQ scores in the borderline to mild intellectual disability range, with boys slightly more cognitively impaired than girls.[21,22] Overall, the mean IQ of individuals who have VCFS is in the low to mid 70s, with approximately 25% to 40% of individuals having an IQ in the range of intellectual disability. Children who have VCFS show considerable improvement in language functioning after the characteristic delays in the toddler period but retain deficits in higher-order language skills, as manifested by lowered scores on specific tests of language functioning.[21] Nonverbal IQ scores of children who have VCFS, however, often are lower than verbal IQ scores, because children who have VCFS also have deficits in abstract, nonverbal reasoning, and visual-spatial processing; executive functioning deficits also are common.[22] The measured intelligence of substantial numbers of individuals who have VCFS is in the low average or average range. Cases of VCFS in which overall intelligence is not in the disabled range along with those of few or only mild physical anomalies are less likely to be FISH tested for VCFS, when patients present with a VCFS-related psychiatric disorder.

First recognition of the significant psychiatric symptoms associated with VCFS did not occur until the 1990s. Research studying psychiatric and behavioral traits of VCFS developed rapidly only after confirmatory FISH diagnostic testing enabled the systematic study of cohorts of children homogeneous for the 22q11.2 microdeletion. After this came the identification by FISH testing of previously unrecognized cases of microdeletion in populations of psychiatrically disordered adults who had schizophrenia and who had congenital medical defects characteristic of VCFS.[17,23] Psychiatric disorders in children were noted first, as FISH testing was applied mostly to very young children who had characteristic congenital defects.

Children who have VCFS have high rates of psychiatric disorder and behavioral disturbance, and there is evidence that this increased rate of disorder represents a primary behavioral phenotype rather than a secondary effect of lowered IQ.[7,8,24–28] Common problems are overactivity and impulsivity, many fears and phobias, emotional lability, shyness, and poor social skills.[8,17] Attention-deficit/hyperactivity disorder (ADHD) is the most common psychiatric diagnosis in children who have VCFS, with rates between 25% and 46% reported.[8,26,27] Mood disorders, including depression and, occasionally, bipolar spectrum disorders, also are common, with rates of major depression reported between 12% and 20%.[25–27] High rates of anxiety disorders, especially specific phobias, occur in 27% to 61% of children who have VCFS.[26,27]

Somewhat more controversial is the diagnosis of pervasive developmental disorders/autism spectrum disorder. In recent studies, these have been reported to occur in between 14% and 50% of children who have VCFS, with use, for the first time, of appropriate and reliable assessment for autism spectrum disorders.[29,30] These reports focus attention on the social phenotypic traits observed in VCFS and raise complex questions about how to link or compare a homogeneous, biologically validated disorder, such as VCFS, with a behaviorally defined cluster of disorders or traits that lacks biologic validation, such as the autism spectrum disorders.[6] The controversy is whether or not VCFS cases meeting research diagnostic criteria for autism spectrum disorders are accounted for more appropriately in terms of their cognitive phenotype (poor language and executive functioning, social anxiety, and the social deficits characteristic of ADHD) or the schizotypal features that are prodromal to schizophrenia in many of these youngsters.[31,32] In any case, if this high rate of autism-like symptoms is replicated in future studies, gene-brain-behavior relationships in VCFS inevitably will be studied as one of the genetically based human models for studying the core deficits that define the autism spectrum disorders.

Childhood-onset schizophrenia or schizoaffective disorder occurs in approximately 6% of children who have VCFS[33] and becomes more prevalent by midadolescence. Baker and Skuse, studying late adolescents who had VCFS and matched controls, found ongoing high rates of ADHD, anxiety disorders, and mood disorders in the subjects who had VCFS.[34] Thirty-six percent of the VCFS subjects experienced episodes of intense irritability or mood lability whereas almost half of them experienced fleeting psychotic-like experiences, including transient delusional thoughts and auditory and visual hallucinations. Most of the VCFS subjects led impoverished social lives, characterized by withdrawal and poor social skills exacerbated by peer rejection.[34] Vorstman and colleagues[30] studied 60 children and adolescents, between the ages of 9 and 20, who had VCFS. Sixteen of these youngsters reported auditory hallucinations or delusions, seven of them reporting associated distress (and diagnosed as psychotic) and two of whom showing strong evidence of decline in functioning. Overall, 29.7% showed some form of psychotic thinking whereas 11.7% met diagnostic criteria for schizophreniform disorder. The mean age of onset for thought disorder symptoms was 14.2 years.

Gothelf and colleagues[9,35] performed a 5-year follow-up study of the cohort of children who had VCFS reported initially by Feinstein. At follow-up, 32.1% of the adolescents from this original sample (mean age 17.4 years) had developed psychotic disorders (schizophreniform disorders). Baseline subthreshhold thought disorder, symptoms of anxiety or depression, lower baseline verbal IQ, and catechol-O-methyltransferase (COMT) genotype (homozygous met allele) predicted 61% of the variance. The influence in patients who have VCFS of homozygosity for the COMT met allele (low acting) and the resultant higher prefrontal dopamine as a risk factor aggravating psychotic outcome recently has been replicated.[36]

Shprintzen and colleagues,[37,38] in 1992 and 1994, first diagnosed schizophrenia or schizoaffective disorder based on following early subjects who had clinically diagnosed VCFS who were tested using cytogenetic FISH when it first became available. The series of findings that followed this, however, involved studying patient populations who had schizophrenia but no previous workup for VCFS by using FISH testing. Using this approach, Karayiorgou and coworkers[39] found two schizophrenic patients who had VCFS. Gothelf and colleagues[23] then developed a more focused approach by first identifying from a larger sample of patients who had schizophrenia those who had heart or palate defects and then studying the refined sample with FISH testing. They were able to identify three subjects who had VCFS among a pool of 20. Bassett and Chow[40,41] pursued this strategy in a larger sample and found that approximately 1% to 2% of all patients diagnosed with schizophrenia had the 22q11.2 deletion syndrome. Conversely, it is now well established that between 20% and 30% of all individuals who have VCFS have or will develop schizophrenia by late adolescence or early adulthood.[8,42,43]

FRAGILE X SYNDROME AND FRAGILE X–ASSOCIATED TREMOR/ATAXIA SYNDROME

FXS is the most common heritable neurodevelopmental disorder.[2,44] It is caused by a cytosine-guanine-guanine (CGG) repeat expansion mutation on the FMR1 gene. located on the long arm of the X chromosome.[2,45–48] Its pattern of inheritance is sex linked. The prevalence of FXS, in which the full mutation is present, is approximately 1 per 4000 live births for boys and between 1 per 6000 and 1 per 8000 for girls.[49,50] Recent findings indicate, however, that many problems, including developmental disability, psychiatric disorders, maturity-onset neurologic cognitive disorders, and premature ovarian failure, are found in individuals who have partial mutations.[43,51] The prevalence of the partial mutation in the general population is 1 in 130 to 250 females and 1 in 250 to 810 men.[48,52–54]

The FMR1 gene is an unstable region of the human genome. The triplicate repeat expansion of the FMR1 gene is dynamic, in that the normal number of CGG repeats found in the gene is approximately 6 to 44, with a mode of 29 or 30; however, at the upper end of the normal range, instability begins to appear, with an increased risk for expansion of the number of repeats from generation to generation into what is termed the premutation range (55–200).[43,54] The premutation FMR1 gene has an escalating tendency to expand into the full mutation, which is at approximately 200 or more CGG repeats. Individuals who have partial mutations are called carriers, because of the increased likelihood that further triplicate repeat expansion will cause a full mutation in their offspring. Full mutation FMR1 alleles generally are hypermethylated and silenced, producing no FMR protein.[48] This results in the FXS.

Men who have FXS almost invariably are affected severely, with lower FMR protein, related to having only one X chromosome. Females are affected more variably, as determined in individual cases by which of the X chromosomes is imprinted (silenced). If the full mutation X chromosome is imprinted, then FMR protein still may be produced by the remaining normal X chromosome. Mosaicism, with autosomal cells variably imprinted or even variably mutated, adds further to the continuum of severity expressed in men and women, but in particular women. Although the mechanism of FMR inactivation in FXS is hypermethylation of the full mutation allele, premutation alleles result in elevated mRNA levels that partially block protein production in proportion to the size of the repeat. Therefore, individuals who have the premutation (carriers) also are vulnerable to the neurophysiologic consequences of reduced autosomal FMR protein.[51] The laboratory diagnosis of FXS and the premutation is made by Southern blot or, more recently, by polymerase chain reaction.[55]

Boys who have FXS have a distinctive physical phenotype with some associated medical vulnerability. External physical features often include an elongated face, large prominent ears, a prominent jaw, strabismus, a high arched palate, dental malocclusion, a single palmar crease, kyphoscoliosis, pectus excavatum, macro-orchidism, and pes planus,[44,46,56] although these features are only variably present and should not become the basis for a diagnosis. There also is an increased risk for cardiac mitral valve prolapse and dilation of the aortic root.

Almost all boys who have FXS have IQs in the range of intellectual disability, generally in the moderate range. Developmental delays are present from early in development, with speech and motor skills lagging. Because FXS rarely is diagnosed at birth (unless a parent is a likely carrier or a sibling has been diagnosed previously), slow early development is the trigger for genetic testing, often not occurring until 35 months or later.[57] Late identification and the consequent late introduction of remedial therapies are concerning particularly because boys who have FXS show a downward trajectory on standardized measures of intelligence and adaptive functioning, compared with normal controls, that continues through early adolescence. This poor developmental trajectory reflects slower cognitive and adaptive progress compared with normally developing children rather than an absolute loss of skills.[57–61] By school age, boys who have FXS show aberrant speech patterns characterized by rapid speech rate, poor intelligibility, dyspraxia, poor syntax development, perseverative speech, and impaired pragmatics of communication.[44] Although there is considerable development of expressive language in many boys who have FXS, nonverbal cognitive deficits in the domains of visual-spatial abilities, visual-motor coordination, short-term memory, and visual-motor coordination are most prominent.

The cognitive phenotype of girls who have FXS is wider in range, related to the variable dose of FMR resulting from two X chromomes, mosaicism, and so forth. One third to one half of female patients who have FXS have IQs in the range of intellectual disability.[62–65] Unfortunately, the generally milder pattern of deficits results in an average age of diagnosis for FXS girls up to age 8.[64] The most pronounced cognitive disabilities in female FXS patients are visual-spatial processing deficits, executive functioning deficits, poor mathematical skill, and attentional problems.[62]

The psychiatric and behavioral phenotype for boys who have FXS is specific and well documented. The syndrome involves hyperactivity and distractibility (particularly in the school-age period), irritability, repetitive stereotyped movements, pronounced gaze aversion, and social anxiety.[44,66–68] Face-to-face gaze is associated with hyper-arousal and high levels of stress.[6,69,70] These symptoms are not correlated with IQ in individuals who have FXS. There is a clear overlap in the behavioral phenotype for FXS with the diagnostic criteria for autism, with estimates of 25% to 47% meeting criteria for autism.[71–78] Only 2% to 7% of all cases of autism have the fragile X mutation, however.[78] It is difficult to compare the diagnostic overlap of a biologically validated disorder stemming from a gene mutation, such as FXS, with a Diagnostic and Statistical Manual of Mental Disorders diagnosis based on a cluster of symptoms with hundreds of genetic risk factors and no biologic validation;[71] however, there can be little doubt that the FXS is a neurogenetic model for one pathway to autism, and the data also are suggestive for ADHD.

Female patients who have FXS have their own distinctive psychiatric phenotype. Even girls who have FXS and who have normal IQs manifest high rates of social anxiety, depressed mood, social withdrawal, and theory of mind deficits, and some, at all levels of IQ, meet criteria for autism or an autism spectrum disorder.[62,79] Many female patients who have FXS also have attentional problems associated with poor organizational skills and impulsivity.[62,79] In addition to phenotypic features overlapping with autism and ADHD, FXS in female patients also may be a neurodevelopmental model for mood dysregulation, in particular chronic depressed mood.[80,81]

Although FXS is caused by a full mutation on the FMR1 gene (greater than 200 CGG repeats), it is becoming increasingly clear that even the premutation condition (55–200 CGG repeats), what used to be referred to as the carrier state, is not benign. Recent clinical research documents that at least some children who have the premutation state have cognitive deficits, behavioral problems, mood and anxiety problems, and autism spectrum disorders.[82,83] Of equal interest is a steady accumulation of findings that there are highly significant and prevalent medical and cognitive problems and psychiatric problems caused by the premutation state in adults, especially older male adults.[43,48,84–86] Given that the prevalence of the premutation state in the general population is approximately 1 per 130 to 1 per 800,[48] a prevalence much greater than that of the full mutation, it is clear that, whenever a child who has FXS is diagnosed, clinicians must take into account and evaluate the potential health consequences for all family members who could be premutation carriers and consider fragile X screening and genetic counseling for those family members. Furthermore, as reviewed later, fragile X testing should be considered for those types of medical, neurocognitive, and psychiatric problems that are known to be highly associated with the fragile X premutation state.

Several reports document that social deficits, autism spectrum disorders, and attention problems are found in some children who have the fragile X premutation.[87,88] In a recent study, Farzin and colleagues[82] studied a group of boys who presented for evaluation of significant behavioral problems and were found to have the premutation. These probands were compared with a second group of boys, who were identified by pedigree analysis and cascade testing in fragile X families after a proband was found to have FXS or the permutation, and a third group of boys consisted of control siblings who were tested and found to not have the premutation. They found a significantly higher rate of autism spectrum disorders and symptoms of ADHD in the boys who had premutation alleles who presented as clinical probands. Seventy-nine percent of the clinically ascertained boys who had the premutation allele met criteria for an autism spectrum disorder. In contrast, only 8% of the control siblings who did not have the premutation met diagnostic criteria for an autism spectrum disorder. The premutation boys who were found by family tree testing of relatives of the probands had a significantly higher rate of autism than the control siblings. These findings replicated other studies that had found a high rate of social deficits in male premutation carriers and confirm that fragile X premutation status confers increased risk for autism spectrum disorder. What is not yet known is the relative risk factor for autism spectrum disorder in the total population of premutation carriers.

A recent national survey of families of children who have FXS found that premutation boys were more likely to be diagnosed with developmental delays, attentional problems, aggression, seizures, anxiety, and autism. Girls who had the premutation were more likely to suffer from attention problems, shyness, social anxiety, depression, and developmental delay.[89] A national survey of mothers of children who had FXS and who were premutation carriers found they were more likely to suffer from chronic major depressive disorders, lifetime panic disorder, and agoraphobia, anxiety, and developmental delay when compared with normal controls.[83]

Fragile X premutation carrier adults are subject to significant medical issues. The most straightforward is premature ovarian failure, which occurs in approximately 21% of premutation carriers compared with approximately 1% in the general population.[85] Fragile X–associated tremor/ataxia syndrome (FXTAS) is now recognized as a major neurologic, neurocogntive, and psychiatric problem in older men who are premutation carriers.[85] This condition appears in approximately 17% of male premutation carriers aged 50 to 59, in 38% in their 60s, and in 47% in their 70s. Movement disorders found in FXTAS consist of cerebellar ataxia, intentional tremor, parkinsonism, peripheral neuropathy, lower limb proximal muscle weakness, dysarthric speech, and autonomic dysfunction.[84] Neurocognitive problems commonly found in FXTAS include deficits in behavioral self-regulation, attentional and working memory problems, deficits in verbal fluency, executive functioning deficits, and impairments in declarative memory and information processing.[43,90]

DOWN SYNDROME

DS is the most common chromosomal syndrome associated with intellectual disability, occurring in 1 in 732 infants.[91] It is seen in nondisjunction (95% of cases) or translocation of chromosome 21 resulting in complete trisomy 21 or mosaicism of trisomy 21.[92] Lockstone and colleagues[93] cited up-regulation of chromosome 21, leading to dysregulation of functionally linked genes involved in development, lipid transport, and cellular proliferation as a cause of many pathologies found in DS. Gene-dosage effects of chromosome 21 cause characteristic changes of reduced cerebellar volume and number of granular cells, defective cortical lamination and reduced cortical neurons, malformed dendritic trees and spines, and abnormal synapses in the DS brain.[94]

DS may be first detected during the second trimester of higher-risk pregnancies (maternal age greater than 35) with a triple screen, involving decreased serum levels of maternal serum α-fetoprotein, increased levels of human chorionic gonatotropin (hCG), and decreased levels of estriol.[95] First-trimester risk assessment is becoming more widely available with detection rates of 87% and increased sensitivity for DS.[96]

Anatomic and medical features in DS are distinctive, involving a small broad head with sparse hair, small upward slanting eyes with epicanthal folds, small nose and ears, and a protruding tongue. Hands have a single transverse palmar crease, deviation of the fifth finger, and abnormally short digits. The pelvis may be hypoplastic, the atlantoaxial joint unstable, and muscles hypotonic. Laxity in joints leads to chronic patellar dislocation, pes planus, and ankle pronation.[97] DS involves cardiovascular, gastrointestinal, genitourinary, hematologic, ophthalmologic, and auditory abnormalities. Atrioventricular septal defects (45%) and ventricular septal defects (35%) are the most common congenital heart lesions.[98] Pulmonary hypertension is seen possibly as the result of the decreased number of alveoli, and celiac disease is prevalent (5%–15%).[99] Congenital and acquired cataracts and strabismus are common visual problems[97] and sensorineural hearing loss is higher than in the general population.[100] Thyroid function abnormalities are found in up to 30% of patients who have DS[101] and type 1 diabetes mellitus and type 2 diabetes mellitus are seen.[102] Immune dysfunction may be the cause of increased infections, cancers (leukemia, lymphoma, and seminomas), and autoimmune diseases in patients who have DS. Seizures appear bimodally, with a peak in infancy, and a second peak after puberty.[97]

Although children who have DS commonly are described as cheerful and friendly, approximately 20% to 40% have behavioral problems, such as aggression and attention problems in childhood, whereas withdrawal, depression, and early-onset dementia are more common problems in adulthood.[103] In a British study of 3065 adults who had learning disabilities, adults who had DS were much less likely to be physically aggressive (6%) than IQ-matched adults (14%).[104] Meyers and Pueschel found 22.1% of 497 patients who had DS to have psychiatric disorders, including 6.1% of children who had ADHD, 11.9% of children who had conduct or oppositional disorders, and 6.1% of adults who had depression.[105] In a study of negative affective expression and coping strategies, Jahromi and colleagues[106] found that children who had DS expressed more frustration and did not ask for help in comparison with typical children, indicating more limited coping skills and capacity for emotional self-regulation. Glenn and Cunningham found routinized and compulsive behaviors at higher levels in children who had DS than in typical children and found them associated with behavioral problems.[107] Prasher and Day found that 9 of 201 adults (4.5%) who had DS met criteria for obsessive-compulsive disorder.[108]

Depression in DS is expressed differently from that in the typical population because it is poorly verbalized. Crying, depressed appearance, hallucinations, and "vegetative symptoms of disinterest with severe withdrawal and mutism, psychomotor retardation, decreased appetite, weight loss, and insomnia are prominent."[109] Dykens[110] found 42% of 36 young patients who had DS (13–29 years) to have psychosis not otherwise specified characterized by frequent auditory and visual hallucinations rather than aggression. Miano and colleagues[111] found lower sleep efficiency of nine children who had DS (mean age 13.8) in that there was reduced rapid eye movement (REM) sleep and higher percentage of stage 1 non-REM (NREM) compared with age-matched normal controls. In a neuropsychologic battery of testing emotion recognition, frontal lobe functioning, and social approach, Porter and colleagues[112] determined that the inappropriate approach behavior of people who have DS likely is the result of frontal lobe impairment.

The decrement in intellectual skills found in DS is variable with the majority of individuals falling in the mild to moderate range of mental retardation. In updated studies on the cognitive characteristics of DS, relative weaknesses consistently are found associated with expressive language, syntactic processing, and verbal working memory.[113] Nash and Snowling evaluated verbal fluency in children who had DS with age-matched controls and found that the children had less efficient retrieval strategies pointing to executive deficits rather than problems with language processes.[114] Typically, microencephaly is observed in DS. Carter and colleagues[115] observed selective reduction of frontal and parietal gray matter volumes in MRI studies of 15 children and adolescents who had DS compared with age-matched controls. Groen and colleagues[116] found in children who had DS that those who had a stronger hand preference had better language and memory skills, which could not be explained by differences in nonverbal cognitive ability or hearing loss.

Cognitive issues often may evolve in to early-onset Alzheimer dementia (AD). It may be indicated to screen for mosaicism with FISH in selected patients who have mild developmental delay and those who have AD of young onset. Ringman and colleagues did so in the case of a 55-year-old man who had probable early-onset AD and mild developmental delay without prior diagnosis of DS and found trisomy 21 in 10% of peripheral lymphocytes.[117]

Down Syndrome and Autism

Recently, Lowenthal and colleagues[118] sampled 180 subjects who had DS and found 15.8% met criteria for a pervasive developmental disorder with 5.58% meeting criteria for autism—rates double those in past studies. Approximately 50% of the children who had concurrent autism and DS had a pattern of symptom development characteristic of autistic regression and involving substantial loss of language skills. Castillo and colleagues[119] found that autistic regression occurs more commonly and at a later age in children who have DS when compared with autistic children who do not have

DS. Children who have concurrent DS and autism spectrum disorder have lower IQs, bizarre stereotypic behavior, anxiety, and social withdrawal.[120] In DS with autism spectrum disorder (n = 15), white matter in the cerebellum and brainstem was hyperplastic relative to those who had DS alone and is correlated positively with severity of stereotypies.[115]

Treatment Specifically for Down Syndrome

Recently, Rachidi and Lopes[94] found that treatment of DS mouse model Ts65Dn with γ-aminobutryic acid type A (GABAA) antagonists allowed postdrug rescue of cognitive defects, indicating a hopeful direction in clinical therapies for intellectual disability in children who have DS. The GABAA antagonist picrotoxin, at nonepileptic doses, recently showed considerable promise in aTs65Dn mouse model for DS, resulting in lasting improvement in cognition.[121] Rivastigmine, a cholinesterase inhibitor, targeting the cholinergic deficiency found in DS, shows promise in improving cognitive functioning in DS. Heller and colleagues[122] found significant improvement in overall adaptive function, attention, memory, and language domains in 11 subjects who have DS (aged 10–17) treated with rivastigmine for 20 weeks, with transient mild adverse events typically noted with cholinesterase inhibitors. Donepezil, another cholinesterase inhibitor, also has been used to target cognition in DS by Spiridigliozzi and colleagues[123] and found promising for improving memory and language in a 22-week, open-label trial in seven children who had DS. Ellis and colleagues[124] did not find antioxidant (selenium [10 mg], zinc [5 mg, vitamin A [0.9 mg], vitamin E [100 mg], and vitamin C [50 mg]) or folinic acid (0.1 mg) therapy useful in a randomized placebo controlled trial of 156 infants who had DS (younger than 7 months) treated for 18 months and evaluated for development and biochemical markers.

PRADER-WILLI SYNDROME

PWS is a chromosomal disorder, occurring in approximately 1 in 10,000 to 15,000 births. The specific chromosomal defect consists of a missing paternally imprinted portion of chromosome 15. Approximately 70% of individuals who have PWS have a deletion of the region 15q11-13 on the paternally contributed chromosome15, whereas approximately 20% of the remainder have uniparental (maternal) disomy, thus having two intact chromosome 15s of maternal origin while lacking the paternal contribution.[125] Between 1% and 5% of cases have both copies of chromosome 15 intact, with maternal and paternal contributions present, but there is a mutation in the imprinting center that results in abnormal gene expression.[126] This occurs as a result of chromosome 15 translocations or from microdeletions or epimutations of the imprinting center in the 15q11-q13 region.[127] Diagnosis is made with a high-resolution karyotype and is followed by methylation studies specific for PWS.[128]

PWS has a characteristic and dramatic behavioral, cognitive, and physical phenotype. Babies who have PWS may first present with failure to thrive, requiring supplemental tube feedings. Later in childhood they demonstrate insatiable polyphagia, likely arising from hypothalamic dysfunction in the satiety center. Children and adults who have PWS have short stature, are extremely overweight secondary to their intense overeating, and have other congenital abnormalities, including hypogonadism, myopia, strabismus, delayed puberty, mental retardation, and learning disabilities.

As children who have PWS grow, the food-seeking behavior becomes increasingly difficult to control, involving temper tantrums, begging, lying, stealing, taking food from garbage, and attempts to eat frozen, raw, or even pet food.[126] These youngsters have high pain thresholds, sleep disturbances, and skin picking. Treatment involves regular physical activity and strict restriction of access to food. Patients must be monitored for hypoventilation and pulmonary infections secondary to hypotonia. Obstructive sleep apnea syndrome in infants and children who have PWS is common and creates additional risk for delayed mental development.[129] Treatment with growth hormone should be considered. Recently, Bertella and colleagues[130] found that growth hormone–initiated in adult patients who had PWS and continued for 24 months improved quality of life and psychologic well-being. Additionally, Hoybye found that sustained growth hormone treatment of 5 years in nine adults favorably changed body mass (more lean muscle and less body fat).[131] Eiholzer and colleagues[132] found that timely application of hCG to treat hypogonadism in six prepubertal boys who had PWS promoted virilization and normalized muscle mass without detrimental effects on behavior.

Benarroch and colleagues[126] found children who have PWS to be stubborn, insisting on sameness, and inflexible, probably because of impaired executive function and low performance in sequential processing. Ogura and colleagues[133] found that patients who have PWS experience symptoms similar to those who have frontotemporal dementia (as measured by assessment questionnaire), suggesting dysfunction in orbitofrontal cortices and anterior temporal lobes in PWS. Additionally, individuals who have PWS with maternal uniparental disomy as the cause of PWS are at greater risk for autistic symptomatology than those who have paternal deletions of 15q11-q13. They have bizarre rituals and compulsive behaviors, such as playing with feces, skin picking, and anal and vaginal digging.[126] Within the deletion subtypes, Zarcone and colleagues[134] found individuals who had the long type I 15q deletion had more compulsions regarding personal cleanliness (ie, excessive bathing or grooming), and their compulsions were more difficult to interrupt and interfered with social activities more than the other subtypes. In contrast, individuals who had the short type II 15q deletion were more likely to have compulsions related to specific academic areas (ie, re-reading, erasing answers, and counting objects or numbers).

Affect in individuals who have PWS is poorly regulated, resulting in mood swings, frustration, and explosive behavior. In 15% to 17% of persons who have PWS, hypomanic episodes of increased goal-directed behavior and irritability are sufficiently prolonged and profound to justify a diagnosis of mood disorder.[135] Boer and colleagues[136] reported a prevalence of 28% for severe affective disorders with psychotic features (paranoid delusions without hallucinations) in adolescents nearly exclusively associated with uniparental disomy or imprinting genetic types.

TURNER'S SYNDROME

Turner's syndrome (TS) is among the most common sex chromosome aneuploidies (1:2000) and is associated with a loss of the X chromosome resulting in the karyotype 45,XO or a mosaic of 45,XO and 46,XX. The prototypical female patient who has TS has webbed neck, short stature, aortic coarctation, impaired glucose tolerance, autoimmune thyroid disease, hypertension, gonadal dysgenesis, and ovarian failure.[137] At initial diagnosis, it is medically important for patients to have a cardiology consultation, renal ultrasound, audiology evaluation, scoliosis/kyphosis evaluation, ophthalmologic evaluation, orthodontic evaluation, thyroid screen, celiac screen, bone-mineral density scan, and ovarian function evaluation.[138] It also is important to follow progression through puberty and to follow social skill progression. Endocrinology consult can be considered to evaluate the use of growth hormone for augmenting stature.[139] In adolescence, estrogen replacement therapy is the standard recommended treatment.

Girls who have TS have a behavioral phenotype characterized by increased shyness and social anxiety, attention deficits, and hyperactivity.[140,141] In exploring whether or not the social difficulties were the result of family factors rather than genetic sequelae, Mazzocco and colleagues[142] compared nine girls who had TS to their unaffected sisters and found higher ratings of social and attentional problems relative to their unaffected sisters, implying that social dysfunction possibly is a phenotypic element in TS and not due to family environment. On average, women who have TS tend to have a lower level of sexual functioning. Recently, Sheaffer and colleagues[143] found that height and years of education correlated positively with sexual function and partner status whereas age, neck webbing, testosterone levels, age of puberty, hearing loss, and parental origin of the single normal X chromosome did not seem to contribute to sexual function. Women who had TS and were in a partner relationship had relatively normal overall sexual function, but the majority of unpartnered women had low-level sexual functioning. Some women who have TS have increased psychiatric issues. Catinari and colleagues[144] report mild psychotic features that respond to antipsychotic medication, prominent anxiety symptoms, and later life–onset of labile mood.

In TS, there also is a subtle but distinctive neurocognitive phenotype. Girls and women who have TS usually have normal global intellectual function and good verbal skills but characteristically impaired nonverbal abilities (attention, working memory, visual-spatial, visual-perceptual, visual-motor, motor function, and executive function [planning and organizing]).[141] Recently, Messina and colleagues[145] evaluated 33 girls who had TS, ranging from 6 to 18 years old, and found that TS girls as a group may have a slightly reduced full-scale IQ, with verbal IQ significantly higher than performance IQ. Although many children who have TS do well in school, some have resulting academic difficulties at school secondary to visual-spatial cognitive deficits and poor mathematics skills. Murphy and Mazzocco found that 18 TS girls had mathematic learning disabilities especially in visual-spatial cognition relative to their peers.[146] Ross and colleagues[141] suggest that motor speed and verbal memory are improved with the standard estrogen treatment but that tasks involving a spatial component or attention requiring self-monitoring and control of impulsivity are insensitive to estrogen and that those difficulties persist into adulthood.

Extensive neuroimaging research has been performed to better understand the nature of the neurocognitive phenotype of TS. Functional MRI (fMRI) and volumetric MRI studies have found parietal lobe anomalies bilaterally,[147] deficits in frontal striatal and frontal parietal circuits,[148] and reduced areas of the pons, cerebellar vermis lobules VI and VII, and the genu of the corpus callosum[149] as possible explanations for deficits in visuospatial and visuomotor deficits, executive functioning, and interhemispheric spatial processing. Neural pruning mechanisms may be linked to imprinting, as Kesler and colleagues[150] found in 30 female patients (7.6–33.3 years old) who had TS. Those who had maternally derived X chromosome demonstrated more aberrant superior temporal gyrus volumes (involved in language capacities) in gray matter compared with those who had paternally derived X chromosome. Additionally, Kesler and colleagues[151] found larger left amygdala gray matter volumes and disproportionately reduced right hippocampal volumes suggesting that X-linked morphology changes in these regions may be related to the social cognition and memory deficits in TS. Recently, Holzapfel and colleagues[152] found increases in fractional anisotropy values (a measure of degree of myelination) and white matter density in language-related areas of the inferior parietal and temporal lobes in 10 girls who had TS, implicating alterations in white matter pathways in TS. TS subjects seem to have incongruent responses to difficult tasks. In fMRI studies using spatial orientation tasks,

Kesler and colleagues[153] found less activation in the parietal-occipital regions and impaired recruiting of frontal areas as task demands increased in 13 subjects who had TS as compared with their age-matched controls. Although arithmetic performance in 15 female patients who had TS was comparable to their age-matched controls, Kesler and colleagues[154] found that they recruited additional resources in the frontal and parietal regions during easy tasks demonstrating inefficient responses to escalating task difficulty. The deficiencies suggest that the brain in TS is structurally and functionally impaired as a result of the loss of X-linked genetic products.

KLINEFELTER'S SYNDROME

Klinefelter's syndrome (KS) was first noted in 1942 in patients who had small testes, gynecomastia, and hypogonadism. It is a common sex chromosome disorder (1:500–1000)[155] in which the male karyotype has the abnormal addition of an X chromosome, 47,XXY.[156] The sex chromosomal aneuploidies may vary to include 48,XXYY or 48,XXXY at a decreased frequency of 1 per 17,000 to 1 per 50,000 male births.[157] Only 25% of the expected number of individuals who have KS are diagnosed, and most are diagnosed after puberty.[158] Traditionally, a person who has KS is described as "tall, with narrow shoulders, broad hips, sparse body hair, gynecomastia, small testicles, androgen deficiency, azoospermia and decreased verbal intelligence."[158] Definitive diagnosis is made with cytogenetic analysis and almost all patients suffer from infertility.[159]

Infants may present with developmental delay, small phallus, or hypospadias.[157] Zeger and coworkers[160] performed a cross-sectional study of 55 boys who had KS, aged 2.0 to 14.6 years, at an outpatient center to determine common phenotypes and found that they commonly had reduced penile length and small testes in childhood. Boys who have KS may be identified before puberty by tall stature, decreased penile length, clinodactyly, hypotonia, and speech-language deficits. Androgen replacement therapy should begin at approximately age 12 and dosed to maintain age-appropriate serum concentrations of testosterone, estradiol, follicle-stimulating hormone, and luteinizing hormone.[161] If not diagnosed in childhood, adolescents who have KS initially may present with delay of puberty, whereas adults may present with infertility or breast malignancy.[157] Each additional X is associated with a decrease of approximately 15 IQ points, a decline in expressive language skills, and increasingly pronounced physical differences.[157,162] Testosterone replacement corrects the androgen deficiency (libido, bone mineral density, and muscle-bulk) but not infertility. Patients may use intracytoplasmic sperm injection successfully for procreation with the increased risk for transmitting chromosomal errors to their offspring due to higher rates of sex chromosomal hyperploidy and autosomal aneuploidies in their spermatozoa.[163]

KS is associated with higher rates of psychiatric symptoms and deficiencies in cognitive domains. Boks and colleagues[164] report an increase in prevalence of psychiatric disorders, including psychotic disorders in a sample of patients who had KS. Autistic features, such as avoidant eye contact, restricted affect, rigid patterns of play, and social deficits, were noted by Jha and colleagues in two boys who had KS boys (47,XXY and 48,XXYY).[165] Ross and colleagues[166] studied 50 boys who had KS (4.1–17.8 years old) to expand the cognitive phenotype via neuropsychologic measures. Although there was impairment of higher-level language, vocabulary and meaningful language understanding abilities were intact. Motor difficulties were pronounced especially in strength and running speed. The younger boys were unable to sustain attention but did not have impulsivity. Neither genetic factors examined nor previous testosterone treatment accounted for variation in the cognitive phenotype in KS. Vawter and colleagues[167] found overexpressed genes on the extra X chromosome in KS correlated with poor verbal IQ, which may have been responsible for language impairment.

On MRI, Giedd and colleagues[168] discovered that the cortex was significantly thinner in the left inferior frontal, temporal, and superior motor regions with sparing of parietal regions in 42 XXY male subjects age-matched (5–26 years old) against 87 healthy XY male subjects. All are consistent with impairment in language. On fMRI, van Rijn and colleagues[169] found reduced hemispheric specialization for language processing as a result of decreased functional asymmetry in the superior temporal gyrus. They suggest that this deficiency implicates disorganization of thought and language similar to that seen in the schizophrenia spectrum. Rezaie and colleagues[170] also found decreased brain asymmetry throughout the frontal lobes in men who had KS suggesting that the sex chromosomes may influence brain asymmetry in development.

47,XYY AND 48,XXYY

Although KS is the more common sex chromosome aneuploidy in men, the addition of the Y chromosome (47,XYY) also is frequent. Early studies of sex chromosome aneuploidies were based on prison inmates, and the 47,XYY karyotype was associated with violence and aggressiveness. In 1981, Schroder and colleagues[171] reported an increased proportion of sexual crimes of 47,XYY men as compared with other sex chromosomal aneuploidies (ie, XXY). In mouse studies, Park and colleagues[172] found that mice with additional copies of the male sex chromosome had shorter latency to mount, thrust, and achieve ejaculation relative to normal male mice and male mice with additional X chromosomes, which implicates the role of the sex chromosomes in sexual behaviors.

The physical phenotype of 48,XXYY karyotype is commonly a tall, euchanoid men who have long legs, sparse body hair, small testicles and penis, hypergonadotropic hypogonadism, and gynecomastia.[157] They are prone to peripheral vascular disease resulting in leg ulcers and varicosities.[157] Occasionally, 47,XYY may be found in children who have pervasive developmental disorder (2/40)[173] or in children who have autism (1/57).[174] In a retrospective study of 69 subjects who had normal intelligence and who had sex chromosome aberrations, speech delays were common in nearly all abnormal sex karyotypes (47,XYY, 47,XXY, and 47,XXX), except in TS (45,X). Hyperactivity was frequent in 47,XYY and TS but not in those who had a 47,XXX or 47,XXY karyotype.[175] Tartaglia and colleagues[176] studied 95 men who had the rare XXYY syndrome (1:18,000–1:40,000) finding substantial rates of ADHD (72.2%), mood disorders (46.8%), increased autism spectrum disorders (28.3%), intellectual disability (26%), and tic disorders (18.9%). Common medical problems in 48,XXYY included allergies and asthma, congenital heart defects, radioulnar synostosis, inguinal hernia or cryptorchidism, seizures, DVT, intention tremor, and type 2 diabetes mellitus.

SUMMARY

Tremendous advances in understanding of the human genome over the past 2 decades and the clinical science application of this information to pediatrics, neurology and psychiatry, clinical genetics, and clinical psychology have led to the identification of several genetically based disorders that have distinctive behavioral phenotypes that put people who have these disorders at risk for serious psychiatric disorders. These neurogenetic disorders often have a complex developmental course. Several of these genetic disorders are sufficiently prevalent so that practicing clinicians encounter patients who have had these conditions diagnosed and patients who may never have been diagnosed. Good treatment of these individuals requires accurate diagnosis. This can happen only if clinicians are actively aware of the possibility that some of their patients may have unrecognized genetic disorders presenting as psychiatric symptoms and are knowledgeable about the association between patients' symptoms and their underlying genetic bases. Good treatment of neurogenetic disorders generally includes providing highly salient information to patients and family members about the causes and prognoses for their conditions (including appropriate genetic counseling, when indicated). Although psychiatrists may be able to treat emergent emotional or behavioral symptoms, patients are best served if they can remain for the long haul with a multidisciplinary team of providers who recognize and accept the realities of a lifetime course, the high risk for symptom recurrence, the special need to provide information and support to the families of the patients, and the necessity of coordinating medical and psychiatric care.

REFERENCES

1. Landis S, Insel TR. The "neuro" in neurogenetics. Science 2008;322(5903):821.
2. Reiss A, Dant C. The behavioral neurogenetics of fragile X syndrome: analyzing gene-brain-behavior relationships in child developmental psychopathologies. Dev Psychopathol 2003;15(4):927–78.
3. Jasny BR, Kelner KL, Pennisi E. From genes to social behavior. Science 2008; 322(5903):891.
4. Donaldson ZR, Young LJ. Oxytocin, vasopressin, and the neurogenetics of sociality. Science 2008;32(5903):900–4.
5. Robinson GE, Fernald RD, Clayton DF. Genes and social behavior. Science 2008;322(5903):896–900.
6. Feinstein C, Singh S. Social phenotypes in neurogenetic syndromes. Child Adolesc Psychiatr Clin N Am 2007;16(3):631–47.
7. Gothelf D. Velocardiofacial syndrome. Child Adolesc Psychiatr Clin N Am 2007; 16(3):677–93.
8. Gothelf D, Schaer M, Eliez S. Genes, brain development and psychiatric phenotypes in velo-cardio-facial syndrome. Dev Disabil Res Rev 2008;14:59–68.
9. Gothelf D, Feinstein C, Thompson T, et al. Risk factors for the emergence of psychotic disorders in adolescents with 22q11.2 deletion syndrome. Am J Psychiatry 2007;164(4):663–9.
10. Kirkpatarick JA, DiGeorge AM. Congenital absence of the thymus. Am J Roentgenol Radium Ther Nucl Med 1968;103:32–7.
11. Shprintzen RJ, Goldbert RB, Lewin ML, et al. A new syndrome involving cleft palat, caradiac anomalies, typical facies, and learning disabilities: velo-cardiofacial syndrome. Cleft Palate J 1978;15(1):56–62.
12. Ryan AK, Goodship JA, Wilson DI, et al. Spectrum of clinical features associated with interstitial chromosome 22q11 deletions: a European collaborative study. J Med Genet 1997;34(10):798–804.
13. McDonald-McGinn D, Kirschner R, Goldmuntz E. The Philadelphia story: the 22q11.2deletion:report on 250patients. Genet Couns 1999;10:11–24.
14. Shaikh TH, Kurahashi H, Saitta SC, et al. Chromosome 22-specific low copy repeats and the 22q11.2 deletions syndrome: genomic organization and deletion endpoint analysis. Hum Mol Genet 2000;9(4):489–501.

15. Botto L, May K, Fernhoff P, et al. A population-based study of the 22q11.2 deletion: phenotype, incidence, and contribution to major birth defects in the population. Pediatrics 2003;112:101–7.
16. Marino B, Mileto F, Digilio MC. Congential cardiovascular disease and velo-car-dio-facial syndrome. In: Murphy KC, Scambler PJ, editors. Velo-cardio-facial syndrome: a model for understanding microdeletion disorders. Cambridge (UK): Cambridge University Press; 2005. p. 47–82.
17. Eliez S, Feinstein C. Velo-cardio-facial syndrome (deletion 22q11.2): a homoge-neous neurodevelopmental model for schizophrenia. In: Keshavan M, Kennedy J, Murray R, editors. Neurodevelopment and schizophrenia. Cam-bridge: Cambridge University Press; 2004. p. 121–37.
18. Feinstein C, Eliez S. The velocardiofacial syndrome in psychiatry. Curr Opin Psychiatry 2000;13:485–90.
19. Gerdes M, Solot C, Wang PP, et al. Cognitive and behavior profie of preschool children with chromosome 22q11.2 deletion. Am J Med Genet 1999;85:127–33.
20. Solot CB, Gerdes M, Kirschner RE, et al. Communication issues in 22q11.2 deletion syndrome: children at risk. Genet Med 2001;3(1):67–71.
21. Moss E, Batshaw M, Solot C. Psychoeducational profile of the 22q11.2 microde-letion: a complex pattern. J Pediatrics 1999;134:193–8.
22. Antshel KM, Abdulsabur N, Roizen N, et al. Sex differences in cognitive func-tioning in velocardiofacial syndrome (VCFS). Dev Neuropsychol 2005;28(3):849–69.
23. Gothelf D, Frisch A, Munitz H, et al. Velocardiofacial manifestations amd micro-deletions in schizophrenic inpatients. Am J Med Genet 1997;72:455–61.
24. Shprintzen RJ. Velo-cardio-facial syndrome: a distinctive behavioral phenotype. Ment Retard Dev Disabil Res Rev 2000;6(2):142–7.
25. Arnold PD, Siegel-Bartelt J, Cytrynbaum C, et al. Velo-cardio-facial syndrome: implications of microdeletion 22q11 for schizophrenia and mood disorders. Am J Med Genet 2001;105(4):354–62.
26. Feinstein C, Eliez S, Blasey C, et al. Psychiatric disorders and behavioral problems in children with velocardiofacial syndrome: usefulness as phenotypic indicators of schizophrenia risk. Biol Psychiatry 2002;51(4):312–8.
27. Antshel KM, Fremont W, Roizen N, et al. ADHD, major depressive disorder, and simple phobias are prevalent psychiatric conditions in youth with velocardiofa-cial syndrome. J Am Acad Child Adolesc Psychiatry 2006;45:593–603.
28. Jansen PW, Duijff SN, Beemer FA, et al. Behavioral problems in relation to intel-ligence in children with 22q11.2 deletion syndrome: a matched control study. Am J Med Genet A 2007;143(6):574–80.
29. Fine SE, Weissman A, Gerdes M, et al. Autism spectrum disorders and symp-toms in children with molecularly confirmed 22q11.2 deletion syndrome. J Autism Dev Disord 2005;35(4):461–70.
30. Vorstman JA, Morcus M, Duijff SN, et al. The 22q11.2 deletion in children: high rate of autistic disorders and early onset of psychotic symptoms. J Am Acad Child Adolesc Psychiatry 2006;45(9):1104–13.
31. Reirson AM. Psychopathology in 22q11.2 deletion syndrome. (letter to the editor). J Am Acad Child Adolesc Psychiatry 2007;46(8):942.
32. Eliez S. Autism in children with 22q11.2 deletion syndrome. (letter to the editor). J Am Acad Child Adolesc Psychiatry 2007;46(4):433–4.
33. Usiskin S, Nicolson R, Krasnewich D. Velocardiofacial syndrome in childhood-onset schizophrenia. J Am Acad Child Adolesc Psychiatry 1999;38:1536–43.

34. Baker KD, Skuse DH. Adolescents and young adults with 22q11 deletion syndrome: psychopathology in an at-risk group. Br J Psychiatry 2005;186:115–20.
35. Gothelf D, Eliez S, Thompson T, et al. COMT genotype predicts longitudinal cognitive decline and psychosis in 22q11.2 deletion syndrome. Nat Neurosci 2005;8(11):1500–2.
36. Bassett AS, Caluseriu O, Weksberg R, et al. Catechol-O-methyl transferase and expression of schizophrenia in 73 adults with 22q11.2 deletion syndrome. Biol Psychiatry 2007;61(10):1119–20.
37. Shprintzen RJ, Goldberg RB, Golding-Kushner KJ, et al. Late-onset psychosis in the velo-cardio-facial syndrome. Am J Med Genet 1992;42:141–2.
38. Pulver AE, Nestadt G, Goldberg R, et al. Psychotic illness in patients with velo-cardio–facial syndrome ane their relatives. J Nerv Ment Dis 1994;182:476–8.
39. Karayiorgou M, Morris MA, Morrow B, et al. Schizophrenia susceptibiliity associated with interstitial deletions of chromosome 22q11. Proc Natl Acad Sci USA 1995;92:7612–76.
40. Bassett A, Chow E. 22q11 deletion syndrome: a genetic subtype of schizophrenian. Biol Psychiatry 1999;46:882–91.
41. Bassett AS, Chow EW. Schizophrenia and 22q11.2 deletion syndrome. Curr Psychiatry Rep 2008;10(2):148–57.
42. Murphy K, Jones L, Owen M. High rates of schizophrenia in adults with velo-cardio-facial syndrome. Arch Gen Psychiatry 1999;56:940–5.
43. Brega AG, Goodrich G, Bennett RE, et al. The primary cognitive deficit among males with fagile-X-associated tremor.ataxia syndrome (FXTAS) is a dysexecutive. J Clin Exp Neuropsychol 2008;30(8):853–69.
44. Eliez S, Feinstein C. The fragile X syndrome: bridging the gap from gene to behavior. Curr Opin Psychiatry 2001;14:443–9.
45. Bell MJ. A pedigree of mental defect showing sex-linkage. J Neurol Psychiatry 1943;6:154–7.
46. Hagerman RJ. Physical and behavioral phenotype. In: Hagerman R, Cronister A, editors. Fragilel X syndrome: diagnosis, treatment, and research. 2nd edition. Baltimore (MD): Johns Hopkins University Press; 1996. p. 3–87.
47. Verkerk AJ, Pieretti M, Sutcliffe JS. Identification of a gene (FMR-1) containing a CGG repeat coincidenet with a breakpoint cluster region exhibiting length variation in frabile X syndrome. Cell 1991;65(5):905–14.
48. Hagerman RJ, Hagerman PJ. Testing for Fragile X gene mutations throught the life span. JAMA 2008;300(20):2419–21.
49. Crawford D, Meadows K, Newman J. Prevalence and phenotype consequence of FRAXA and FRAXE alleles in a large, ethnically diverse, special educaton-needs population. Am J Hum Genet 1999;2:495–507.
50. Hagerman R. Clinical and molecular aspects of fragile X syndrome. In: Tager-Flusberg H, editor. Neurodevelopmental disorders. Cambridge (MA): MIT Press; 1999. p. 27–42.
51. Hagerman PJ, Hagerman RJ. The fragile X premuation: a maturing perspective. Am J Hum Genet 2004;75:805–16.
52. Rousseau F, Rouillard P, Morel ML, et al. Prevalence of carriers of premutation-size alleles of the FMR1 gene-and implications for the populaton genetics of the fragile X syndrome. Am J Hum Genet 1995;57:1006–18.
53. Dombrowski C, Levesque ML, Morel ML, et al. Premutationand intermediae-size allelels of the FMR1 alleles in 10, 572 males from the general population: loss of an AGG interruption is a late event in the generation of fragile X syndrome alleles. Hum Mol Genet 2002;11:371–8.

54. Song FJ, Barton P, Sleightholme V, et al. Screening for fragile X syndrome: a literature review and modeling study. Health Technol Assess 2003;7(16):1–106.
55. Tassone F, Pan R, Amiri K, et al. A rapid polymerase chain reaction-based screening method for identification of all expanded alleles of the fragile X (FMR1) gene in newborn and high-risk populations. J Mol Diagn 2008;10(1):43–9.
56. Lachiewicz AM, Dawson DV, Spiridigliozzi GA. Physical characteristics of young boys with fragile X syndrome: reasons for difficulties in makng a diagnosis in young males. Am J Med Genet 2000;92:229–36.
57. Bailey D, Hatton D, Skinner M, et al. Early developmental trajectories of males with fragile X syndrome. Am J Ment Retard 1998;103(1):29–39.
58. Fisch G, Carpenter N, Holden JA, et al. Longitudinal assessment of adpative and maladaptive behaviors in fragile X males. Am J Med Genet 1999;83:257–63.
59. Kau A, Reider E, Payne L, et al. Early behavior signs of psychiatric phenotypes in fragile X syndrome. Am J Ment Retard 2000;105:266–99.
60. Reiss AL, Hall SS. Fragile X Syndrome: assessment and treatment implications. Child Adolesc Psychiatr Clin N Am 2007;16(3):663–75.
61. Skinner M, Hooper S, Hatton DD, et al. Mapping nonverbal IQ in young boys with fragile X syndrome. Am J Med Genet 2005;132(1):25–32.
62. Mazzocco MM, Pennington BF, Hagerman RJ. The neurocognitive phenotype of female carriers of fragile X: additional evidence for specificity. J Dev Behav Pediatr 1993;14(5):328–35.
63. Mazzocco MM, Pennington BF, Hagerman RJ. Social cognition skills among females with fragile X. J Autism Dev Disord 1994;24(4):473–85.
64. Wattendorf DJ, Muenke M. Diagnosis and management of fragile X syndrome. Am Fam Physician 2005;72(1):111–3.
65. Maes B, Fryns JP, Ghesquiere P, et al. Phenotypic checklist to screen for fragile X syndrome in people with mental retardatopm. Ment Retard 2000;38:207–15.
66. Lachiewicz AM, Spiridigliozzi GA, Gullion CM. Aberrant behavior of young boys wieteh fragile X syndrome. Am J Ment Retard 1994;98:567–79.
67. Baumgardner T, Reiss A, Freund L, et al. Specification of the neurobehavioral phenotype in males with fragile X syndrome. Pediatrics 1995;95:744–52.
68. Einfeld SL, Tonge BJ, Florio T. Behavioral and emotional disturbance in fragile X syndrome. Am J Med Genet 1994;51:386–91.
69. Garrett AS, Menon V, MacKenzie K, et al. Here's looking at you, kid: neural systems underlying face and gaze processing in fragile X syndrome. Arch Gen Psychiatry 2004;61(3):281–8.
70. Hessl D, Blaser B, Dyer-Friedman J, et al. Social behavior and cortisol reactivity in children with fragile X syndrome. J Child Psychol Psychiatry 2006;47(6):602–10.
71. Feinstein C, Reiss A. Autism: the point of view from fragile x studies. J Autism Dev Disord 1998;28(5):393–405.
72. Hatton DD, Sideris J, Skinner M, et al. Autistic behavior in children with fragile X syndrome: prevalence, stability, and the impact of FMRP. Am J Med Genet A 2006;140(17):1804–13.
73. Rogers S, Wehner E, Hagerman R. The behavioral phenotype in fragile X: symptoms of autism in very young children with fragile X syndrome, idiopathic autism, and other developmental disorders. J Dev Behav Pediatr 2001;22:409–17.
74. Turk J, Grahan P. Fragile X syndrome, autism and autistic features. Autism 1997; 1:175–97.
75. Bailey D, Mesibov G, Hatton D, et al. Autistic behavior in young boys with fragile X syndrome. J Autism Dev Disord 1998;28:499–507.

76. Demark J, Feldman M, Holden J. Behavioral relationship between autism and fragile X syndrome. Am J Ment Retard 2003;108:314–26.
77. Kaufmann W, Corell R, Kau A, et al. Autisms spectrum disorder in fragile X syndrome: communication, social ineraction, and specific behaviors. Am J Med Genet 2004;129A:225–34.
78. Hagerman R. Commonalities in the neurobiology between autism and fragile X. J Intellect Disabil Res 2008;52(10):817.
79. Sobesky WE, Taylor AK, Pennington BF, et al. Molecular/clinical correlations in females with fragile X. Am J Med Genet 1996;64(2):340–5.
80. Freund LS, Reiss AL, Abrams MT. Psychiatric disorders associated with fragile X in the young female. Pediatrics 1993;91(2):321–9.
81. hagan CC, Hoeft F, Mackey A, et al. Aberrant neural function during emotion attribution in female subjects with fragile X syndrome. J Am Acad Child Adolesc Psychiatry 2008;47(12):1443–54.
82. Farzin F, Perry H, Hessl D, et al. Autism spectrum disorders and attention-deficit/hyperactivity disorder in boys with the fragile X premutation. J Dev Behav Pediatr 2006;27(2 Suppl):S137–44.
83. Roberts JE, Bailey DB, Mankowski J, et al. Mood and anxiety disorders in females with the FMR1 premutation. Am J Med Genet B Neuropsychiatr Genet 2008.
84. Jacquement S, Hagerman RJ, Seehev MA, et al. Penetrance of the fragile X-associated tremor/ataxia syndrome in a premutation carrier population. JAMA 2004;291(4):460–9.
85. Sherman SL. Premature ovarian failure in the fragile X syndrome. Am J Hum Genet 2000;97:189–94.
86. Hagerman J, Hagerman R. The fragile X premutation: a maturing perspective. Am J Hum Genet 2004;74:805–16.
87. Goodlin-Jones BL, Tassone F, Gane LW, et al. Autism spectrum disorder and the fragigle X premutation. J Dev Behav Pediatr 2004;25:3392–8.
88. Tassone F, Hagerman RJ, Taylor AK, et al. Clinical involvement and protein expression in individuals with the FMR1 premutation. Am J Med Genet 2000; 91:144–52.
89. Bailey DB, Raspa M, Olmsed M, et al. Co-occurring conditions associated with FMR1 gene variations: findings from a national parent survey. Am J Med Genet 2008;146A(16):2060–9.
90. Grigsby J, Brega AG, Engle K, et al. Cognitive profile of fragile X premutation carriers with and without fragile X-associated tremor/ataxia syndrome. Neuropsychology 2008;22:48–60.
91. Sherman SL, Allen EG, Bean LH, et al. Epidemiology of Down syndrome. Ment Retard Dev Disabil Res Rev 2007;13(3):221–7.
92. Baum RA, Nash PL, Foster JE, et al. Primary care of children and adolescents with down syndrome: an update. Curr Probl Pediatr Adolesc Health Care 2008;38(8):241–61.
93. Lockstone HE, Harris LW, Swatton JE, et al. Gene expression profiling in the adult down syndrome brain. Genomics 2007;90(6):647–60.
94. Rachidi M, Lopes C. Mental retardation and associated neurological dysfunctions in Down syndrome: a consequence of dysregulation in critical chromosome 21 genes and associated molecular pathways. Eur J Paediatr Neurol 2008;12(3):168–82.
95. Wildschut HI, Peters TJ, Weiner CP. Screening in women's health, with emphasis on fetal Down's syndrome, breast cancer and osteoporosis. Hum Reprod Update 2006;12(5):499–512.

96. Reddy UM, Wapner RJ. Comparison of first and second trimester aneuploidy risk assessment. Clin Obstet Gynecol 2007;50(2):442–53.
97. Davidson MA. Primary care for children and adolescents with Down syndrome. Pediatr Clin North Am 2008;55(5):1099–111, xi.
98. Freeman SB, Taft LF, Dooley KJ, et al. Population-based study of congenital heart defects in Down syndrome. Am J Med Genet 1998;80(3):213–7.
99. Cooney TP, Thurlbeck WM. Pulmonary hypoplasia in Down's syndrome. N Engl J Med 1982;307(19):1170–3.
100. Roizen NJ, Wolters C, Nicol T, et al. Hearing loss in children with Down syndrome. J Pediatr 1993;123(1):S9–12.
101. Tuysuz B, Beker DB. Thyroid dysfunction in children with Down's syndrome. Acta Paediatr 2001;90(12):1389–93.
102. Van Goor JC, Massa GG, Hirasing R. Increased incidence and prevalence of diabetes mellitus in Down's syndrome. Arch Dis Child 1997;77(2):186.
103. Visootsak J, Sherman S. Neuropsychiatric and behavioral aspects of trisomy 21. Curr Psychiatry Rep 2007;9(2):135–40.
104. Tyrer F, McGrother CW, Thorp CF, et al. Physical aggression towards others in adults with learning disabilities: prevalence and associated factors. J Intellect Disabil Res 2006;50(Pt 4):295–304.
105. Myers BA, Pueschel SM. Psychiatric disorders in persons with Down syndrome. J Nerv Ment Dis 1991;179(10):609–13.
106. Jahromi LB, Gulsrud A, Kasari C. Emotional competence in children with Down syndrome: negativity and regulation. Am J Ment Retard 2008;113(1):32–43.
107. Glenn S, Cunningham C. Typical or pathological? Routinized and compulsive-like behaviors in children and young people with Down syndrome. Intellect Dev Disabil 2007;45(4):246–56.
108. Prasher VP, Day S. Brief report: obsessive-compulsive disorder in adults with Down's Syndrome. J Autism Dev Disord 1995;25(4):453–8.
109. Myers BA, Pueschel SM. Major depression in a small group of adults with Down syndrome. Res Dev Disabil 1995;16(4):285–99.
110. Dykens EM. Psychiatric and behavioral disorders in persons with Down syndrome. Ment Retard Dev Disabil Res Rev 2007;13(3):272–8.
111. Miano S, Bruni O, Elia M, et al. Sleep phenotypes of intellectual disability: a polysomnographic evaluation in subjects with Down syndrome and fragile-X syndrome. Clin Neurophysiol 2008;119(6):1242–7.
112. Porter MA, Coltheart M, Langdon R. The neuropsychological basis of hypersociability in Williams and Down syndrome. Neuropsychologia 2007;45(12):2839–49.
113. Silverman W. Down syndrome: cognitive phenotype. Ment Retard Dev Disabil Res Rev 2007;13(3):228–36.
114. Nash HM, Snowling MJ. Semantic and phonological fluency in children with Down syndrome: atypical organization of language or less efficient retrieval strategies? Cogn Neuropsychol 2008;25(5):690–703.
115. Carter JC, Capone GT, Kaufmann WE. Neuroanatomic correlates of autism and stereotypy in children with Down syndrome. Neuroreport 2008;19(6):653–6.
116. Groen MA, Yasin I, Laws G, et al. Weak hand preference in children with down syndrome is associated with language deficits. Dev Psychobiol 2008;50(3):242–50.
117. Ringman JM, Rao PN, Lu PH, et al. Mosaicism for trisomy 21 in a patient with young-onset dementia: a case report and brief literature review. Arch Neurol 2008;65(3):412–5.

118. Lowenthal R, Paula CS, Schwartzman JS, et al. Prevalence of pervasive developmental disorder in Down's syndrome. J Autism Dev Disord 2007;37(7):1394–5.
119. Castillo H, Patterson B, Hickey F, et al. Difference in age at regression in children with autism with and without Down syndrome. J Dev Behav Pediatr 2008;29(2): 89–93.
120. Carter JC, Capone GT, Gray RM, et al. Autistic-spectrum disorders in Down syndrome: further delineation and distinction from other behavioral abnormalities. Am J Med Genet B Neuropsychiatr Genet 2007;144B(1):87–94.
121. Fernandez F, Morishita W, Zuniga E, et al. Pharmacotherapy for cognitive impairment in a mouse model of Down syndrome. Nat Neurosci 2007;10(4):411–3.
122. Heller JH, Spiridigliozzi GA, Crissman BG, et al. Safety and efficacy of rivastigmine in adolescents with Down syndrome: a preliminary 20-week, open-label study. J Child Adolesc Psychopharmacol 2006;16(6):755–65.
123. Spiridigliozzi GA, Heller JH, Crissman BG, et al. Preliminary study of the safety and efficacy of donepezil hydrochloride in children with Down syndrome: a clinical report series. Am J Med Genet A 2007;143A(13):1408–13.
124. Ellis JM, Tan HK, Gilbert RE, et al. Supplementation with antioxidants and folinic acid for children with Down's syndrome: randomised controlled trial. BMJ 2008; 336(7644):594–7.
125. Dykens EM, Roof E. Behavior in Prader-Willi Syndrome: relationship to genetic subtypes and age. J Child Psychol Psychiatry 2008;49(9):1001–8.
126. Benarroch F, Hirsch HJ, Genstil L, et al. Prader-Willi Syndrome: medical prevention and behavioral challenges. Child Adolesc Psychiatr Clin N Am 2007;16(3): 695–708.
127. Bittel DC, Butler MG. Prader-Willi syndrome: clinical genetics, cytogenetics and molecular biology. Expert Rev Mol Med 2005;7(14):1–20.
128. Wattendorf DJ, Muenke M. Prader-Willi syndrome. Am Fam Physician 2005; 72(5):827–30.
129. Festen DA, Wevers M, de Weerd AW, et al. Psychomotor development in infants with Prader-Willi syndrome and associations with sleep-related breathing disorders. Pediatr Res 2007;62(2):221–4.
130. Bertella L, Mori I, Grugni G, et al. Quality of life and psychological well-being in GH-treated, adult PWS patients: a longitudinal study. J Intellect Disabil Res 2007;51(Pt 4):302–11.
131. Hoybye C. Five-years growth hormone (GH) treatment in adults with Prader-Willi syndrome. Acta Paediatr 2007;96(3):410–3.
132. Eiholzer U, Grieser J, Schlumpf M, et al. Clinical effects of treatment for hypogonadism in male adolescents with Prader-Labhart-Willi syndrome. Horm Res 2007;68(4):178–84.
133. Ogura K, Shinohara M, Ohno K, et al. Frontal behavioral syndromes in Prader-Willi syndrome. Brain Dev 2008;30(7):469–76.
134. Zarcone J, Napolitano D, Peterson C, et al. The relationship between compulsive behaviour and academic achievement across the three genetic subtypes of Prader-Willi syndrome. J Intellect Disabil Res 2007;51(Pt 6):478–87.
135. Vogels A, De Hert M, Descheemaeker MJ, et al. Psychotic disorders in Prader-Willi syndrome. Am J Med Genet A 2004;127A(3):238–43.
136. Boer H, Holland A, Whittington J, et al. Psychotic illness in people with Prader Willi syndrome due to chromosome 15 maternal uniparental disomy. Lancet 2002;359(9301):135–6.
137. Jones KL, Smith DW. Smith's recognizable patterns of human malformation. 6th edition. Philadelphia: Elsevier Saunders; 2006.

138. Bondy CA. Care of girls and women with Turner syndrome: a guideline of the Turner Syndrome Study Group. J Clin Endocrinol Metab 2007;92(1):10–25.
139. Loscalzo ML. Turner syndrome. Pediatr Rev 2008;29(7):219–27.
140. Siegel PT, Clopper R, Stabler B. The psychological consequences of Turner syndrome and review of the National Cooperative Growth Study psychological substudy. Pediatrics 1998;102(2 Pt 3):488–91.
141. Ross JL, Stefanatos GA, Kushner H, et al. Persistent cognitive deficits in adult women with Turner syndrome. Neurology 2002;58(2):218–25.
142. Mazzocco MM, Baumgardner T, Freund LS, et al. Social functioning among girls with fragile X or Turner syndrome and their sisters. J Autism Dev Disord 1998; 28(6):509–17.
143. Sheaffer AT, Lange E, Bondy CA. Sexual function in women with Turner syndrome. J Womens Health (Larchmt) 2008;17(1):27–33.
144. Catinari S, Vass A, Heresco-Levy U. Psychiatric manifestations in Turner Syndrome: a brief survey. Isr J Psychiatry Relat Sci 2006;43(4):293–5.
145. Messina MF, Zirilli G, Civa R, et al. Neurocognitive profile in Turner's syndrome is not affected by growth impairment. J Pediatr Endocrinol Metab 2007;20(6):677–84.
146. Murphy MM, Mazzocco MM. Mathematics learning disabilities in girls with fragile X or Turner syndrome during late elementary school. J Learn Disabil 2008;41(1):29–46.
147. Brown WE, Kesler SR, Eliez S, et al. A volumetric study of parietal lobe subregions in Turner syndrome. Dev Med Child Neurol 2004;46(9):607–9.
148. Haberecht MF, Menon V, Warsofsky IS, et al. Functional neuroanatomy of visuospatial working memory in Turner syndrome. Hum Brain Mapp 2001;14(2): 96–107.
149. Fryer SL, Kwon H, Eliez S, et al. Corpus callosum and posterior fossa development in monozygotic females: a morphometric MRI study of Turner syndrome. Dev Med Child Neurol 2003;45(5):320–4.
150. Kesler SR, Blasey CM, Brown WE, et al. Effects of X-monosomy and X-linked imprinting on superior temporal gyrus morphology in Turner syndrome. Biol Psychiatry 2003;54(6):636–46.
151. Kesler SR, Garrett A, Bender B, et al. Amygdala and hippocampal volumes in Turner syndrome: a high-resolution MRI study of X-monosomy. Neuropsychologia 2004;42(14):1971–8.
152. Holzapfel M, Barnea-Goraly N, Eckert MA, et al. Selective alterations of white matter associated with visuospatial and sensorimotor dysfunction in turner syndrome. J Neurosci 2006;26(26):7007–13.
153. Kesler SR, Haberecht MF, Menon V, et al. Functional neuroanatomy of spatial orientation processing in Turner syndrome. Cereb Cortex 2004;14(2):174–80.
154. Kesler SR, Menon V, Reiss AL. Neuro-functional differences associated with arithmetic processing in Turner syndrome. Cereb Cortex 2006;16(6):849–56.
155. Bojesen A, Juul S, Gravholt CH. Prenatal and postnatal prevalence of Klinefelter syndrome: a national registry study. J Clin Endocrinol Metab 2003;88(2):622–6.
156. Bradbury JT, Bunge RG, Boccabella RA. Chromatin test in Klinefelter's syndrome. J Clin Endocrinol Metab 1956;16(5):689.
157. Visootsak J, Graham JM Jr. Klinefelter syndrome and other sex chromosomal aneuploidies. Orphanet J Rare Dis 2006;1:42.
158. Bojesen A, Gravholt CH. Klinefelter syndrome in clinical practice. Nat Clin Pract Urol 2007;4(4):192–204.
159. Smyth CM, Bremner WJ. Klinefelter syndrome. Arch Intern Med 1998;158(12): 1309–14.

160. Zeger MP, Zinn AR, Lahlou N, et al. Effect of ascertainment and genetic features on the phenotype of Klinefelter syndrome. J Pediatr 2008;152(5):716–22.
161. Kocar IH, Yesilova Z, Ozata M, et al. The effect of testosterone replacement treatment on immunological features of patients with Klinefelter's syndrome. Clin Exp Immunol 2000;121(3):448–52.
162. Linden MG, Bender BG, Robinson A. Sex chromosome tetrasomy and pentasomy. Pediatrics 1995;96(4 Pt 1):672–82.
163. Lanfranco F, Kamischke A, Zitzmann M, et al. Klinefelter's syndrome. Lancet 2004;364(9430):273–83.
164. Boks MP, de Vette MH, Sommer IE, et al. Psychiatric morbidity and X-chromosomal origin in a Klinefelter sample. Schizophr Res Jul 2007;93(1–3):399–402.
165. Jha P, Sheth D, Ghaziuddin M. Autism spectrum disorder and Klinefelter syndrome. Eur Child Adolesc Psychiatry 2007;16(5):305–8.
166. Ross JL, Roeltgen DP, Stefanatos G, et al. Cognitive and motor development during childhood in boys with Klinefelter syndrome. Am J Med Genet A 2008; 146A(6):708–19.
167. Vawter MP, Harvey PD, DeLisi LE. Dysregulation of X-linked gene expression in Klinefelter's syndrome and association with verbal cognition. Am J Med Genet B Neuropsychiatr Genet 2007;144B(6):728–34.
168. Giedd JN, Clasen LS, Wallace GL, et al. XXY (Klinefelter syndrome): a pediatric quantitative brain magnetic resonance imaging case-control study. Pediatrics 2007;119(1):e232–40.
169. van Rijn S, Aleman A, Swaab H, et al. Effects of an extra X chromosome on language lateralization: an fMRI study with Klinefelter men (47,XXY). Schizophr Res 2008;101(1–3):17–25.
170. Rezaie R, Daly EM, Cutter WJ, et al. The influence of sex chromosome aneuploidy on brain asymmetry. Am J Med Genet B Neuropsychiatr Genet 2008.
171. Schroder J, de la Chapelle A, Hakola P, et al. The frequency of XYY and XXY men among criminal offenders. Acta Psychiatr Scand 1981;63(3):272–6.
172. Park JH, Burns-Cusato M, Dominguez-Salazar E, et al. Effects of sex chromosome aneuploidy on male sexual behavior. Genes Brain Behav 2008;7(6): 609–17.
173. Nicolson R, Bhalerao S, Sloman L. 47,XYY karyotypes and pervasive developmental disorders. Can J Psychiatry 1998;43(6):619–22.
174. Herman GE, Henninger N, Ratliff-Schaub K, et al. Genetic testing in autism: how much is enough? Genet Med 2007;9(5):268–74.
175. Hier DB, Atkins L, Perlo VP. Learning disorders and sex chromosome aberrations. J Ment Defic Res 1980;24(1):17–26.
176. Tartaglia N, Davis S, Hench A, et al. A new look at XXYY syndrome: medical and psychological features. Am J Med Genet A 2008;146A(12):1509–22.

Review of Pediatric Attention Deficit/ Hyperactivity Disorder for the General Psychiatrist

Christopher J. Kratochvil, MD[a,*], Brigette S. Vaughan, MSN, APRN[a], Amy Barker, MD[b], Lindsey Corr, MD[b], Ashley Wheeler, MD[b], Vishal Madaan, MD[b]

KEYWORDS

- Attention • Hyperactivity • Impulsivity • ADHD
- Treatment • Diagnosis

Attention deficit/hyperactivity disorder (ADHD) is a common and impairing psychiatric condition, affecting significant numbers of children and adolescents. General psychiatrists serve, both by choice and out of necessity, in the assessment and treatment of children and adolescents who have ADHD and in the education of patients and their families. For many clinicians, however, there are numerous unanswered questions regarding the diagnosis and therapeutic interventions for ADHD. This article provides general psychiatrists with a practical overview and update on the assessment, diagnosis, and treatment of pediatric ADHD.

Background information, recent relevant research, current evidence-based practice guidelines, and tips for clinical practice are reviewed in this article. The information is presented in a question-answer format.

HOW COMMON IS ATTENTION DEFICIT/HYPERACTIVITY DISORDER?

ADHD is one of the most common psychiatric disorders in pediatrics. Conservative estimates report ADHD prevalence rates of 3% to 7% in children,[1] with other estimates

Dr. Kratochvil is supported by NIMH Grant 5K23MH06612701A1; receives grant support from Eli Lilly, McNeil, Shire, Abbott, and Somerset; is a consultant for Eli Lilly, AstraZeneca, Abbott, and Pfizer; and receives study drugs for an NIMH-funded study from Eli Lilly.
[a] Division of Child and Adolescent Psychiatry, Department of Psychiatry, University of Nebraska Medical Center, 985581 Nebraska Medical Center, Omaha, NE 68198-5581, USA
[b] Division of Child and Adolescent Psychiatry, Department of Psychiatry, Creighton University/ University of Nebraska Medical Center, Omaha, NE 68198-5581, USA
* Corresponding author.
E-mail address: ckratoch@unmc.edu (C.J. Kratochvil).

as high as 7% to 12%.[2,3] Even if the conservative reports are the most accurate, ADHD is clearly a significant public health issue. Additionally, as many as 60% to 85% of children diagnosed with ADHD continue to meet criteria for the disorder as teenagers, and up to 60% continue to experience symptoms as adults.[4–7] It is critical that clinicians be skilled at identifying and managing this impairing condition.

Although ADHD is most commonly diagnosed between ages 7 and 10 years, symptom presentation and impairment can often be seen in children as young as 3 years of age.[8] Epidemiological studies have shown that 2% to 6% of preschoolers meet diagnostic criteria for ADHD.[8,9] Because inattention, impulsivity, and hyperactivity can all be appropriate behaviors for a young child, making a diagnosis of ADHD requires the degree and impairment of these symptoms to be beyond what is developmentally appropriate.

ADHD is diagnosed more often in boys than girls, with a ratio of about 3:1 in clinical settings.[10] This difference may be attributable at least in part to a referral bias[10] because girls may be less disruptive and more likely than boys to meet criteria for the inattentive subtype. With increasing awareness of the variability in the clinical presentation of ADHD in children, girls are now being diagnosed and treated more frequently.

WHY IS IT IMPORTANT TO TREAT ATTENTION DEFICIT/HYPERACTIVITY DISORDER EARLY AND EFFECTIVELY?

One of the crucial elements for making a diagnosis of ADHD is identifying significant impairment in functioning in at least two settings. Three- to 5-year-old children who have ADHD have been shown to be at increased risk for academic, social, behavioral, and family dysfunction.[11] Affected preschoolers are more likely to need special education services and have increased academic difficulties.[12,13] These young children are also at higher risk for accidents and injuries,[13] aggression,[14] and internalizing symptoms.[15]

Throughout grade school, children who have ADHD demonstrate increased difficulties in peer interactions, academic struggles, and conflicts with parents when compared with children who do not have ADHD. Adolescents who have ADHD continue to face significant challenges. Clinical lore has historically led us to think children who have ADHD simply outgrow the disorder with puberty. We now know, however, that ADHD often persists into adolescence and adulthood and is associated with increased rates of substance use and abuse, motor vehicle accidents, academic and occupational impairments, unplanned pregnancy, and sexually transmitted diseases.[16]

WHAT CAUSES ATTENTION DEFICIT/HYPERACTIVITY DISORDER?

ADHD is a disorder with strong neurobiological underpinnings. In a meta-analysis, Faraone and colleagues[17] estimated the heritability of ADHD to be approximately 76%. Although genetics play a significant role,[17,18] nongenetic factors and environmental exposures, such as prenatal smoking and alcohol use, pre- and neonatal hypoxia, lead exposure, and traumatic brain injury have also been associated with the development of ADHD.[19–22] Additionally, neuroimaging studies have reinforced the biological etiology of the disorder by consistently demonstrating structural and metabolic differences in the brains of individuals who have or do not have ADHD.[23,24]

HOW DOES ATTENTION DEFICIT/HYPERACTIVITY DISORDER TYPICALLY PRESENT IN THE PEDIATRIC POPULATION?

Hyperactivity is the most common presenting symptom for preschool children who have ADHD.[25] Inattention becomes more apparent during the school-aged years because of increased academic demands, although hyperactive and impulsive behaviors frequently persist. Overt physical hyperactivity and impulsivity are often less prominent after puberty.[26] These symptoms may change over time in presentation, in fact persisting as excessive talking, avoidance of situations requiring sitting quietly, recklessness, risk-taking, and poor decision making. Clinicians must be aware of these issues, effectively adapt the current DSM-IV criteria to account for the patient's developmental stage and circumstances, and ultimately develop individualized treatment plans for patients of various ages.[27]

In addition to the core symptoms of ADHD, clinicians should also be alert for other associated difficulties, including academic struggles, difficulty completing work, delays in reading, frequent injuries, and problems interacting with peers, all of which may warrant further evaluation. The frequency with which ADHD occurs in the general population should encourage clinicians working with children and adolescents to have a very low threshold for screening for ADHD.

HOW IS ATTENTION DEFICIT/HYPERACTIVITY DISORDER DIAGNOSED?

Increased awareness and improved detection of ADHD has resulted in an increased number of children being identified with the disorder. Although estimates of the prevalence of ADHD vary, it is clear that it is a common and impairing condition with the potential for negative sequela if left undiagnosed and untreated. Currently there are no blood tests or neuroimaging studies available to diagnose ADHD. A careful systematic assessment by a trained clinician is required. The diagnostic process begins with a comprehensive evaluation, including the child's prenatal and birth history; developmental, medical, and psychiatric history; an evaluation of academic performance; and a review of family and social history. If a diagnosis of ADHD is suspected, the DSM-IV TR criteria for ADHD must be used (**Box 1**).[1] To meet criteria for a diagnosis of ADHD, the child must display at least six of nine inattentive and/or six of nine hyperactive/impulsive symptoms for a minimum of 6 months, with an onset before the age of 7. The symptoms must be inappropriate to the developmental level of the child and also impair his or her ability to function in at least two settings.[1]

A careful review of the 18 diagnostic symptoms of ADHD has been demonstrated to be a reliable means of making a diagnosis of ADHD. Several standardized rating scales can be useful in systematically collecting these data from parents and teachers and so facilitating the diagnostic process (and can be useful later in monitoring symptom control over time) (**Table 1**).

DuPaul's ADHD-IV Rating Scale,[28] for example, is an 18-item checklist composed of the 18 diagnostic criteria for ADHD. It can be completed and scored within a few minutes, and is useful for identifying the presence and severity of target symptoms at baseline and longitudinally monitoring outcomes during treatment.[29,30] The norms provided with the scale help the clinician to compare the child's symptoms with children of the same gender and age range. Various Conners' Rating Scales[21,22,31,32] are available, including short and long forms, with parent and teacher formats. These scales have been normed on large populations, and some are quite extensive and comprehensive. Clinicians in practice may also find scales such as the SNAP-IV and the Vanderbilt ADHD Rating Scales particularly useful, given their availability in the public domain at no charge. These scales also offer the ability to assess symptoms across domains, including inattention, hyperactivity/impulsivity, oppositional and conduct problems, anxiety, and depression. The Vanderbilt scales contain subscales for academic and behavioral performance.[29,30] Numerous rating scales are available, so clinicians are encouraged to identify a small number of scales that work well in their

---

Box 1

Diagnostic criteria for attention deficit/hyperactivity disorder

The diagnosis of ADHD requires the presence of six (or more) of symptoms of inattention or hyperactivity/impulsivity for at least 6 months. The symptoms should have an onset before age 7 years and should cause impairment in social, academic, or occupational functioning.

Inattention

Often fails to give close attention to details or makes careless mistakes in schoolwork, work, or other activities

Often has difficulty sustaining attention in tasks or play activities

Often does not seem to listen when spoken to directly

Often does not follow through on instructions and fails to finish schoolwork, chores, or duties in the workplace (not due to oppositional behavior or failure to understand instructions)

Often has difficulty organizing tasks and activities

Often avoids, dislikes, or is reluctant to engage in tasks that require sustained mental effort (such as schoolwork or homework)

Often loses things necessary for tasks or activities (eg, toys, school assignments, pencils, books, or tools)

Is often easily distracted by extraneous stimuli

Is often forgetful in daily activities

Hyperactivity/impulsivity

Often fidgets with hands or feet or squirms in seat

Often leaves seat in classroom or in other situations in which remaining seated is expected

Often runs about or climbs excessively in situations in which it is inappropriate (in adolescents or adults, may be limited to subjective feelings of restlessness)

Often has difficulty playing or engaging in leisure activities quietly

Is often "on the go" or often acts as if "driven by a motor"

Often talks excessively

Often blurts out answers before questions have been completed

Often has difficulty awaiting turn

Often interrupts or intrudes on others (eg, butts into conversations or games)

Adapted from American Psychiatric Association. Diagnostic and statistical manual of mental disorders. 4th edition, text revision. Washington, DC: American Psychiatric Association; 2000; with permission.

---

clinical setting and to routinely use them in patient care. Rating scales alone, however, are not sufficient to make a diagnosis of ADHD. A full clinical evaluation is necessary to assess the ADHD symptoms within a global clinical and developmental context.

Practice parameters from the American Academy of Child and Adolescent Psychiatry (AACAP)[33] and the American Academy of Pediatrics (AAP)[34] offer comprehensive guidelines for assessing, managing, and monitoring ADHD in pediatric patients. Both groups used data from the National Institutes of Mental Health–funded Multimodal Treatment Study of ADHD (MTA)[35] and the Preschool ADHD Treatment Study (PATS)[36] to support their recommendations for a thorough diagnostic evaluation, collaborative treatment planning, and multimodal management of ADHD, which generally includes careful yet strategic pharmacotherapy.

Table 1
Commonly used attention deficit/hyperactivity disorder rating scales

Scale	Price/Availability (as of 9/29/08)	Ages (y)	Details
ADHD Rating Scale-IV	$45 for manual and rating scales; http://www.guilford.com	5–18	18 items Parent and teacher versions English and Spanish
Swan, Nolan, and Pelham-IV (SNAP-IV)	Available free at http://www.adhd.net	5–11	90 items Parent and teacher versions
Swanson, Kotkin, Agler, M-Flynn, and Pelham (SKAMP)	Available free at http://www.jabfm.org/cgi/content/full/19/2/195	7–12	13 items Clinician rated in classroom setting
Conners' Rating Scales	$280 for complete CBRS-R (Comprehensive Behavior Rating Scales) parent, teacher, and adolescent user's package with 25 scales of each; 25 additional forms $35 $500 for available complete software program and forms. Available at http://www.mhs.com	3–17; self-report 12–17	Parent (80-item long; 27-item short) Teacher (59-item long; 28-item short) Self-report (87-item long; 27-item short) Available in English, Spanish, and French
NICHQ Vanderbilt Assessment Scale	Available free at http://NICHQ/Topics/ChronicConditions/ADHD/Tools	6–12	43-item teacher report 55-item parent report
Strengths and Weaknesses of ADHD Symptoms and Normal Behavior (SWAN)	Available free at http://www.adhd.net	5–11	18-item parent report
Brown Attention-Deficit Disorder Scales	$225 for starter kit; 25 additional ready-score forms $65; Available at http://www.harcourtassessment.com	3–18; self-reports available for 8–18	3–7-y-olds: 44-item parent and teacher reports 8–12-y-olds: 50-item parent, teacher, and self-report 12–18-y-olds: 40-item self-report

WHAT OTHER DISORDERS SHOULD BE CONSIDERED IN THE DIFFERENTIAL DIAGNOSIS OF A CHILD WHO HAS SUSPECTED ATTENTION DEFICIT/HYPERACTIVITY DISORDER?

Various other disorders and conditions might masquerade as ADHD. A child who has developmental disabilities, learning disorders, or cognitive limitations may be unable to complete certain academic tasks, be unable to focus because he or she may not understand the task, and may become disruptive out of frustration. A child who has poor vision or poor hearing might present with symptoms overlapping those of ADHD, and so these impairments should be ruled out. Depressive and anxiety disorders frequently present with poor concentration, psychomotor agitation, or disruptive behaviors. (The former two symptoms are among the diagnostic criteria for major depressive disorder and generalized anxiety disorder.) Pediatric bipolar disorder may present with increased distractibility, talkativeness, intrusiveness, and decreased sleep. Inattention, poor concentration, hyperactivity, and distractibility can also be markers for substance abuse. Medical problems, such as hyperthyroidism, partial complex seizures, or lead toxicity can mimic ADHD. Additionally, behaviors that are characteristic of normal childhood development may be misinterpreted as ADHD if not considered in an age-appropriate context.

HOW FREQUENTLY IS ATTENTION DEFICIT/HYPERACTIVITY DISORDER COMORBID WITH OTHER PSYCHIATRIC DISORDERS?

Perhaps one of the most compelling reasons for a comprehensive psychiatric evaluation is the frequency of comorbidity with ADHD. Even when a diagnosis of ADHD is certain, the examination is only partially complete, because nearly two thirds of children diagnosed with ADHD have at least one comorbid psychiatric diagnosis. The MTA study included the largest and best characterized ADHD population to date, and demonstrated that only 31% of participants had ADHD alone, whereas 40% also met criteria for oppositional defiant disorder, 38% for anxiety/mood disorders, 14% for conduct disorder, and 11% for tic disorders.[35] A comprehensive assessment can better inform treatment selection and prioritization. Diagnostic reassessment should be considered whenever adequate response to initial treatment is not achieved, or treatment effectiveness is lost despite adherence to the treatment plan.

WHAT DO WE KNOW ABOUT THE TREATMENTS FOR ATTENTION DEFICIT/ HYPERACTIVITY DISORDER?
Educating the Patient and Family

The National Initiative for Children's Healthcare Quality (NICHQ) recommends that children who have ADHD and their families receive ongoing support and education as a foundation to individualized treatment planning.[37,38] A multitude of reliable educational resources are available for patients, parents, and teachers to facilitate the educational component of the treatment plan (**Box 2**).

Behavioral Interventions

Behavioral therapies for ADHD (such as parent training), child-focused treatments (such as behavioral modification and social skills training), and school-based interventions should be included as part of an effective ADHD management plan. The AACAP[33] and AAP[34] recommend that behavioral interventions be attempted before starting medication in preschool children or children who have mild symptoms. Studies have demonstrated that although they offer some benefit, behavioral interventions may have limited effectiveness as a monotherapy for treating ADHD, particularly when

---

Box 2
Web sites and attention deficit/hyperactivity disorder resources for families

Organizational Web sites

American Academy of Child and Adolescent Psychiatry: http://www.aacap.org

American Academy of Pediatrics: http://www.aap.org

Attention Deficit Disorder Resources: http://www.addresources.org

Children and Adults with Attention-Deficit/Hyperactivity Disorder: http://www.chadd.org

National Resource Center on AD/HD: http://www.help4adhd.org

Family resources

A guide to ADHD and to medication for ADHD: http://www.ParentsMedGuide.org

ADHD—A Guide for Families: http://www.aacap.org/cs/adhd_a_guide_for_families/
resources_for_families_adhd_a_guide_for_families

The Disorder named ADHD: http://www.help4adhd.org/documents/WWK1.pdf

Parenting a Child with ADHD: http://www.help4adhd.org/documents/WWK2.pdf

Managing Medication for Children and Adolescents with AD/HD: http://www.help4adhd.org/
documents/WWK3.pdf

Facts for Families: http://www.aacap.org/cs/root/facts_for_families/facts_for_families

---

symptoms are severe. For children who have significantly impairing ADHD, behavioral interventions are only one component of a more extensive treatment plan.

The MTA study randomized school-aged children to intensive behavioral therapy, pharmacotherapy with systematically delivered methylphenidate, or a combination of the two. Core ADHD symptoms were significantly improved in the pharmacotherapy and combined treatment groups; however, there was no significant difference in response between the pharmacotherapy groups that did and those that did not receive behavioral therapy. Medication seems to have the most significant impact on core ADHD symptoms.[35]

The MTA study found that the addition of behavioral interventions to pharmacotherapy increased parent and teacher satisfaction with treatment and improved the child's interpersonal relationships. On average the children who received behavioral interventions required lower doses of medication.[35]

Pharmacotherapy

Strong evidence exists to support the role of pharmacotherapy in the treatment of pediatric ADHD.[39] The stimulant medications have efficacy data dating back to the 1930s and were well established as effective treatments for ADHD by the 1970s. Since that time, the safety and efficacy database on these agents has grown, and our notion of the "typical" patient who has ADHD as a school-aged child has expanded to include preschoolers and adolescents.[34,39–42] There has also been an increase in data supporting the usefulness of nonstimulant agents for ADHD in the past 10 years.[34,39–43]

WHAT GUIDANCE IS AVAILABLE REGARDING THE SELECTION, INITIATION, TITRATION, AND MONITORING OF ATTENTION DEFICIT/HYPERACTIVITY DISORDER PHARMACOTHERAPY?
Stimulants

Although there are more than a dozen US Food and Drug Administration (FDA)–approved stimulant medications that are currently available, all are derivatives of either methylphenidate or amphetamine. The stimulants act by enhancing the neurotransmission of dopamine, and to a lesser extent, norepinephrine.[39] The stimulants have one of the highest response rates in all of psychopharmacology, with approximately two of every three patients treated with either methylphenidate or amphetamine responding.[33] Both methylphenidate and amphetamine have extensive data supporting their safety and efficacy and their onset and duration of action. Much of the research over the past decade has been focused on improving the delivery system of the stimulant medications to extend the duration of action beyond the approximately 4 hours seen with immediate-release preparations. The availability of multiple formulations of these medications (short, intermediate, and long acting) and various administration options (eg, sprinkle capsules, chewable tablets, liquids, transdermal patches) allows for treatment to be tailored to the needs of individual patients (**Tables 2** and **3**).

When choosing a stimulant medication, factors such as past treatment history, family's preference, clinician's experience and comfort, family history of response, duration of effect, and family resources should be considered. A long-acting methylphenidate or dextroamphetamine-based formulation is generally initially recommended, although for younger children an immediate-release methylphenidate may be a good option while establishing a target dose. For patients who have problems with swallowing, preparations such as Ritalin LA, Adderall XR, Focalin XR, or Metadate CD may be a consideration. These medications come as capsules that can be opened, with microbeads that can be sprinkled into food, such as applesauce. It is important that any of the sustained-release preparations not be chewed, because the delayed-release mechanism of these medications requires the beads or the capsule/tablet to remain intact.

Another option is the methylphenidate transdermal patch (Daytrana), which can be used for children who have swallowing difficulties, those who experience stomach discomfort with oral preparations, or to individualize the duration of action by removing the patch when no longer required. Parents should be warned, however, about the risk for contact dermatitis and the theoretical risk for systematic sensitization with the patch. A recent addition, lisdexamfetamine (Vyvanse), is a dextroamphetamine-based prodrug that is activated in the gut by cleaving lysine off of an amphetamine molecule. It is theorized that because this medication is activated in the gut its abuse potential may be limited, because it may have limited bioavailability if used through alternate routes, such as intravenously or nasally.

Atomoxetine

Atomoxetine (Strattera) is the only nonstimulant medication FDA approved for the treatment of ADHD (**Table 4**). It selectively blocks reuptake at the noradrenergic neurons, and is the only approved ADHD medication that is not a Schedule II drug. Atomoxetine is dosed according to body weight and should generally be initiated at 0.5 mg/kg/d (given in a single dose or divided and administered BID) and titrated to a target of 1.2 mg/kg/d over about 2 weeks. The maximum FDA-approved dose is 1.4 mg/kg/d or 100 mg, whichever is less. Unlike the stimulant medications, which have a rapid onset of action, peak efficacy of atomoxetine may not occur for 2 to 6 weeks or longer. Symptom control is also more sustained, however, which may be helpful to children before the morning medication is absorbed, or in the evening.

Off-Label Attention Deficit/Hyperactivity Disorder Medications

The alpha2-adrenergic medications clonidine (Catapres) and guanfacine (Tenex) are typically second-line agents or adjunctive treatment with stimulants. Clonidine is not typically as effective as the stimulants; however, it has been shown to reduce

Table 2
US Food and Drug Administration–approved methylphenidate attention deficit/hyperactivity disorder pharmacotherapies

Medication (Trade Name)	FDA Approval	Available Preparations	Usual Starting Dose	Max Recommended Dose/d
Methylphenidate (Ritalin)	≥Age 6 y	Immediate-release tablet (5, 10, 20 mg)	5 mg	60 mg
Methylphenidate (Methylin)	≥Age 6 y	Immediate-release tablet (5, 10, 20 mg), chewable tablet (2.5, 5, 10 mg), and solution (5 mg/5 mL; 10 mg/5 mL)	5 mg	Lesser of 2 mg/kg/d or 60 mg
D-methylphenidate (Focalin)	Ages 6 to 17 y	Immediate-release tablet (2.5, 5, 10 mg)	2.5 mg BID	Lesser of 1 mg/kg/d or 20 mg
Methylphenidate (Ritalin SR)	≥Age 6 y	Tablet (must be swallowed whole); (20 mg)	10 mg	60 mg
Methylphenidate (Metadate ER)	≥Age 6 y	Tablet (must be swallowed whole); (10, 20 mg)	10 mg	Lesser of 2 mg/kg/d or 60 mg
Methylphenidate (Methylin ER)	≥Age 6 y	Tablet (must be swallowed whole); (10, 20 mg)	10 mg	60 mg
Methylphenidate (Metadate CD)	≥Age 6 y	Beaded capsule (may be opened and sprinkled); (10, 20, 30, 40, 50, 60 mg); 30% immediate release and 70% 3 h later	20 mg	Lesser of 2 mg/kg/d or 60 mg
Methylphenidate (Ritalin LA)	≥Age 6 y	Beaded capsule (may be opened and sprinkled); (10, 20, 30, 40 mg); 50% immediate release and 50% 4 h later	20 mg	60 mg
D-methylphenidate (Focalin XR)	≥Age 6 y	Beaded capsule (may be opened and sprinkled); (5, 10, 15, 20 mg); 50% immediate release and 50% 4 h later	5 mg	Lesser of 1 mg/kg/d or 30 mg
Methylphenidate (Concerta)	≥Age 6 y	Capsule (must be swallowed whole) (18, 27, 36, 54 mg); replicates tid dosing of immediate release; OROS delivery system: 18% immediate-release outer coating; remainder gradually released osmotically	18 mg	Lesser of 2 mg/kg/d or 72 mg
Methylphenidate (Daytrana)	Ages 6–12 y	Transdermal patch (10, 15, 20, 30 mg); gradually releases methylphenidate; worn up to 9 h/d	10 mg	Lesser of 1 mg/kg/d or 30 mg

Data from Pliszka S. Practice parameter for the assessment and treatment of children and adolescents with attention-deficit/hyperactivity disorder. J Am Acad Child Adolesc Psychiatry 2007;46:894.

Table 3
US Food and Drug Administration–approved amphetamine attention deficit/hyperactivity disorder pharmacotherapies

Medication (Trade Name)	FDA Approval	Available Preparations	Typical Starting Dose	Max Recommended Dose/d
Mixed amphetamine salts (Adderall)	≥ Age 3 y	Immediate-release tablet; (5, 7.5, 10, 12.5, 15, 20, 30 mg)	3–5 y: 2.5 mg qd ≥ 6 y: 5 mg qd–bid	Lesser of 1 mg/kg/d or 40 mg
Amphetamine (Dexedrine)	≥ Age 3 y	Immediate-release tablet (5 mg)	2.5 mg qd	40 mg
Amphetamine (Dextrostat)	≥ Age 6 y	Immediate-release tablet; (5, 10 mg)	5 mg qd–bid	40 mg
Mixed amphetamine salts (Adderall XR)	≥ Age 6 y	Beaded capsule (may be opened and sprinkled); 50% immediate release and 50% 4 h later; (5, 10, 15, 20, 25, 30 mg)	10 mg qd	Lesser of 1 mg/kg or 30 mg
Amphetamine (Dexedrine spansule)	≥ Age 6 y	Beaded capsule; initial immediate-release dose with remainder gradually released (5, 10, 15 mg)	5–10 mg qd–bid	Lesser of 1 mg/kg or 40 mg
Lisdexamfetamine (Vyvanse)	Ages 6–12 y and adults	Capsule; amphetamine with lysine attached, activated in GI tract when lysine is cleaved; (20, 30, 40, 50, 60, 70 mg)	30 mg qd	Lesser of 1 mg/kg or 70 mg

Data from Pliszka S. Practice parameter for the assessment and treatment of children and adolescents with attention-deficit/hyperactivity disorder. J Am Acad Child Adolesc Psychiatry 2007;46:894.

Table 4
US Food and Drug Administration–approved nonstimulant attention deficit/hyperactivity disorder pharmacotherapy

Medication (Trade Name)	FDA Approval	Available Preparations	Typical Starting Dose	Max Recommended Dose/d
Atomoxetine (Strattera)	≥Age 6 y	Capsule; immediate-release; generally dosed qd, but can be dosed bid (10, 18, 25, 40, 60, 80, 100 mg)	<70 kg: 0.5 mg/kg/d for 4 d, then 1 mg/kg/d for 4 d, then 1.2 mg/kg/d; >70 kg: 40 mg/d	Lesser of 1.4 mg/kg or 100 mg

Data from Pliszka S. Practice parameter for the assessment and treatment of children and adolescents with attention-deficit/hyperactivity disorder. J Am Acad Child Adolesc Psychiatry 2007;46:894.

ADHD symptoms co-occurring with tics, aggression, or conduct disorder. It is also commonly used to treat stimulant-induced tics and insomnia. Full effects may not be seen for 4 to 6 weeks. Clonidine is short-acting and thus frequently administered in divided doses. Common side effects include sedation and orthostatic hypotension.[40] To avoid rebound hypertension, slow titration is recommended when discontinuing clonidine. Guanfacine is a more selective α2-adrenergic agonist with less sedation and a longer duration of action.[39] An extended-release guanfacine recently received a letter of approvability from the FDA for the treatment of ADHD.

Bupropion (Wellbutrin, Zyban), a dopaminergic and noradrenergic antidepressant, has been shown to be effective for ADHD and may also be beneficial for nicotine dependence and comorbid depression. Common side effects include irritability, decreased appetite, and insomnia.[39] Bupropion is contraindicated in patients who have seizures and eating disorders. Patients taking bupropion should be monitored for suicidal ideation.

The AAP practice parameters[34] and the Texas Children's Medication Project[44] recommend stimulants as the first-line psychopharmacologic treatment of ADHD, especially when no comorbid conditions are present. Atomoxetine (Strattera) is considered an initial medication option for ADHD in patients who have comorbid anxiety, an active substance abuse problem, or tics. Atomoxetine may also be preferred if the patient experiences problematic side effects to stimulants, such as mood lability or tics.[45] A meta-analysis of atomoxetine and stimulant studies revealed that the effect size for atomoxetine was 0.62 compared with 0.91 and 0.95 for immediate-release and long-acting stimulants, respectively.[46] The AACAP[33] guidelines describe atomoxetine, amphetamine, and methylphenidate all as appropriate first-line treatments. The Texas medication project algorithm suggests that in general, a failed trial of one stimulant should be followed by a trial of an agent from the other class of stimulant first before switching over to atomoxetine.[44]

WHAT ARE THE ADVERSE EFFECTS OF ATTENTION DEFICIT/HYPERACTIVITY DISORDER PHARMACOTHERAPIES, AND WAYS TO MANAGE THEM?
Stimulants

Adverse event profiles are comparable for all formulations of the stimulant medications.[41] Delayed sleep onset, decreased appetite, weight loss, headache, stomach upset, and increased heart rate and blood pressure are common. Emotional outbursts and irritability have also been reported in younger children.[47] Many of these problems can be managed by selecting alternate formulations with shorter durations of action to minimize effects on sleep and evening appetite, modifying administration schedules, using a slow titration schedule, or by giving the medication with food in the case of stomach upset. Common suggestions for managing anorexia include instructing the parent to allow the child to eat when hungry, not limit meals to a set schedule, and to supplement calories using foods with high nutritional value throughout the day whenever possible. Managing insomnia can be challenging for families and clinicians. If addressing sleep hygiene, changing the medication administration schedule, or changing to alternate formulations does not improve the delay in sleep onset, use of an agent to assist with sleep (clonidine, melatonin, and so forth) may be warranted.

Atomoxetine

Common side effects of atomoxetine include sedation, loss of appetite, nausea, vomiting, irritability, and headaches. Irritability and mood lability may be even more significant in young children treated with atomoxetine.[48] A more gradual titration, and consideration of divided dosing, may improve tolerability by reducing sedation and irritability. If sedation is problematic, dosing at bedtime, particularly early in treatment, may be helpful. Potential nausea and vomiting are typically avoided by administering the medication with food.

Growth and Attention Deficit/Hyperactivity Disorder Pharmacotherapies

Growth suppression is one of the most common concerns expressed by parents when discussing the potential initiation of medication for ADHD. Concerns about the effects of amphetamine and methylphenidate-based psychostimulants on growth may have initially stemmed from their well-documented anorexic effects, but have subsequently been validated in clinical trials. Meta-analyses conducted by Faraone and colleagues[49] demonstrated statistically significant delays in height and weight with stimulant treatment. Data pooled from 22 studies of stimulants demonstrated height deficits, suggesting slower growth than expected. With time, however, height velocity seems to normalize. The studies also found deficits in weight in children treated with stimulants. This effect also seems to normalize with time. Faraone's data showed that the weight deficits were more significant than the deficits seen in height ($P = .002$). Swanson and colleagues[50] presented similar data, suggesting that children treated with stimulants grow more slowly and seem to gain less weight than expected, but also theorized that there may be differences in growth trajectories for children who have ADHD in general.

Based on a qualitative meta-analysis, Faraone and colleagues suggested that the effects on weight and height may be dose-dependent. Further, there was no apparent difference in the growth effects between methylphenidate and amphetamine, and cessation of treatment seemed to normalize growth. This normalization of growth with breaks over the summer or with drug discontinuation has been demonstrated in several studies;[51–54] although analysis of data from the MTA study[55] showed that discontinuation of methylphenidate treatment did not reverse losses in expected height, but did have a beneficial effect on weight gain.

Interestingly, atomoxetine has also been clearly linked with changes in height and weight trajectories.[56] Although for the group as a whole this seems to resolve when followed longitudinally, even with ongoing treatment it is clear that all patients treated with pharmacotherapy require careful monitoring. Adjustments to doses and dosing schedules should be considered, and caloric supplementation encouraged, as indicated. For patients who do not respond to these interventions, drug holidays may be warranted.

Cardiovascular Concerns

Recent attention has been focused on the rare but serious issue of sudden cardiac death in pediatric patients treated with ADHD pharmacotherapy. After careful examination the AAP came out with a policy statement in August, 2008, which stated that "…there have been no studies or compelling clinical evidence to demonstrate that the likelihood of sudden death is higher in children receiving medications for ADHD than that in the general population. It has not been shown that screening ECGs before starting stimulants have an appropriate balance of benefit, risk, and cost-effectiveness for general use in identifying risk factors for sudden death. Until these questions can be answered, a recommendation to obtain routine ECGs for children receiving ADHD medications is not warranted."[57]

At this time the AAP recommends a careful assessment of all children, particularly those initiating medications for ADHD, by collecting a targeted cardiac history (eg, previously detected cardiac disease, palpitations, syncope, or seizures; family history of sudden death in children or young adults; hypertrophic cardiomyopathy; long QT syndrome) and completing a physical examination, including a careful cardiac examination. If concerns arise based on the history or physical examination, an ECG should be obtained, and additional consultation with a pediatric cardiologist may be indicated before treatment with stimulants or atomoxetine. All children treated with medications for ADHD should have their pulse and blood pressure monitored before and during treatment.[33,34]

Atomoxetine—Suicidality and Hepatic Issues

Atomoxetine has a black box warning pertaining to suicidality. Although the number was small, a meta-analysis of 12 pediatric studies demonstrated 0.4% of children and adolescents taking atomoxetine experienced suicidal thoughts or behaviors, compared with none of those taking placebo. Although there were no completed suicides in these studies, educating patients and their families of the potential risk and warning signs is important. There have also been rare occurrences of liver toxicity reported. The few individuals who did experience the liver injury recovered after the medication was discontinued. Nonetheless, patients should be educated as to this risk and warning signs for hepatic dysfunction (eg, jaundice, urticaria, dark urine).

Monitoring

The clinician may use one of the readily available rating scales, such as ADHD-IV, Vanderbilt, or SNAP-IV, to establish a baseline and monitor the effectiveness of the medication. The patient's weight, height, blood pressure, and pulse should also be monitored, preferably at every visit. At present, the AACAP does not recommend a mandatory baseline EEG, psychological testing, or ECG before starting a stimulant or atomoxetine, or baseline liver function tests before initiating atomoxetine (Strattera). These decisions are made on an individual basis by the clinician and the patient's family.

WHAT IS IMPORTANT TO KNOW ABOUT THE TREATMENT OF PRESCHOOL CHILDREN WHO HAVE ATTENTION DEFICIT/HYPERACTIVITY DISORDER?

Apart from obtaining a detailed history and thorough examination, assessment of developmental milestones is particularly important in the evaluation of the pre-schooler, because many developmental disorders are associated with attentional problems and hyperactivity.[33] In addition, temperament difficulties, learned behavioral responses, parent–child relationship problems, and anxiety may all present with ADHD-like symptoms. Although pharmacotherapy in this population has been increasing, growing data suggest that mild or moderate cases should still generally be treated initially with parent training and behavioral modification techniques. The efficacy of stimulant medications in treating ADHD in preschool-aged children has been more variable than seen in older children,[58] and reports of side effects are increased (eg, sadness, irritability, clinginess, insomnia, and anorexia).[47,59] The PATS study examined immediate-release methylphenidate in 3- to 5-year-olds who suffered from significant dysfunction due to ADHD.[36] Only children who did not demonstrate adequate response following a 10-week parent-training program were eligible for the medication phase of the study. A total of 165 children were randomized to treatment. Methylphenidate demonstrated a graded dose response, with the mean best total daily dose 14.2 ± 8.1 mg/d or 0.7 ± 0.4 mg/kg/d, which is lower than the mean of 1.0 mg/kg/d found to be optimal in the MTA study with school-aged children. Effect sizes in PATS were smaller than those observed in MTA subjects.[36] Pharmacokinetic data obtained in PATS indicated that because clearance of a single dose of methylphenidate in preschoolers is longer than the same dose-by-weight in school-aged children, younger, smaller patients may respond to lower doses with less frequent administration.[60]

There are no controlled data available on the use of atomoxetine in preschool-aged children.

WHAT IS IMPORTANT TO KNOW ABOUT THE TREATMENT OF ADOLESCENTS WHO HAVE ATTENTION DEFICIT/HYPERACTIVITY DISORDER?

In a longitudinal study of 358 clinically referred subjects who had ADHD, 27.9% of those who were on medication at some point in their lives, usually starting treatment by age 10, had stopped taking medication by age 11, and 67.9% had discontinued pharmacotherapy by age 15.[61] Treatment adherence frequently decreases in adolescence, although the consequences of untreated ADHD can be just as significant, if not more so, as those in younger children (ie, motor vehicle accidents, unplanned pregnancy, sexually transmitted diseases, substance abuse, legal problems, school drop-out).[62] Despite the frequent discontinuation of treatment, however, stimulant medications continue to show efficacy for about 70% of adolescents, demonstrating dose-dependent improvements in behavioral and cognitive symptoms.[45,63] Beneficial effects and short-term side effects of stimulants seem comparable to those seen in school-aged children.[64] Atomoxetine has been demonstrated to be of clear benefit in the adolescent population also.[65,66]

In light of the potential benefit of treating adolescents who have ADHD, and the potential for negative sequelae without intervention, it is important to partner with the teens in their treatment planning. Several aspects of pharmacotherapy management may be specific to adolescents. Their schedules often include evening activities, such as extracurricular programs, studying, and work, so dosing adjustments may be required to manage symptoms over longer periods of time. Driving at night and participation in activities in which supervision is limited and impulsive behaviors may have significant consequences all support the need for extended coverage. This coverage may require a long-acting stimulant alone or in combination with a short-acting stimulant at the end of the day, or perhaps treatment with a nonstimulant to provide coverage throughout the waking hours. Growing rates of substance use concerns may also lead to alterations in treatment strategies to limit availability of agents with greater substance abuse potential, such as the immediate-release stimulants. Sustained-release preparations or nonstimulants may help to mitigate some of the abuse potential.

By working together, the likelihood of treatment adherence and optimal outcomes is increased.

SUMMARY

ADHD is well known to be a common condition in children, with increasing awareness of its presence in preschoolers and adolescents. Given the potential for functional impairment over time, it is important for psychiatrists to be able to identify and accurately diagnose ADHD, make appropriate decisions regarding treatment, educate those involved, and carefully monitor the safety and effectiveness of the treatment. By partnering with the patient, the family, and the school, ADHD can be consistently identified and effectively treated, leading to improved outcomes for affected children and their families.

REFERENCES

1. American Psychiatric Association: diagnostic and statistical manual of mental disorders fourth edition text revision. Washington, DC: American Psychiatric Association; 2000.
2. Mental health in the United States. Prevalence of diagnosis and medication treatment for attention-deficit/hyperactivity disorder—United States. MMWR Morb Mortal Wkly Rep 2003;54(842):842–7.
3. Woodruff TJ, Axelrad DA, Kyle AD, et al. Trends in environmentally related childhood illnesses. Pediatrics 2004;113:1133–40.
4. Barkley RA, Fischer M, Edelbrock CS, et al. The adolescent outcome of hyperactive children diagnosed by research criteria: I. An 8-year prospective follow-up study. J Am Acad Child Adolesc Psychiatry 1990;29:546–7.
5. Barkley RA, Fischer M, Smallish L, et al. The persistence of attention-deficit/hyperactivity disorder into young adulthood as a function of reporting source and definition of disorder. J Abnorm Psychol 2002;111:279–89.
6. Biederman J, Faraone S, Milberger S, et al. A prospective 4-year follow-up study of attention-deficit hyperactivity and related disorders. Arch Gen Psychiatry 1996; 53:437–46.
7. Kessler RC, Adler LA, Barkley R, et al. Patterns and predictors of attention-deficit/hyperactivity disorder persistence into adulthood: results from the national comorbidity survey replication. Biol Psychiatry 2005;57:1442–51.
8. Lavigne JV, Gibbons RD, Christoffel KK, et al. Prevalence rates and correlates of psychiatric disorders among preschool children. J Am Acad Child Adolesc Psychiatry 1996;35:204–14.
9. Angold A, Erkanli A, Egger HL, et al. Stimulant treatment for children: a community perspective. J Am Acad Child Adolesc Psychiatry 2000;39:975–84.
10. Biederman J, Kwon A, Aleardi M, et al. Absence of gender effects on attention deficit hyperactivity disorder: findings in nonreferred subjects. Am J Psychiatry 2005;162:1083–9.
11. DuPaul GJ, McGoey KE, Eckert TL, et al. Preschool children with attention-deficit/hyperactivity disorder: impairments in behavioral, social, and school functioning. J Am Acad Child Adolesc Psychiatry 2001;40:508–15.
12. Lahey BB, Pelham WE, Loney J, et al. Three-year predictive validity of DSM-IV attention deficit hyperactivity disorder in children diagnosed at 4–6 years of age. Am J Psychiatry 2004;161:2014–20.

13. Lahey BB, Pelham WE, Stein MA, et al. Validity of DSM-IV attention-deficit/hyperactivity disorder for younger children. J Am Acad Child Adolesc Psychiatry 1998; 37:695–702.

14. Connor DF, Edwards G, Fletcher KE, et al. Correlates of comorbid psychopathology in children with ADHD. J Am Acad Child Adolesc Psychiatry 2003;42:193–200.

15. Cunningham CE, Boyle MH. Preschoolers at risk for attention-deficit hyperactivity disorder and oppositional defiant disorder: family, parenting, and behavioral correlates. J Abnorm Child Psychol 2002;30:555–69.

16. Barkley RA. Attention-deficit hyperactivity disorder: a handbook for diagnosis and treatment. 3rd Edition. New York: Guilford Press; 2006.

17. Faraone SV, Perlis RH, Doyle AE, et al. Molecular genetics of attention-deficit/ hyperactivity disorder. Biol Psychiatry 2005;57:1313–23.

18. Willcutt EG, Doyle AE, Nigg JT, et al. Validity of the executive function theory of attention-deficit/hyperactivity disorder: a meta-analytic review. Biol Psychiatry 2005;57:1336–46.

19. Castellanos FX, Lee PP, Sharp W, et al. Developmental trajectories of brain volume abnormalities in children and adolescents with attention-deficit/hyperactivity disorder. JAMA 2002;288:1740–8.

20. Biederman J. Attention-deficit/hyperactivity disorder: a selective overview. Biol Psychiatry 2005;57:1215–20.

21. Biederman J, Faraone SV. Attention-deficit hyperactivity disorder. Lancet 2005; 366:237–48.

22. Kreppner JM, O'Connor TG, Rutter M. Can inattention/overactivity be an institutional deprivation syndrome? J Abnorm Child Psychol 2001;29:513–28.

23. Voeller KK. Attention-deficit hyperactivity disorder (ADHD). J Child Neurol 2004; 19:798–814.

24. Durston S, Hulshoff Pol HE, Schnack HG, et al. Magnetic resonance imaging of boys with attention-deficit/hyperactivity disorder and their unaffected siblings. J Am Acad Child Adolesc Psychiatry 2004;43:332–40.

25. Hardy KK, Kollins SH, Murray DW, et al. Factor structure of parent- and teacher-rated ADHD symptoms in preschoolers in the preschoolers with ADHD treatment study (PATS). Journal of Child and Adolescent Psychopharmacology 2007;17:621–34.

26. Krause J, Krause KH, Dresel SH, et al. ADHD in adolescence and adulthood, with a special focus on the dopamine transporter and nicotine. Dialogues Clin Neurosci 2006;8:29–36.

27. Vaughan BS, Wetzel MW, Kratochvil CJ. Beyond the "typical" patient: treating attention-deficit/hyperactivity disorder in preschoolers and adults. Int Rev Psychiatry 2008;20:143–9.

28. DuPaul GJ, Power TJ, Anastopoulos AD, et al. ADHD Rating Scale-IV: checklists, norms, and clinical interpretations. New York, NY: Guilford Press; 1998.

29. Collett BR, Ohan JL, Myers KM. Ten-year review of rating scales. V: scales assessing attention-deficit/hyperactivity disorder. J Am Acad Child Adolesc Psychiatry 2003;42:1015–37.

30. Madaan V, Daughton J, Lubberstedt B, et al. Assessing the efficacy of treatments for ADHD: overview of methodological issues. CNS Drugs 2008;22:275–90.

31. Conners CK, Sitarenios G, Parker JD, et al. The revised Conners' Parent Rating Scale (CPRS-R): factor structure, reliability, and criterion validity. J Abnorm Child Psychol 1998;26:257–68.

32. Conners CK, Sitarenios G, Parker JD, et al. Revision and restandardization of the Conners Teacher Rating Scale (CTRS-R): factor structure, reliability, and criterion validity. J Abnorm Child Psychol 1998;26:279–91.

33. Pliszka S. Practice parameter for the assessment and treatment of children and adolescents with attention-deficit/hyperactivity disorder. J Am Acad Child Adolesc Psychiatry 2007;46:894–921.

34. American Academy of Pediatrics: clinical practice guideline: treatment of the school-aged child with attention-deficit/hyperactivity disorder. J Pediatri 2001; 108:1033–44.

35. MTA Cooperative Group: a 14-month randomized clinical trial of treatment strategies for attention-deficit/hyperactivity disorder. The MTA Cooperative Group. multimodal treatment study of children with ADHD. Archives of General Psychiatry 1999;56:1073–86.

36. Greenhill L, Kollins S, Abikoff H, et al. Efficacy and safety of immediate-release methylphenidate treatment for preschoolers with ADHD. J Am Acad Child Adolesc Psychiatry 2006;45:1284–93.

37. Bodenheimer T, Wagner EH, Grumbach K. Improving primary care for patients with chronic illness. JAMA 2002;288:1775–9.

38. Bodenheimer T, Wagner EH, Grumbach K. Improving primary care for patients with chronic illness: the chronic care model, Part 2. JAMA 1909;288:1909–14.

39. Biederman J, Spencer TJ. Psychopharmacological interventions. Child Adolesc Psychiatr Clin N Am 2008;17:439–58.

40. Brown RT, Amler RW, Freeman WS, et al. Treatment of attention-deficit/hyperactivity disorder: overview of the evidence. Pediatrics 2005;115:e749–757.

41. Greenhill LL, Pliszka S, Dulcan MK, et al. Practice parameter for the use of stimulant medications in the treatment of children, adolescents, and adults. J Am Acad Child Adolesc Psychiatry 2002;41:26S–49S.

42. Pliszka SR, Liotti M, Bailey BY, et al. Electrophysiological effects of stimulant treatment on inhibitory control in children with attention-deficit/hyperactivity disorder. J Child Adolesc Psychopharmacol 2007;17:356–66.

43. Madaan V, Kinnan S, Daughton J, et al. Innovations and recent trends in the treatment of ADHD. Expert Rev Neurother 2006;6:1375–85.

44. Pliszka SR, Crismon ML, Hughes CW, et al. The Texas Children's Medication Algorithm Project: revision of the algorithm for pharmacotherapy of attention-deficit/hyperactivity disorder. J Am Acad Child Adolesc Psychiatry 2006;45:642–57.

45. Biederman J, Spencer T, Wilens T. Evidence-based pharmacotherapy for attention-deficit hyperactivity disorder. Int J Neuropsychopharmacol 2004;7:77–97.

46. Faraone S. Understanding the effect size of ADHD medications: implications for clinical care. Medscape Psychiatry & Mental Health 2003;8:2.

47. Wigal T, Greenhill L, Chuang S, et al. Safety and tolerability of methylphenidate in preschool children with ADHD. Journal of the American Academy of Child and Adolescent Psychiatry 2006;45:1294–303.

48. Kratochvil CJ, Vaughan BS, Mayfield-Jorgensen ML, et al. A pilot study of atomoxetine in young children with attention-deficit/hyperactivity disorder. J Child Adolesc Psychopharmacol 2007;17:175–85.

49. Faraone SV, Biederman J, Morley CP, et al. Effect of stimulants on height and weight: a review of the literature. Journal of the American Academy of Child and Adolescent Psychiatry 2008;47:994–1009.

50. Swanson JM, Ruff DD, Feldman PD, et al. Characterization of growth in children with ADHD. In: Annual Meeting of the American Academy of Child and Adolescent Psychiatry, Toronto Canada; 2005.

51. Gittelman R, Landa B, Mattes J, et al. Methylphenidate and growth in hyperactive children: a controlled withdrawal study. Archives of General Psychiatry 1988;45: 1127–30.

52. Kaffman M, Sher A. Bar-Sinai N: MBD children-variability in developmental patterns or growth inhibitory effects of stimulants? Israel Annals of Psychiatry and Related Disciplines 1979;17:58–66.

53. Klein RG, Mannuzza S. Hyperactive boys almost grown up. III. Methylphenidate effects on ultimate height. Arch Gen Psychiatry 1988;45:1131–4.

54. Safer D, Allen R, Barr E. Growth rebound after termination of stimulant drugs. J Pediatri 1975;86:113–6.

55. National Institute of Mental Health Multimodal Treatment Study of ADHD follow-up: changes in effectiveness and growth after the end of treatment. Pediatrics 2004;113:762–9.

56. Spencer TJ, Newcorn JH, Kratochvil CJ, et al. Effects of atomoxetine on growth after 2-year treatment among pediatric patients with attention-deficit/hyperactivity disorder. Pediatrics 2005;116:e74–80.

57. Perrin JM, Friedman RA, Knilans TK. Cardiovascular monitoring and stimulant drugs for attention-deficit/hyperactivity disorder. Pediatrics 2008;122:451–3.

58. Connor DF. Preschool attention deficit hyperactivity disorder: a review of prevalence, diagnosis, neurobiology, and stimulant treatment. J Dev Behav Pediatr 2002;23:S1–9.

59. Firestone P, Musten LM, Pisterman S, et al. Short-term side effects of stimulant medication are increased in preschool children with attention-deficit/hyperactivity disorder: a double-blind placebo-controlled study. J Child Adolesc Psychopharmacol 1998;8:13–25.

60. Wigal SB, Gupta S, Greenhill L, et al. Pharmacokinetics of methylphenidate in preschoolers with attention-deficit/hyperactivity disorder. J Child Adolesc Psychopharmacol 2007;17:153–64.

61. Charach A, Ickowicz A, Schachar R. Stimulant treatment over five years: adherence, effectiveness, and adverse effects. J Am Acad Child Adolesc Psychiatry 2004;43:559–67.

62. Barkley RA. Driving impairments in teens and adults with attention-deficit/hyperactivity disorder. Psychiatr Clin North Am 2004;27:233–60.

63. Evans SW, Pelham WE, Smith BH, et al. Dose-response effects of methylphenidate on ecologically valid measures of academic performance and classroom behavior in adolescents with ADHD. Exp Clin Psychopharmacol 2001;9:163–75.

64. Smith BH, Pelham WE, Gnagy E, et al. Equivalent effects of stimulant treatment for attention-deficit hyperactivity disorder during childhood and adolescence. J Am Acad Child Adolesc Psychiatry 1998;37:314–21.

65. Wilens TE, Kratochvil C, Newcorn JH, et al. Do children and adolescents with ADHD respond differently to atomoxetine? J Am Acad Child Adolesc Psychiatry 2006;45:149–57.

66. Wilens TE, Newcorn JH, Kratochvil CJ, et al. Long-term atomoxetine treatment in adolescents with attention-deficit/hyperactivity disorder. J Pediatr 2006;149:112–9.

Anxiety Disorders and Posttraumatic Stress Disorder Update

Andrea M. Victor, PhD*, Gail A. Bernstein, MD

KEYWORDS

- Pediatric anxiety disorders • Separation anxiety disorder
- Generalized anxiety disorder • Social phobia
- Obsessive-compulsive disorder
- Posttraumatic stress disorder

Anxiety disorders are one of the most prevalent categories of pediatric psychopathology.[1] There is a range of prevalence estimates based on the type of epidemiologic study that is completed. Short assessment intervals and single collection points result in the lowest prevalence estimates. Childhood prevalence studies of having any anxiety disorder show that 3-month estimates range from 2.2% to 8.6%[2,3] and 6-month estimates range from 5.5% to 17.7%.[4,5] In contrast, retrospective studies with older adolescents and adults that use a lifetime interval typically report higher prevalence estimates. Lifetime prevalence estimates range from 8.3% to 27%.[6] Because pediatric anxiety disorders are relatively common, there is an increasing interest in understanding the research and clinical issues related to the presentation and treatment of these disorders.

Anxiety disorders are diagnosed throughout the life span. *The Diagnostic and Statistical Manual of Mental Disorders, Fourth Edition, Text Revision* (DSM-IV-TR)[7] criteria are similar for youth and adults; however, there are some notable differences that need to be considered when diagnosing anxiety disorders in children and adolescents. **Table 1** provides a summary of the differences in diagnostic criteria for pediatric anxiety disorders.

SEPARATION ANXIETY DISORDER
Clinical Presentation

The key feature of separation anxiety disorder (SAD) is excessive anxiety about separation from primary attachment figures (eg, parents, grandparents). Children with SAD fear that harm will come to themselves or their attachment figures when separated. Other symptoms include distress at the time of separation, somatic complaints

Division of Child & Adolescent Psychiatry, University of Minnesota Medical School, 2450 Riverside Avenue, F256/2B West, Minneapolis, MN 55454, USA
* Corresponding author.
E-mail address: avictor@umn.edu (A.M. Victor).

Psychiatr Clin N Am 32 (2009) 57–69
doi:10.1016/j.psc.2008.11.004
0193-953X/08/$ – see front matter © 2009 Elsevier Inc. All rights reserved.

Table 1
DSM-IV-TR criteria differences for anxiety disorders in youth

Anxiety Disorder	Differences in Criteria for Youth
Generalized anxiety disorder	Requires only one associated symptom.
Social phobia	Children must have the ability to develop age appropriate friendships Children must endorse anxiety with adults and peers Anxiety may be shown through crying, tantrums, freezing, or shrinking from social situations Children do not need to recognize that the fear is excessive or unreasonable
Obsessive-compulsive disorder	Children do not need to recognize that the obsessions and compulsions are excessive or unreasonable
Posttraumatic stress disorder	Response to the traumatic event may be expressed through agitated or disorganized behavior rather than extreme fear, helplessness, or horror Traumatic event may be re-experienced through the use of repetitive play about the trauma Children may have scary dreams without recognizable content that is related to the event Children may re-enact trauma-specific details

when separation occurs or is anticipated, nightmares with themes of separation, shadowing parents in the home, and sleeping with family members.[7] Children with SAD commonly refuse to attend school and are reluctant to go other places without their parents. To be diagnosed with SAD, symptoms must be more intense than expected for the child's developmental level, be present for at least 4 weeks, have an onset before 18 years of age, and cause significant distress or impairment. A distinguishing feature of SAD is that the child's anxiety is alleviated when with parents, whereas in other anxiety disorders, the presence of an attachment figure has minimal effect on symptom presentation.[8]

SAD is common in youth with a prevalence rate of 3% to 5%.[9,10] It is more likely to occur in children compared with adolescents. Onset is typically at 7 to 9 years of age.[9,11] Common comorbid diagnoses include generalized anxiety disorder (GAD), specific phobia, attention-deficit hyperactivity disorder (ADHD), and social phobia (SP).[12]

Course and Outcome

SAD can be short-lived or chronic and persistent. Last and colleagues[13] followed children in an anxiety clinic prospectively for 3 to 4 years and found that SAD had the highest remission rate (95.7%) of all the anxiety disorders. In another prospective study, young children in a community sample were assessed at age 3 ($n = 60$) and 3.5 years later ($n = 44$) to evaluate the stability of SAD.[14] At baseline, the children were classified as having clinical, subclinical, or nonclinical levels of separation anxiety. Children who met full diagnostic criteria for SAD compared with those with subclinical or nonclinical status were more likely to have comorbid disorders and high levels of internalizing symptoms. In addition, parents of children with clinical SAD experienced high levels of internalizing symptoms and general distress. At follow-up, many children showed a decline in separation anxiety symptoms and moved in the direction of subclinical or nonclinical status. The investigators suggested family and parental characteristics (eg, inconsistency in limit setting) predict lower likelihood of remission of SAD. Foley and colleagues[15] assessed the short-term outcome of SAD in a community sample of twins (ages 8 to 17). At an average follow-up period of 18 months, SAD had remitted in 80% of the children. Persistent SAD was predicted by oppositional defiant disorder, impairment because of ADHD, and maternal marital dissatisfaction. Children with persistent SAD were significantly more likely than children with remitted SAD to develop a new depressive disorder within 18 months.

SAD is a risk factor for development of anxiety and depressive disorders in adulthood. A controversy exists in the literature as to whether SAD increases the vulnerability for several anxiety disorders or specifically for panic disorder. Data from the Oregon Adolescent Depression Project[9] were used to determine the risk that SAD confers for new disorders in adulthood. Teenagers were evaluated at age 16, including retrospective reports of childhood psychopathology. They were assessed twice during adolescence and twice as adults. Most teenagers with a history of SAD developed new disorders as adults. The major outcomes were panic disorder (25%) and depression (75%). Several studies have demonstrated that SAD is a risk factor for a variety of anxiety disorders, not specifically panic disorder.[16] In a 7-year follow-up study of children treated for an anxiety disorder, children with SAD compared with children with GAD or SP were more likely to have other anxiety disorders, but not specifically panic disorder.[16]

The association between SAD and future psychopathology does not indicate causality. While SAD may be causal for later psychiatric disorders, it is also possible that SAD and adult panic disorder and depression are caused by a common underlying vulnerability. "If the latter is true, then it may also be true that SAD is a marker for severity of the underlying vulnerability."[9]

GENERALIZED ANXIETY DISORDER
Clinical Presentation

GAD is a relatively new diagnosis in children and adolescents. In the DSM-III-R[17] a diagnosis of GAD required a minimum age of 18 years. Instead, youth with excessive worry were diagnosed with overanxious disorder (OAD). OAD was omitted from the DSM-IV[18] and the age restriction was removed from the GAD diagnostic criteria. DSM-IV-TR criteria for GAD are similar for youth when compared with adults, with one exception. The differentiating factor is that youth are only required to endorse one associated symptom (ie, restlessness, fatigue, difficulty concentrating, irritability, muscle aches or tension, or sleep difficulties), and three are required for a diagnosis of GAD in adults (see **Table 1**). Common domains of worry in children with GAD include health of significant others, personal performance, family matters, and world issues.[19]

Because the number of associated symptoms differentiates DSM-IV-TR criteria for GAD in children and adults, this domain has been an area of interest. Research has consistently shown that youth diagnosed with GAD typically endorse more than one associated symptom.[19,20] Three studies[19,21,22] show that restlessness is the most common and muscle tension is the least common associated symptom endorsed by youth with GAD.

There are limited data on the prevalence of GAD in youth, as it was not diagnosed in children and adolescents until the DSM-IV. The prevalence rate of OAD in early adolescents was estimated at approximately 3%.[23,24] The National Comorbidity Survey, which included individuals ranging in age from 15 to 54 years old, provided GAD prevalence rates from 1.6% current to 5.1% lifetime.[25]

GAD is often comorbid with other psychiatric disorders. Masi and colleagues[20] found that 93% of clinically referred youth with a diagnosis of GAD ($n = 157$) had at least one comorbid disorder. A similar rate of comorbidity of 86% was found in a non-clinical sample of 49 youth diagnosed with GAD.[19] There were differences in the pattern of comorbidity between the clinical and nonclinical samples. Depression was diagnosed in 56% of the clinical sample and was the most common comorbid disorder. In contrast, it was only present in 4% of the nonclinical sample and other anxiety disorders were the most common comorbid disorders. Other anxiety disorders were also common in the clinical sample: specific phobia (42%), SAD (31.8%), SP (28%), obsessive-compulsive disorder (OCD) (19.7%), and panic disorder (16.6%). Externalizing disorders (ie, ADHD, oppositional defiant disorder, conduct disorder) occurred in 21% of the clinical sample diagnosed with GAD.

Course and Outcome

GAD has a bimodal age of onset with an early onset occurring during childhood and adolescence and a later onset during adulthood.[25] Childhood-onset GAD is usually associated with a greater degree of psychopathology and a chronic course with fluctuations in symptom severity.[26,27] Children with GAD and a comorbid diagnosis of depression often have a poorer prognosis, greater symptom severity, and longer duration of symptoms when compared with children without comorbid depression.[28]

Because of high comorbidity rates between GAD and depression, there is speculation as to whether these are two distinct disorders. Researchers have suggested that GAD may be a subsyndrome to major depressive disorder (MDD) because of "sequential comorbidity," in which GAD typically precedes MDD.[29] Other researchers theorize that the disorders have "cumulative comorbidity," meaning that the disorders tend to occur during a lifetime but not in a simultaneous manner.[29] Moffitt and colleagues[29] completed a prospective study following 1,037 participants 3 years to 32 years of age. Results showed a strong cumulative comorbidity from 11 to 32 years of age. Forty-eight percent of participants with MDD had a history of an anxiety disorder and 72% of participants with anxiety had a history of MDD. Findings did not provide strong evidence for sequential comorbidity because GAD was diagnosed first in 42% of participants and MDD was diagnosed first in 32% of participants. These results show a strong relationship between GAD and MDD; however, more longitudinal studies are needed to better understand the association.

SOCIAL PHOBIA
Clinical Presentation

Before the DSM-IV, SP was not diagnosed in children and adolescents. Youth who endorsed anxiety and avoidance of engaging with unfamiliar people were commonly diagnosed with avoidant disorder of childhood or adolescence. This diagnosis was excluded from the DSM-IV; children and adolescents who fear social and performance situations are now diagnosed with SP.

Diagnostic criteria for SP in youth are similar to adult criteria, with a few minor clarifications that take into account developmental differences between adults and children (see **Table 1**). The primary characteristic of SP is the same across all ages. Individuals with SP experience fear regarding social and performance situations because of anxiety that they will act in an embarrassing way. Children with SP often have poor social skills and have difficulty initiating and maintaining interpersonal relationships.[30,31] Beidel and colleagues[30] found that in a clinical sample of 50 children (7–13 years old) with SP, 75% reported having few or no friends and 50% were not involved in extracurricular activities. SP also seems to have an impact on children's functioning in the classroom. Muris and Meesters[32] found that higher SP symptoms in a nonclinical sample of children (10–12 years old) was associated with poorer general classroom functioning, increased difficulty with peer relationships, and lower self-esteem. Bernstein and colleagues[31] examined classroom functioning in a nonclinical sample of children with SP (7–10 years old) based on teacher reports. Results showed that children with greater severity of SP symptoms had poorer social and leadership skills. In addition, there was an association between the severity of SP symptoms and school difficulties: as SP severity increased, attention and learning problems also increased.

The rate of lifetime SP in a community sample of adolescents was found to be 1.6%,[33] and substantially higher at 14.9% in a clinical sample of children.[11] Mean age of onset for social phobia in clinical samples ranges from 11 to 12 years of age[11,34] and the rate of SP increases with age.[33] Essau and colleagues[33] found that the most commonly feared situations in adolescents were performing in front of others, public speaking, and engaging in conversations. The most frequent anxiety endorsed by these adolescents was the fear that something would happen to cause them to be embarrassed.

Beidel and colleagues[30] found that 60% of children with SP met criteria for another Axis I disorder. Thirty-six percent of the comorbid disorders were other anxiety disorders. The most common comorbid disorders included the following: 10% of children had GAD, ADHD, or specific phobia; 8% had selective mutism; and 6% had an affective disorder.

Course and Outcome

A prospective longitudinal study that followed adolescents until 34 years of age showed that a diagnosis of SP during adolescence significantly increases the individual's risk for later onset depression.[35] Approximately 50% of participants with SP met criteria for a depressive disorder during the follow-up period, which placed them at a twofold risk compared with individuals without a diagnosis of SP. Several factors and SP characteristics were found to be associated with an increased risk for subsequent depression. The contributing factors were parental anxiety or major depression, female gender, childhood behavioral inhibition, and having more than two other anxiety disorders. The contributing SP characteristics were increased level of impairment, persistence of symptoms, and greater degree of severity.

In addition to the high rate of depressive disorders found in individuals diagnosed with SP, there is also a high rate of comorbidity of SP and substance use disorders.[36] Buckner and colleagues[37] found that adolescents who were diagnosed with SP were more likely to be diagnosed with alcohol dependence and cannabis dependence during a follow-up period that ended at 30 years of age when compared with adolescents who did not have a diagnosis of SP. Furthermore, the data provide evidence that SP in adolescents seems to be a unique risk factor for the development of subsequent substance dependence disorders. Because of the high comorbidity rates of subsequent depressive and substance dependence disorders, SP places youth at risk for long-term problems across domains of education, social relationships, and employment.

OBSESSIVE-COMPULSIVE DISORDER
Clinical Presentation

DSM-IV-TR requires either obsessions or compulsions to meet criteria for OCD.[7] Obsessions are recurrent intrusive thoughts, images, or impulses that cause excessive anxiety or distress. Compulsions are repetitive behaviors or mental acts that the individual feels compelled to perform in response to an obsession. To be diagnosed with OCD, the individual must experience excessive distress, engage in obsessions or compulsions for greater than 1 hour per day, or experience functional impairment related to the OCD. Young children do not necessarily recognize their obsessions and compulsions as senseless or excessive.

Prevalence of OCD in children and adolescents ranges from 1% to 4%.[38,39] The male-to-female ratio is approximately 3:2 in youth and changes to a slight female predominance in adulthood.[40] Common comorbid conditions are tic disorders, other anxiety disorders, ADHD, pervasive developmental disorder, and depression.[41]

Almost all children and adolescents with OCD have both obsessions and compulsions. One study showed that 93% of children with OCD experience multiple obsessions and 100% engage in multiple compulsions.[42] In a series of 70 consecutive cases of early onset OCD, the most common obsessions were concern about dirt or germs, danger to self or family, and symmetry; the most common compulsions were excessive washing, repeating rituals, and checking behaviors.[43]

Children with OCD present with a variety of obsessions and compulsions. Stewart and colleagues[44] used a principal component analysis to identify factors from the Children's Yale-Brown Obsessive-Compulsive Scale (CY-BOCS)[45] in a sample of 231 children and adolescents with OCD. The CY-BOCS is a semistructured interview that assesses severity of OCD symptoms and includes a checklist of the types of obsessions and compulsions experienced. Four factors were identified as strongly associated with the presentation of pediatric OCD and accounted for 60% of the symptom variance: preoccupation with contamination/cleaning/aggressive/somatic, symmetry/ordering/repeating/checking, sexual/religious themes, and hoarding.[44] There is evidence that suggests a similar four-factor structure is applicable across the lifespan.[46] A dimensional approach is useful in understanding the heterogeneity in OCD.[44]

Course and Outcome

There is a bimodal pattern to age of onset in OCD, with one peak in childhood and a second in adulthood. Age of onset for pediatric OCD is typically around 10 years, with a range from 7.5 to 12.5 years.[40] In youth, the mean age at identification is 2.5 years after onset of the disorder. This delay may be in part due to the secretive nature of the symptoms in many children.

In a meta-analysis of 16 pediatric samples ($n = 521$ participants) followed for 1 to 15.6 years, with the average period to follow-up of 5.7 years, a substantial number of children with OCD achieved remission of symptoms.[47] In the pooled sample, 59% of participants no longer met criteria for the OCD diagnosis and 40% did not show any evidence of residual OCD symptoms at follow-up. Predictors of persistence of OCD diagnosis included earlier age of onset, longer duration of illness at ascertainment, and a history of inpatient hospitalization.[47]

Pediatric Autoimmune Neuropsychiatric Disorders Associated with Streptococcal Infections

A small subgroup of children with OCD or tics has been classified as having pediatric autoimmune neuropsychiatric disorders associated with streptococcal infections (PANDAS).[48] This subset of children experiences a sudden onset of OCD or motor tics in association with group A streptococcal infections (eg, "strep throat"). Diagnostic criteria for PANDAS include: (1) presence of OCD or tics, (2) prepubertal onset, (3) abrupt onset or episodic course of symptom severity, (4) exacerbations associated with streptococcal infections, and (5) exacerbations associated with neurologic abnormalities (eg, hyperactivity, choreiform movements).[48] There is an increased rate of comorbid neuropsychiatric symptoms in children with PANDAS, including separation anxiety, impulsivity, hyperactivity, enuresis, and deterioration in handwriting.[48,49] Although streptococcal infections are believed to be involved in the etiologic pathway leading to OCD in children with PANDAS, the mechanism is still under investigation. Research suggests that circulating autoimmune antibodies that cross-react with neuronal structures (particularly the basal ganglia) may play a key role in the pathogenesis of PANDAS.[50]

Case Example

Peter is an 11-year-old boy presenting with a two-year history of intrusive, obsessive thoughts and compulsive, ritualistic behaviors. The obsessions began at around 9 years of age with concern about contamination of food. Peter would not eat anything that a family member had touched. Before preparing food, Peter required that his mother put on a clean outfit and thoroughly wash her hands. If he observed his mother touch the kitchen countertop or cough or sneeze during meal preparation, he demanded that she change clothes and wash her hands again. If she did not comply, Peter would not eat the food she prepared.

One of Peter's prominent intrusive thoughts was that meat was not thoroughly cooked. He asked his mother multiple times whether she had cooked the meat long enough. He worried that that he or a family member might contract mad cow disease and die if the meat was not completely cooked. He refused to eat at restaurants because of his concerns about contamination and whether meat was completely cooked. He did not eat the hot lunch at school and brought his own lunch instead. Peter washed his hands multiple times during the day, using large amounts of soap and spending up to 30 minutes washing at a time. If he was interrupted, he restarted the compulsion that consisted of washing each hand an even number of times.

Obsessions and compulsions were causing substantial impairment. Peter was often late to school because of the excessive time he spent engaged in washing and grooming rituals. He walked two blocks to school. On his way to school, he felt compelled to pick up candy and gum wrappers and other paper scraps and stuff them into his pockets. This also contributed to his tardiness. He was having difficulty concentrating on schoolwork and homework because of his obsessive thoughts. After returning home from school, Peter emptied his pockets. He hoarded the paper scraps in his closet and under the bed. Total time spent in obsessions and compulsions was approximately 5 hours per day. He had lost 6 pounds because of his restricted eating.

There was no history of psychiatric assessments or interventions for OCD. Initially, Peter was very secretive about his symptoms. Medical history was noncontributory. The OCD symptoms came on gradually and onset and exacerbations were not associated with streptococcal infections. Family psychiatric history was positive for an older brother with OCD and Tourette's disorder, a paternal aunt with OCD, and Peter's father, who had obsessive tendencies.

Mental status examination revealed a preadolescent boy who was neatly dressed and groomed. He would not shake hands with the examiner. Peter's hands were noticeably red, dry, and chapped because of frequent handwashing. He opened the door to the examination room using a Kleenex so his hand did not touch the knob and he appeared worried about sitting in the chair, but did so after encouragement from his mother. Mood was described by his mother as "nervous and irritable" and affect was anxious. He was embarrassed to talk about his symptoms. Thought content was remarkable for intrusive thoughts. There were no suicidal or homicidal ideations. There was no evidence of psychosis. No motor tics, vocal tics, or hyperactivity were observed. Insight was limited. Peter did not view his obsessions and compulsions as irrational or unreasonable.

Peter was diagnosed with OCD with a Global Assessment of Functioning score of 48. Because of the severity of his symptoms, a multimodal approach including cognitive-behavioral therapy (CBT) for OCD and a selective serotonin reuptake inhibitor (SSRI) was recommended. Peter and his parents agreed to participate in CBT, as well as initiate an SSRI. Peter was gradually titrated to a therapeutic dose of the SSRI. In the meantime, he actively participated in weekly CBT sessions that provided him and his parents with skills to manage and reduce his obsessions and compulsions. Peter and his parents were provided with psychoeducation about OCD. Peter then learned and implemented cognitive modification, relaxation skills, and exposure and response prevention to resist his compulsive behaviors and manage his obsessive thoughts. With the combination of an SSRI and CBT, Peter noticed a reduction in the frequency and severity of his obsessions and compulsions. Over time, he was able to eat foods prepared by his mother without requiring her to wash and change her clothes before meal preparation and was able to throw away candy wrappers and other papers that he hoarded under his bed and in the closet. Eventually, Peter stopped picking up trash on the way to school and he spent less time engaged in washing his hands.

POSTTRAUMATIC STRESS DISORDER
Clinical Presentation

Clinical presentation of posttraumatic stress disorder (PTSD) in older children and adolescents is similar to that in adults. Older children and adolescents have a better understanding of the traumatic experiences and the long-term consequences than children.[51] Additionally, they have the cognitive abilities to describe symptoms of re-experiencing, avoidance, numbing, and dissociation. Carrion and colleagues[52] assessed the frequency and intensity of PTSD symptoms in children ranging from 7 to 14 years of age. The most frequent symptoms included: 83% engaged in avoidance of thoughts, feelings, and conversations associated with the trauma; 70% had distressing recollections and the inability to recall important aspects of the traumatic event; and 64% reported problems concentrating. Children rated irritability and anger, distressing dreams, and detachment from others as the most intense symptoms.

Clinical presentation of PTSD in young children tends to be markedly different than that in older children, adolescents, and adults. Young children are less likely to demonstrate emotional numbing and avoidance, which is likely because of the complicated cognitive introspection that is required.[51] Young children are more likely to exhibit overt aggression, destructive behavior, and repetitive play about the traumatic event. Because of these developmental differences in clinical presentation, it is less likely that young children will meet DSM-IV-TR criteria for PTSD.

Alternative criteria that are more developmentally appropriate to diagnose PTSD in infants and younger children have been proposed and are being evaluated.[53–55] Many of the adult PTSD symptoms depend on higher-level cognitive functions (ie, memory, abstract thinking, emotional processing, language).[54] The criteria being investigated for younger children are less dependent on verbalizations and rely more on behavioral observations. The alternative criteria do not require young children to demonstrate an intense fear response during the traumatic event. The re-experiencing criteria emphasize posttraumatic play and play reenactment of the traumatic event. Young children are not required to exhibit avoidance behaviors related to the traumatic event or beliefs regarding a shortened future and recall of the event is not assessed. Instead, it is proposed that young children demonstrate a numbing of responsiveness through constricted play, socially withdrawn behavior, and restricted range of affect. Young children need to show increased arousal similar to DSM-IV-TR criteria. The proposed criteria include an additional domain, which is related to the development of new fears and aggression (ie, separation anxiety, fear of toileting alone, fear of the dark). The duration of the symptoms is still at least 1 month; however, the symptoms do not need to cause significant distress or impairment. These proposed criteria are not part of the DSM-IV-TR at this time.

Prevalence of pediatric PTSD was studied in the Great Smoky Mountains Study (GSMS), which is a longitudinal community study of childhood psychopathology that included 1,420 youths ranging in age from 9 to 16 years. At 16 years of age, 67.8% of participants reported exposure to at least one traumatic event and the trauma occurred more often during adolescence, as compared with childhood.[56] Of the participants exposed to trauma, 40.4% met criteria for a psychiatric disorder, compared with 25.5% of participants who were not exposed to trauma. Only 0.5% of the sample met full criteria for PTSD; however, higher rates of subclinical PTSD and painful recall were endorsed. Subclinical PTSD (ie, one symptom of painful recall, hyperarousal, and avoidance) was present in 2.2% of the youth and painful recall was present in 9.1% of the youth.

The occurrence of PTSD in a community sample of older adolescents is shown to be higher than reported in the GSMS that included younger children. From a sample of 384 adolescents with an average age of 17.9 years, 43% reported experiencing a traumatic event.[57] Of these participants, 14.5% met full DSM-III-R criteria for PTSD (ie, 6.3% of total sample). The median age of onset of PTSD was 16 years. The rate of trauma did not significantly differ between males and females; however, females were six times more likely to meet criteria for PTSD. Adolescents diagnosed with PTSD were seven times more likely to develop another psychiatric disorder (most commonly major depression or substance dependence) compared with adolescents with no trauma exposure and four times more likely compared with other adolescents who experienced trauma but did not meet criteria for PTSD.

Course and Outcome

Risk factors associated with the development of PTSD in youth are based on factors before the trauma, related to the trauma, and following the trauma. Parental psychopathology and family conflict significantly increase the risk of youth experiencing a traumatic event.[58] Other risk factors related to the youth's life before the trauma include: history of poor social support and adverse life events, parental poverty, history of childhood maltreatment, poor family functioning, family history of psychiatric disorders, introversion or extreme behavioral inhibition, female gender, younger age, poor health, and history of psychiatric disorder.[59,60]

Risk factors for PTSD associated with the traumatic experience include the degree of trauma exposure and the parent's and child's subjective sense of danger.[61] Witnessing a threat to a primary caregiver during infancy, childhood, and adolescence is related to an increase in total number of PTSD symptoms.[62] Lack of social support, continued negative life events, parental reactions, and lack of posttrauma intervention are risk factors associated with poor outcome after the trauma.[61]

SUMMARY

Anxiety disorders are commonly diagnosed in children and adolescents. Prevalence rates range from 2% to 27%, depending on the length of the assessment interval.

Therefore, it is important to identify and treat pediatric anxiety disorder to reduce the long-term consequences. Although anxiety disorders often have similar clinical presentations in youth and adults, it is critical to understand the differences that may occur across the lifespan.

ACKNOWLEDGMENTS

The authors would like to thank Heidi Fall and Bonnie Allen, administrative assistants in the Division of Child and Adolescent Psychiatry, for their help in preparing the manuscript.

REFERENCES

1. Costello EJ, Egger HL, Angold A. The developmental epidemiology of anxiety disorders: phenomenology, prevalence, and comorbidity. Child Adolesc Psychiatr Clin N Am 2005;14(4):631–48, vii.
2. Costello EJ, Angold A, Burns BJ, et al. The great smoky mountains study of youth. Goals, design, methods, and the prevalence of DSM-III-R disorders. Arch Gen Psychiatry 1996;53(12):1129–36.
3. Simonoff E, Pickles A, Meyer JM, et al. The Virginia twin study of adolescent behavioral development. Influences of age, sex, and impairment on rates of disorder. Arch Gen Psychiatry 1997;54(9):801–8.
4. Beals J, Piasecki J, Nelson S, et al. Psychiatric disorder among American Indian adolescents: prevalence in northern plains youth. J Am Acad Child Adolesc Psychiatry 1997;36(9):1252–9.
5. Costello EJ, Angold A, Keeler GP. Adolescent outcomes of childhood disorders: the consequences of severity and impairment. J Am Acad Child Adolesc Psychiatry 1999;38(2):121–8.
6. Lewinsohn PM, Gotlib IH, Lewinsohn M, et al. Gender differences in anxiety disorders and anxiety symptoms in adolescents. J Abnorm Psychol 1998; 107(1):109–17.
7. American Psychiatric Association. Diagnostic and statistical manual of mental disorders, fourth edition, text revision. Washington, DC: American Psychiatric Association; 2000.
8. Suveg C, Aschenbrand SG, Kendall PC. Separation anxiety disorder, panic disorder, and school refusal. Child Adolesc Psychiatr Clin N Am 2005;14(4):773–95.
9. Lewinsohn PM, Holm-Denoma JM, Small JW, et al. Separation anxiety disorder in childhood as a risk factor for future mental illness. J Am Acad Child Adolesc Psychiatry 2008;47(5):548–55.
10. Shear K, Jin R, Ruscio AM, et al. Prevalence and correlates of estimated DSM-IV child and adult separation anxiety disorder in the National comorbidity survey replication. Am J Psychiatry 2006;163(6):1074–83.
11. Last CG, Perrin S, Hersen M, et al. DSM-III-R anxiety disorders in children: sociodemographic and clinical characteristics. J Am Acad Child Adolesc Psychiatry 1992;31(6):1070–6.
12. Verduin TL, Kendall PC. Differential occurrence of comorbidity within childhood anxiety disorders. J Clin Child Adolesc Psychol 2003;32(2):290–5.
13. Last CG, Perrin S, Hersen M, et al. A prospective study of childhood anxiety disorders. J Am Acad Child Adolesc Psychiatry 1996;35:1502–10.
14. Kearney CA, Sims KE, Pursell CR, et al. Separation anxiety disorder in young children: a longitudinal and family analysis. J Clin Child Adolesc Psychol 2003;32(4): 593–8.

15. Foley DL, Pickles A, Maes HM, et al. Course and short-term outcomes of separation anxiety disorder in a community sample of twins. J Am Acad Child Adolesc Psychiatry 2004;43(9):1107–14.

16. Aschenbrand SG, Kendall PC, Webb A, et al. Is childhood separation anxiety disorder a predictor of adult panic disorder and agoraphobia? A seven-year longitudinal study. J Am Acad Child Adolesc Psychiatry 2003;42(12):1478–85.

17. American Psychiatric Association. Diagnostic and statistical manual of mental disorders, third edition. Washington, DC: American Psychiatric Association; 1987.

18. American Psychiatric Association. Diagnostic and statistical manual of mental disorders, fourth edition. Washington, DC: American Psychiatric Association; 1994.

19. Layne AE, Bernat DH, Victor AM, et al. Generalized anxiety disorder in a nonclinical sample of children: symptom presentation and predictors of impairment. J Anxiety Disord 2008; 10.1016/j.janxdis.2008.08.003, in press.

20. Masi G, Millepiedi S, Mucci M, et al. Generalized anxiety disorder in referred children and adolescents. J Am Acad Child Adolesc Psychiatry 2004;43(6):752–60.

21. Kendall PC, Pimentel SS. On the physiological symptom constellation in youth with generalized anxiety disorder (GAD). J Anxiety Disord 2003;17(2):211–21.

22. Tracey SA, Chorpita BF, Douban J, et al. Empirical evaluation of DSM-IV generalized anxiety disorder criteria in children and adolescents. J Clin Child Psychol 1997;26(4):404–14.

23. Anderson JC, Williams S, McGee R, et al. DSM-III disorders in preadolescent children. Prevalence in a large sample from the general population. Arch Gen Psychiatry 1987;44(1):69–76.

24. Bowen RC, Offord DR, Boyle MH. The prevalence of overanxious disorder and separation anxiety disorder: results from the Ontario child health study. J Am Acad Child Adolesc Psychiatry 1990;29(5):753–8.

25. Wittchen HU, Zhao S, Kessler RC, et al. DSM-III-R generalized anxiety disorder in the national comorbidity survey. Arch Gen Psychiatry 1994;51(5):355–64.

26. Bell-Dolan DJ, Last CG, Strauss CC. Symptoms of anxiety disorders in normal children. J Am Acad Child Adolesc Psychiatry 1990;29(5):759–65.

27. Hoehn-Saric R, Hazlett RL, McLeod DR. Generalized anxiety disorder with early and late onset of anxiety symptoms. Compr Psychiatry 1993;34(5):291–8.

28. Masi G, Mucci M, Favilla L, et al. Symptomatology and comorbidity of generalized anxiety disorder in children and adolescents. Compr Psychiatry 1999; 40(3):210–5.

29. Moffitt TE, Harrington H, Caspi A, et al. Depression and generalized anxiety disorder: cumulative and sequential comorbidity in a birth cohort followed prospectively to age 32 years. Arch Gen Psychiatry 2007;64(6):651–60.

30. Beidel DC, Turner SM, Morris TL. Psychopathology of childhood social phobia. J Am Acad Child Adolesc Psychiatry 1999;38(6):643–50.

31. Bernstein GA, Bernat DH, Davis AA, et al. Symptom presentation and classroom functioning in a nonclinical sample of children with social phobia. Depress Anxiety 2008;25(9):752–60.

32. Muris P, Meesters C. Symptoms of anxiety disorders and teacher-reported school functioning of normal children. Psychol Rep 2002;91(2):588–90.

33. Essau CA, Conradt J, Petermann F. Frequency and comorbidity of social phobia and social fears in adolescents. Behav Res Ther 1999;37(9):831–43.

34. Strauss CC, Last CG. Social and simple phobias in children. J Anxiety Disord 1993;7:141–52.

35. Beesdo K, Bittner A, Pine DS, et al. Incidence of social anxiety disorder and the consistent risk for secondary depression in the first three decades of life. Arch Gen Psychiatry 2007;64(8):903–12.

36. Grant BF, Hasin DS, Blanco C, et al. The epidemiology of social anxiety disorder in the United States: results from the national epidemiologic survey on alcohol and related conditions. J Clin Psychiatry 2005;66(11):1351–61.

37. Buckner JD, Schmidt NB, Lang AR, et al. Specificity of social anxiety disorder as a risk factor for alcohol and cannabis dependence. J Psychiatr Res 2008;42(3):230–9.

38. Rapoport JL, Inoff-Germain G, Weissman MM, et al. Childhood obsessive-compulsive disorder in the NIMH MECA study: parent versus child identification of cases. Methods for the epidemiology of child and adolescent mental disorders. J Anxiety Disord 2000;14(6):535–48.

39. Valleni-Basile LA, Garrison CZ, Jackson KL, et al. Frequency of obsessive-compulsive disorder in a community sample of young adolescents. J Am Acad Child Adolesc Psychiatry 1994;33(6):782–91.

40. Geller D, Biederman J, Jones J, et al. Is juvenile obsessive-compulsive disorder a developmental subtype of the disorder? A review of the pediatric literature. J Am Acad Child Adolesc Psychiatry 1998;37(4):420–7.

41. Geller DA. Obsessive-compulsive and spectrum disorders in children and adolescents. Psychiatr Clin North Am 2006;29(2):353–70.

42. Geller DA, Biederman J, Faraone S, et al. Developmental aspects of obsessive compulsive disorder: findings in children, adolescents, and adults. J Nerv Ment Dis 2001;189(7):471–7.

43. Swedo SE, Rapoport JL, Leonard H, et al. Obsessive-compulsive disorder in children and adolescents. Clinical phenomenology of 70 consecutive cases. Arch Gen Psychiatry 1989;46(4):335–41.

44. Stewart SE, Rosario MC, Brown TA, et al. Principal components analysis of obsessive-compulsive disorder symptoms in children and adolescents. Biol Psychiatry 2007;61(3):285–91.

45. Scahill L, Riddle MA, McSwiggin-Hardin M, et al. Children's Yale-Brown obsessive compulsive scale: reliability and validity. J Am Acad Child Adolesc Psychiatry 1997;36(6):844–52.

46. Stewart SE, Rosario MC, Baer L, et al. Four-factor structure of obsessive-compulsive disorder symptoms in children, adolescents, and adults. J Am Acad Child Adolesc Psychiatry 2008;47(7):763–72.

47. Stewart SE, Geller DA, Jenike M, et al. Long-term outcome of pediatric obsessive-compulsive disorder: a meta-analysis and qualitative review of the literature. Acta Psychiatr Scand 2004;110(1):4–13.

48. Swedo SE, Leonard HL, Garvey M, et al. Pediatric autoimmune neuropsychiatric disorders associated with streptococcal infections: clinical description of the first 50 cases. Am J Psychiatry 1998;155(2):264–71.

49. Murphy ML, Pichichero ME. Prospective identification and treatment of children with pediatric autoimmune neuropsychiatric disorder associated with group A streptococcal infection (PANDAS). Arch Pediatr Adolesc Med 2002;156(4):356–61.

50. Dale RC, Heyman I, Giovannoni G, et al. Incidence of anti-brain antibodies in children with obsessive-compulsive disorder. Br J Psychiatry 2005;187:314–9.

51. Dyregrov A, Yule W. A review of PTSD in children. Child Adolesc Psychiatry Ment Health 2006;11:176–84.

52. Carrion VG, Weems CF, Ray R, et al. Toward an empirical definition of pediatric PTSD: the phenomenology of PTSD symptoms in youth. J Am Acad Child Adolesc Psychiatry 2002;41(2):166–73.

53. Scheeringa MS, Peebles CD, Cook CA, et al. Toward establishing procedural, criterion, and discriminant validity for PTSD in early childhood. J Am Acad Child Adolesc Psychiatry 2001;40(1):52–60.
54. Scheeringa MS, Zeanah CH, Drell MJ, et al. Two approaches to the diagnosis of posttraumatic stress disorder in infancy and early childhood. J Am Acad Child Adolesc Psychiatry 1995;34(2):191–200.
55. Scheeringa MS, Zeanah CH, Myers L, et al. New findings on alternative criteria for PTSD in preschool children. J Am Acad Child Adolesc Psychiatry 2003;42(5): 561–70.
56. Copeland WE, Keeler G, Angold A, et al. Traumatic events and posttraumatic stress in childhood. Arch Gen Psychiatry 2007;64(5):577–84.
57. Giaconia RM, Reinherz HZ, Silverman AB, et al. Traumas and posttraumatic stress disorder in a community population of older adolescents. J Am Acad Child Adolesc Psychiatry 1995;34(10):1369–80.
58. Costello EJ, Erkanli A, Fairbank JA, et al. The prevalence of potentially traumatic events in childhood and adolescence. J Trauma Stress 2002;15(2):99–112.
59. Davidson JRT, Foa EB. Posttraumatic stress disorder: DSM-IV and beyond. Washington, DC: American Psychiatric Press; 1993.
60. Lonigan CJ, Phillips BM, Richey JA. Posttraumatic stress disorder in children: diagnosis, assessment, and associated features. Child Adolesc Psychiatr Clin N Am 2003;12(2):171–94.
61. Pynoos RS, Nader K. Mental health disturbances in children exposed to disaster: prevention intervention strategies. In: Goldston SE, Yager J, Heinicke CM, et al, editors. Preventing Mental Health Disturbances in Childhood. 1st edition. Washington, DC: American Psychiatric Press; 1990. p. 211–33.
62. Scheeringa MS, Wright MJ, Hunt JP, et al. Factors affecting the diagnosis and prediction of PTSD symptomatology in children and adolescents. Am J Psychiatry 2006;163(4):644–51.

Diagnostic Issues in Childhood Bipolar Disorder

Robert Horst, MD[a,b],*

KEYWORDS

- Child • Adolescent • Bipolar • Diagnosis
- Irritability • Aggression • ADHD • Phenotype

In his early descriptions, Kraepelin observed that manic depression, although commonly presenting after puberty, can and does occur in children and adolescents.[1] Yet, despite this early insight, the field of psychiatry largely discounted the existence of bipolar disorder (BD) in children and viewed adolescent-onset BD as uncommon until recently.[2] Evidence demonstrating that a significant number of adults with BD report symptom onset before age 19 has led to an explosion in the recognition of childhood BD over the past decade.[1] Children and adolescents, including preschoolers, are being diagnosed with BD in rapidly increasing numbers.[1,3,4] The criteria for mania are being adjusted in children and adolescents to accommodate various presentations of emotional dysregulation into the paradigm of BD. For example, children with nonspecific symptoms of aggression, irritability, recklessness, and mood lability are being diagnosed with BD.[1] It has yet to be seen whether these presentations will develop in adulthood into what we have traditionally considered to be BD. This blurring of the diagnostic lines has led to significant controversy in the field of child and adolescent psychiatry. Currently there is little agreement on issues, such as the validity of the cardinal symptoms of elated mood and grandiosity, the role of irritability, whether mood episodes are episodic or continuous, the considerable overlap in symptoms with other childhood psychiatric disorders, and the validity of subthreshold presentations.[5] This article introduces current thinking about this controversial diagnosis through two case examples.

[a] Department of Psychiatry, University of California at Davis, 2230 Stockton Boulevard, Sacramento, CA 95817, USA
[b] Sacramento County Child and Adolescent Psychiatry Services, 3331 Power Inn Road, Suite 140, Sacramento, CA 95826, USA
* Corresponding author. Sacramento County Child and Adolescent Psychiatry Services, 3331 Power Inn Road, Suite 140, Sacramento, CA 95826.
E-mail address: horstr@saccounty.net

Psychiatr Clin N Am 32 (2009) 71–80
doi:10.1016/j.psc.2008.11.005
0193-953X/08/$ – see front matter © 2009 Elsevier Inc. All rights reserved.

psych.theclinics.com

CASE 1
Vignette

Jill is a 13-year-old girl who presents to your general psychiatry office in rural Colorado. Jill's mother has BD-I. She is currently in treatment and stable under your care. As there are no child psychiatrists within driving distance of Jill's home town and you are the sole general psychiatrist in the community, you agree to evaluate Jill. You complete a comprehensive evaluation, including interviews with Jill and her family, review of a teacher rating scale, and review of background information, including a physical examination revealing no medical problems.

You find that Jill started having trouble last year after failing multiple math tests. Her parents report that around that time Jill seemed to lose motivation to do well in school, started isolating herself more, sleeping a lot, and appearing sluggish. The family started Jill in counseling and she seemed to be improving. However, about one-and-a-half weeks ago Jill's parents noticed that she was up late at night writing songs and playing her guitar. When they confronted Jill on this they found she had been up most of the night for the previous 3 days. Despite this lack of sleep, Jill appeared to have an excessive amount of energy during the day. Her parents were pleased that she no longer seemed depressed, but the way Jill was acting in the previous week and a half was significantly out of character for her. Jill's teacher rating scales, which were completed within the previous week, indicated that Jill was struggling with paying attention in class, was frequently unable to sit still, and was getting into numerous conflicts with her peers.

In meeting with Jill, you find her to be quite energetic and somewhat hyperverbal on examination. On discussion, you find that she has been practicing her guitar all night long because she believes she is destined to become a world famous musician within the next year. You also find that Jill has never had any guitar lessons in the past nor has she ever played in any kind of a band. She is not having suicidal thoughts and does not report any psychotic symptoms. There are no parental concerns that Jill may be using drugs or alcohol, and Jill denies any such use.

Discussion

Jill's case illustrates the classic presentation of BD in childhood. Jill has a positive family history of BD and presents with symptoms that meet the *Diagnostic and Statistical Manual of Mental Disorders, Fourth Edition* (DSM-IV) criteria for mania: that is, a greater than one week history of grandiosity, decreased need for sleep, excessive talkativeness, and increase in goal-directed activities.[6] In addition, Jill has a premorbid history of a depressive episode. The genetic underpinnings of BD are well established and heritability has been estimated at over 80%.[5] Twin, adoption, and family studies all support a strong genetic component to the disorder.[1] The presence of developmentally inappropriate grandiosity and a markedly decreased need for sleep are unique symptoms of mania that differentiate it from other psychiatric disorders.[1] The lack of confounding, potentially causative factors, such as substance abuse, are important, as is the episodic nature of Jill's symptoms. This history fits into our paradigm of BD in adulthood and has been defined as the "narrow" phenotype of childhood BD. Recent evidence based on a prospective National Institute of Mental Health (NIMH)-funded study by Geller and colleagues suggests the narrow phenotype of childhood BD is continuous with adult BD.[7] However, this narrow phenotype presentation is not likely what is responsible for the marked increase in numbers of children diagnosed with BD.

CASE 2
Vignette

After starting Jill on a mood stabilizer with consequent improvement in symptoms, the family is so impressed with your skills in treating children that they refer a family friend and their 11-year-old boy, Jack, to you. As with Jill, you perform a complete evaluation, which yields the following:

Jack's parents describe Jack as very energetic and stubborn since birth. He was diagnosed with attention-deficit hyperactivity disorder (ADHD) in Kindergarten and has been on various stimulants prescribed by his pediatrician with varying degrees of success. Last year, however, the situation took a turn for the worse for Jack and his family. Jack became progressively more irritable and would "blow up" when faced with seemingly minor stressors, such as being asked to clear his plate from the table. He would shift from being just fine to out of control and angry in a manner of seconds. He has been suspended from school for aggressive behaviors on at least three occasions in the past 6 months and is in danger of expulsion. Although his sleep routine has always been a struggle because of his insistent and repeated attempts to stay up late and play, Jack has continued to sleep about 8 to 9 hours on most nights. He has not been engaging in self-harm behaviors but his parents are very concerned, because he has made statements that he wished he were dead on two occasions when he was upset about not getting his way.

As you probe deeper into the family's history you find that Jack's father had an alcohol problem 5 years ago, at which time he physically abused Jack and his siblings. Child Protective Services were involved, and Jack's father completed substance abuse treatment and anger management classes. Jack's father has been clean from alcohol ever since, and you do not have concerns that there is any current abuse in the home. You are unable to elicit any family history of mental illness in blood relatives.

Discussion

Jack's case illustrates what has been referred to as the "broad" spectrum of BD in children, and this is where much of the controversy in the field lies. Questions around the validity of diagnosing BD in this context and whether these children will grow up to have the same illness classically described in adults are clinically meaningful and remain unanswered. In the following sections, this broad spectrum presentation will be explored, expounding on important and controversial topics in diagnosing BD in youth, such as the role of irritability, episodic versus continuous symptoms, hallmark symptoms, and the relationship of BD with ADHD.

IRRITABILITY AND AGGRESSION IN BD

Irritability is a nonspecific symptom common to a myriad of childhood psychiatric disorders. It is included in the DSM-IV criteria for such diverse diagnoses as disruptive behavior disorders, major depressive disorder, generalized anxiety disorder, and posttraumatic stress disorder.[6] Irritability is also commonly present in numerous additional psychiatric syndromes in children, including ADHD[5,8,9] and autism. Being present in nearly all manic youth to some degree, it is highly sensitive but has very low specificity in the detection of manic youth.[5]

Some researchers believe that chronic severe irritability in youth, accompanied by aggression and volatility, is the predominant mood state in children with BD, with elated or expansive mood playing a secondary role.[5] This controversial stance is countered by others who point out that cross-sectional studies have consistently found a high prevalence of elated or expansive mood in samples of youth with BD.[5]

These differences may be a result of researchers using different inclusion criteria. Overall, because of its lack of diagnostic specificity, irritability appears to be inadequate in making a diagnosis of mania in youth.[9]

EPISODIC VERSUS CONTINUOUS SYMPTOMS

The issue of whether BD must necessarily involve an episodic course has been addressed in both the child and adult literature. The classic thinking that adults with BD have complete interepisode recovery is now being called into question. Children presenting with mixed episodes have been described as often experiencing chronic symptoms that represent their baseline.[10–12] Geller has described a group of children with BD who present with chronic, continuous rapid-cycling, with long duration of episodes and with low rates of interepisode remission.[1] Some groups of researchers describe children suffering from chronic manic symptoms, with mean durations of episodes up to 3 to 4 years, while others describe children with mixed states combined with complex cycling patterns between depression and mania. Still others report chronic mixed states lasting for years, with rapid cycling between mania and depression as frequently as several times per day.[5] This cycling of mood multiple times within the course of a day, or greater than 365 episodes per year, has been defined as "ultradian" cycling and has been found to be present in 77% of one sample of children with BD.[1,8,13] Ultradian cycling is commonly referred to as "mood swings" or "mood lability."[1,7,8] "Ultrarapid" cycling is defined as 5 to 364 episodes in a year and was found in 10% of a sample of children diagnosed with BD.[1,8,13] The general consensus is that BD in youth is more chronic and refractory to treatment than BD in adulthood, with many youth presenting with chronic problems regulating their mood, emotions, and behavior in response to stress and conflict.[1] However, some researchers argue that an episodic course is a key feature of BD that should be present to make the diagnosis, and that the diagnosis should not be made if mood episodes are not clearly demarcated.[5] While there are some researchers who believe that BD in children and adolescents can follow a chronic, continuous course, an episodic course continues to be a reasonable requirement for a conservative approach and increases the probability of making an accurate BD diagnosis.[5]

HALLMARK SYMPTOMS

Hallmark symptoms are symptoms that must be present for a diagnosis to have validity. The primary example of hallmark symptoms is the requirement that either depressed mood or anhedonia be present to meet DSM-IV criteria for a major depressive episode.[6] The DSM-IV does not currently include a similar hallmark symptom paradigm for diagnosing a manic episode. As such, an individual can have an irritable mood and no grandiosity and still meet full DSM-IV criteria for mania.

For example, a child who presents with a week-long history of irritability, distractibility, excessive talkativeness, increased goal-directed activity, and excessive risk-taking is considered to be in a manic episode by DSM-IV criteria.[6] This approach may be too loose and could lead to the misdiagnosis of some children with BD, who may in fact be suffering from other psychiatric disorders, such as severe ADHD.

Geller, in her NIMH study on BD in children and adolescence, refined her criteria for mania by requiring either elated/euphoric mood or grandiosity to be included in her cohort.[7] In other words, a child who presents with irritability as a primary mood state would have to have evidence of grandiosity to be diagnosed with BD. As in any area of child psychiatry, it is imperative to consider the child's developmental stage when evaluating a child with suspected BD using this approach. Normal childhood boasting, imaginary play portraying powerful figures, overactivity, and youthful indiscretions should not be considered as evidence of BD. In addition, the context in which the symptoms occur needs to be considered, as normally developing children may exhibit many of the same symptoms to varying degrees in certain situations or environments.[5] In general, to be included in making a diagnosis of BD, a symptom should be pervasive and impairing. Although compelling, more studies are needed to solidify the use of grandiosity and elated/euphoric mood as hallmark symptoms of BD.[5,7,9]

Marked sleep disturbance has also been posited as a hallmark symptom of BD.[1] Frequently present in adult samples of mania, marked sleep disturbance appears to be less common in children, present in less than 50% of cases.[1] Hyperactivity, irritability, and dangerous play are more generic symptoms that are less likely to differentiate BD from other childhood psychiatric disorders.[1]

BD AND ADHD

The differentiation between BD and ADHD in children can be challenging. There is strong overlap between the disorders, with studies estimating that up to 80% of children with BD also have ADHD.[5] The reasons for this strong relationship are not entirely clear, although they may be related to similar risk factors, with ADHD representing an early presentation of BD in some children, early misdiagnosis of BD as ADHD, or misdiagnosing BD in a child who has severe ADHD. Geller, in a widely cited study, found that symptoms of grandiosity, elated mood, hypersexuality (in the absence any history of sexual abuse or exposure to sexual activity), flight of ideas, and decreased need for sleep differentiated children with BD from children with ADHD alone.[13,14] She found irritability to be common in both cohorts, lending further support to the notion that irritability has low specificity in the diagnosis of BD.[13,14]

A child with ADHD should be suspected of having BD if symptoms begin after age 10 or appear abruptly in an otherwise healthy child.[15] Other factors that increase the likelihood of BD in a child diagnosed with ADHD include ADHD symptoms that come and go with changes in mood, severe mood swings, temper tantrums or rages, hallucinations or delusions, a strong family history of BD, or a lack of symptom response to stimulants in a child who previously responded positively to them.[15]

DIFFERENTIAL DIAGNOSIS

In addition to the above diagnostic considerations, a broader differential diagnosis of Jack's presenting symptoms must be considered. Jack's nonspecific presentation of chronic irritability and mood reactivity in the context of a history of abuse is fairly common in some clinical samples and can represent numerous different childhood psychiatric disorders. A savvy practitioner will probe much deeper into the history of Jack's symptoms to make this differentiation, including following Jack longitudinally and using collateral sources. ADHD, as discussed above, is an important consideration, as are other mood disorders, disruptive behavior disorders, pervasive developmental disorders, schizophrenia, substance abuse, posttraumatic stress disorder, a developing borderline personality disorder, and symptoms secondary to a medication or drug of abuse or a general medical condition.[5,8] Finally, developmentally appropriate symptoms and normal variations in mood need to be included on the differential.[5] Practitioners are advised to use caution in attributing symptoms to mania unless there is a clear temporal association with elevated, expansive or irritable mood.[5]

A particularly important consideration in the diagnosis of BD in children is the presence of another mood disorder. BD is thought to be on a continuum with other mood disorders based on severity, pervasiveness, and presence or absence of mania. Adjustment disorder with depressed mood is characterized as a response to a clear stressor that is mild and time limited.[16] The continuum advances through minor depression classified as depression not otherwise specified (NOS), dysthymia, and major depression with increasing degrees of severity.[16] The presence of mania is what defines BD. To a clinician, determining where a child fits on this continuum can be much more difficult than this straightforward description implies. However, the differentiation between unipolar depression and BD is of paramount importance, as the treatment is quite different. Children with unipolar depression misdiagnosed with BD are not only exposed to the significant side-effect profiles associated with mood stabilizing medication, but their symptoms may not improve without treatment aimed specifically at unipolar depression. On the other hand, any child who presents with a unipolar depression should be carefully assessed for any history of mania, given the risk of antidepressant-induced mania and the increased risk of having a BD, particularly if the depressive episode is characterized by rapid-onset, psychomotor retardation, or psychotic features.[1] Other factors that increase the risk of BD in a child presenting with depression include a positive family history of affective disorder, especially BD, and a history of antidepressant-induced manic symptoms.[1]

COMORBIDITY

In addition to considering the differential diagnosis, practitioners must also be cognizant of the role of comorbidity in childhood-onset BD. Comorbidity in children with BD has been found to be extremely high, up to 98% in some samples.[17] ADHD is the disorder most commonly found comorbid with BD, as discussed above. Anxiety disorders are also frequently comorbid, with some estimates ranging from 30% to 70%.[5] There is considerable overlap with behavioral disorders, such as conduct disorder, and rates of substance dependence are high and increase with age.[5]

EPIDEMIOLOGY

Although the prevalence of BD in youth has yet to be adequately established, the disorder is thought to have a lifetime prevalence of approximately 0.4% to 1.6%.[16,18] A recent large survey estimated that 2% of the population has BD-I or BD-II, and another 2.4% has subsyndromal symptoms.[19] Adults with BD report high rates of symptoms beginning before age 20, with some retrospective studies as high as 60%.[5] BD in adulthood occurs equally in males and females, although early-onset cases have been found to be predominantly male, particularly if symptoms begin before age 13.[1] When using a broader definition of BD in youth, estimates of prevalence have been as high as 1%.[20] Given that the lifetime prevalence of BD has been estimated to be 0.4% to 1.6%, a 1% prevalence in children would seem on the high side. This apparent discrepancy could be caused by a number of factors, including a shift downward in the age of onset, an increased ability to recognize the illness earlier, adult prevalence rates being underestimated, or the prevalence of the disorder increasing significantly.[1] It is also possible that given the controversies in the field, BD in children is being misdiagnosed and therefore over-diagnosed.

There is ample evidence from epidemiological studies that the rates of children and adolescents diagnosed with BD are increasing. For example, Blader and Carlson[3] found an almost sixfold increase in population-adjusted rates of hospital discharges of children with a primary diagnosis of BD from 1996 to 2004. Adolescent discharges increased fourfold.[3] While adult rates also increased significantly during this time period, the rates were far more modest, with a rise of 56%.[3] Because the characterization of BD in youth is still in its infancy, reliable incidence and prevalence numbers are not available. The disorder will need to be defined more specifically and the criteria universally agreed upon before this can happen.

The youngest age at which BD presents is still up for debate. Although BD has been diagnosed in preschool-aged children, the validity of this practice has not been established.[1] A consensus group of experts advised the U.S. Food and Drug Administration to only extend medication studies down to age 10, given the challenge of diagnosing children younger than 10 with BD.[1] The first mood episode typically occurs between the ages of 17 and 42, with a median age of onset of 25.[9]

In comparison with adults with BD, in which a depressed mood state predominates, children with BD have been found to have predominant mood states of mania or hypomania.[9] Prepubertal-onset mania may be more common in boys than girls.[21] In a recent study looking at sex differences in youth with BD, boys were found to present more commonly with a manic mood while girls presented more commonly with depressed mood.[22] Older children also presented with higher levels of manic mood than younger children, who presented more commonly with depressed mood.[22] Mixed states are also very common in children and adolescents.[1]

TREATMENT

The treatment of BD in children should be comprehensive and include pharmacotherapy in addition to psychotherapeutic interventions.[1] Family and behavioral issues may be considerable and should be actively addressed.[23] The goal of psychotherapeutic interventions is to ameliorate symptoms, educate the child and family about BD, promote treatment adherence, reduce morbidity and mortality, and promote healthy growth and development.[1]

Most evidence for the efficacy of available psychopharmacologic treatments is extrapolated from adult studies and this is likely appropriate for the more classic presentation or narrow phenotype of BD in children.[1] However, there is limited evidence for the efficacy of mood-stabilizing medication in the broad-phenotype definition of BD in children. Hence, mood-stabilizing medication should be used cautiously and conservatively in this population. Pharmacotherapy with traditional mood stabilizers or atypical antipsychotics is considered the primary treatment of childhood BD.[1] A more detailed discussion of the pharmacotherapeutic treatment of BD is included in the article "Child and Adolescent Psychopharmacology Update" by McVoy and Findling in this issue.

PROGNOSIS

Numerous studies have found the long term prognosis of BD in adolescents to be similar to that of adults, with a few indicating worse outcomes.[1] Overall, the course of early-onset BD appears to be more chronic and refractory to treatment.[1] Of youth presenting with BD, 70% to 100% eventually recover from their episode but up to 80% will experience at least one recurrence in the following 2 to 5 years.[5] For each year of illness the chances of recovery, defined as minimal or no symptoms for at least 8 consecutive weeks, have been estimated to decrease by 10%.[24] Early age of onset, long duration, low socioeconomic status, episodes of mixed symptoms or rapid cycling, psychosis, subsyndromal symptoms, comorbid disorders, exposure to negative life events, and family psychopathology are all factors that have been linked to poor outcomes.[5,24] Low socioeconomic class, exposure to negative life events, and high expressed emotion or low maternal warmth have all been linked to poor outcomes, specifically in children and adolescents.[5,7] In addition, some studies have linked rapid cycling, mixed episodes, comorbid disorders, and family conflicts with a worse prognosis.[8] Early onset of BD before age 12 has been associated with poor outcomes, including comorbid conduct disorder, anxiety disorders, and substance dependence, as well as suicidal behaviors, attempts, and completion.[9]

Youth diagnosed with BD-NOS (akin to the broad spectrum phenotype) as opposed to BD-I or BD-II (akin to the narrow spectrum phenotype) took longer to recover, and their symptoms recurred sooner, perhaps related to a more chronic, subsyndromal course that may be more resistant to the treatments used.[8] In addition, adolescents with persistent and abnormal elevated, expansive, or irritable mood who did not meet full DSM-IV criteria for mania did not go on to meet diagnostic criteria for BD by their early 20s, but did have higher rates of depression and other psychiatric disorders.[25] Overall, the course of BD in children and adults is marked by recurrence, significant impacts on functioning, decreased quality of life, and suicide.[26]

SUMMARY

The cases of Jack and Jill illustrate an important controversy in the field of child and adolescent psychiatry. More and more children are being diagnosed with BD in communities across the United States, and are being prescribed mood stabilizing medications at ever increasing rates. The more controversial, broad-phenotype definition of BD in childhood is likely responsible for the bulk of this growth, often characterized as BD-NOS. This presentation is marked by an earlier onset, increased association with ADHD and oppositional defiance disorder, irritable mood, and chronic symptoms.[27] All of these characteristics decrease diagnostic reliability. In some samples only one-third were found to progress to BD-I or BD-II. Despite this, however, children diagnosed with BD-NOS were found to get the same amount of medications on average as children diagnosed with BD-I or BD-II. More studies are needed to determine if children with the broad phenotype of BD actually have the same disorder we think of as BD in adulthood, have prodromal symptoms, or have some other as yet unidentified disorder of mood dysregulation.[8]

Despite the lack of a consensus on the broad phenotype definition of BD in childhood, the consensus for the narrow-spectrum definition is quite strong.[8,27] Although mania in youth has not yet been conclusively shown to progress to classic adult BP, Geller's recent article demonstrating that a significant proportion of children diagnosed with BD using a narrow-spectrum definition do progress is compelling. In this study 44.4% of adult subjects with BD diagnosed in childhood had an episode of mania in adulthood. This rate is 13 to 44 times higher than population prevalences, supporting the contention that using a careful diagnostic process, one can accurately identify cases of BD in childhood.[7] However, the surge in children being diagnosed with BD raises many questions and it is still not clear what the broad phenotype of BD actually represents. Children who fit the narrow-spectrum definition of BD should be treated as such, and clinicians can feel comfortable that the current state of the science supports the use of mood-stabilizing medication in this population. However, children fitting in to the broad phenotype should be treated more conservatively.

REFERENCES

1. McClellan J, Kowatch R, Findling R, et al. Practice parameter for the assessment and treatment of children and adolescents with bipolar disorder. J Am Acad Child Adolesc Psychiatry 2007;46(1):107–25.

2. Carlson GA. Early onset bipolar disorder: clinical and research considerations. J Clin Child Adolesc Psychol 2005;34(2):333–43.
3. Blader JC, Carlson GA. Increased rates of bipolar disorder diagnoses among U.S. child, adolescent, and adult inpatients, 1996–2004. Biol Psychiatry 2007; 62(2):107–14.
4. Wilens TE, Biederman J, Forkner P, et al. Patterns of comorbidity and dysfunction in clinically referred preschool and school-age children with bipolar disorder. J Child Adolesc Psychopharmacol 2003;13(4):495–505.
5. Birmaher B, Axelson D, Pavuluri M. Bipolar disorder. In: Martin A, Volkmar FR, editors. Lewis' child and adolescent psychiatry: a comprehensive textbook, 4th edition. Baltimore: Lippincott Williams and Wilkins; 2007, p. 513–28.
6. American Psychiatric Association. Diagnostic and statistical manual of mental disorders, 4th edition, Text Revision (DSM-IV-TR). Washington (DC): American Psychiatric Association; 2000.
7. Geller B, Tillman R, Bolhofner K, et al. Child bipolar I disorder: prospective continuity with adult bipolar I disorder; characteristics of second and third episodes; predictors of 8-year outcome. Arch Gen Psychiatry 2008;65(10):1125–33.
8. Pavuluri MN, Birmaher B, Naylor M. Pediatric bipolar disorder: a review of the past 10 years. J Am Acad Child Adolesc Psychiatry 2005;44(9):846–71.
9. Demeter CA, Townsend LD, Wilson M, et al. Current research in child and adolescent bipolar disorder. Dialogues Clin Neurosci 2008;10(2):215–28.
10. Biederman J, Faraone SV, Wozniak J, et al. Further evidence of unique developmental phenotypic correlates of pediatric bipolar disorder: findings from a large sample of clinically referred preadolescent children assessed over the last 7 years. J Affect Disord 2004;82:S45–58.
11. Biederman J, Mick E, Faraone SV, et al. A prospective follow-up study of pediatric bipolar disorder in boys with attention-deficit/hyperactivity disorder. J Affect Disord 2004;82:S17–23.
12. Wozniak J, Biederman J, Kiely K, et al. Mania-like symptoms suggestive of childhood-onset bipolar disorder in clinically referred children. J Am Acad Child Adolesc Psychiatry 1995;34(7):867–76.
13. Geller B, Zimerman B, Williams M, et al. Diagnostic characteristics of 93 cases of a prepubertal and early adolescent bipolar phenotype by gender, puberty and comorbid attention deficit hyperactivity disorder. J Child Adolesc Psychopharmacol 2000;10(3):157–64.
14. Geller B, Warner K, Williams M, et al. Prepubertal and young adolescent bipolarity versus ADHD: assessment and validity using the WASH-U-KSADS, CBCL and TRF. J Affect Disord 1998;51(2):93–100.
15. Birmaher B. New Hope for Children and Adolescents with BP Disorder. New York: Three Rivers Press, a division of Random House, Inc; 2004.
16. Brent DA, Weersing VR. Chapter 5.4.1: Depressive disorders. In: Martin A, Volkmar FR, editors. Lewis' Child and Adolescent Psychiatry: a comprehensive textbook, 4th edition. Baltimore: Lippincott Williams and Wilkins. 2007. p. 503–13.
17. Tillman R, Geller B, Bolhofner K, et al. Ages of onset and rates of syndromal and subsyndromal comorbid DSM-IV diagnoses in a prepubertal and early adolescent bipolar disorder phenotype. J Am Acad Child Adolesc Psychiatry 2003; 42(12):1486–93.
18. Weller EB, Weller RA, Danielyan AK, et al. Mood disorders in adolescents. In: Wiener JM, Dulcan MK, editors. The American Psychiatric Publishing Textbook of child and adolescent psychiatry. 3rd edition. Arlington (VA): American Psychiatric Publishing, Inc.; 2004. p. 437–81.

19. Merikangas KR, Akiskal HS, Angst J, et al. Lifetime and 12-month prevalence of bipolar disorder spectrum disorder in the national comorbidity survey replication. Arch Gen Psychiatry 2007;64(5):543–52.
20. Geller B, Luby J. Child and adolescent bipolar disorder: a review of the past 10 years. J Am Acad Child Adolesc Psychiatry 1997;36(9):1168–76.
21. Weller EB, Weller RA, Danielyan AK, et al. Mood disorders in prepubertal children. In: Wiener JM, Dulcan MK, editors. The American Psychiatric Publishing Textbook of Child and Adolescent Psychiatry. 3rd edition. Arlington (VA): American Psychiatric Publishing, Inc.; 2004. p. 411–35.
22. Duax JM, Youngstrom EA, Calabrese JR, et al. Sex differences in pediatric bipolar disorder. J Clin Psychiatry 2007;68(10):1565–73.
23. Belardinelli C, Hatch JP, Olvera RL, et al. Family environment patterns in families with bipolar children. J Affect Disord 2008;107(1–3):299–305.
24. Birmaher B, Axelson D, Strober M, et al. Clinical course of children and adolescents with bipolar spectrum disorders. Arch Gen Psychiatry 2006;63(2):175–83.
25. Lewinsohn PM, Rohde P, Seeley JR, et al. Treatment of adolescent depression: frequency of services and impact on functioning in young adulthood. Depress Anxiety 1998;7(1):47–52.
26. Miklowitz DJ, Chang KD. Prevention of bipolar disorder in at-risk children: theoretical assumptions and empirical foundations. Dev Psychopathol 2008; 20(3):881–97.
27. Masi G, Perugi G, Millepiedi S, et al. Clinical implications of DSM-IV subtyping of bipolar disorders in referred children and adolescents. J Am Acad Child Adolesc Psychiatry 2007;46(10):1299–306.

Very Early Interventions in Psychotic Disorders

Robinder K. Bhangoo, MD*, Cameron S. Carter, MD

KEYWORDS

• Psychosis • Prodromal • Ultra–high risk • Early intervention

A schizophrenic patient is brought to us. We examine him, and we talk with the relatives. It must be a very common experience of all who are concerned with mental illness to look back and view the subtle changes which have taken place in the personality of the schizophrenic as his illness was developing. Unfortunately, we are usually aware of these changes only in retrospect. The thought must come to all of us—if only the patient had been brought to consultation earlier, we might have been able, by judicious psychotherapy and perhaps with adequate dosage of chlorpromazine, to ward off the illness without the development of psychosis, without the stigma of insanity, without loss of employment, and without any real disruption of home life.

—Ainslie Meares, 1959[1]

It is well accepted that most serious psychiatric conditions begin in adolescence and are characterized by initial symptoms that predate the full manifestation of illness. This early period often consists of nonspecific symptoms, making accurate detection difficult. In fact, classification as "prodromal" is only possible retrospectively, after a patient has developed positive psychotic symptoms. To monitor these patients prospectively, we must identify and follow patients who are at risk for psychosis, understanding that this group may also include false positives who do not go on to develop psychotic illness. Improving detection of at-risk individuals gives us an opportunity to intervene earlier in the course of the disorder, creating a window of opportunity to improve outcome and decrease overall burden of illness.

NICK

Nick is a 14-year-old boy, currently in the eighth grade, who presents with a 3-year history of worsening depression and anxiety precipitated by abuse from his

Department of Psychiatry and Behavioral Sciences, University of California, Davis, 2230 Stockton Boulevard, Sacramento, CA 95817, USA
* Corresponding author.
E-mail address: robinder.bhangoo@ucdmc.ucdavis.edu (R.K. Bhangoo).

Psychiatr Clin N Am 32 (2009) 81–94
doi:10.1016/j.psc.2008.10.003
0193-953X/08/$ – see front matter © 2009 Elsevier Inc. All rights reserved.

stepfather.[†] Nick's mother describes a normal pregnancy and delivery and says that Nick was an easy baby with a "sweet temperament" who reached his milestones on time. As a young child, Nick was "happy and outgoing" and had no behavioral or emotional problems until the age of 11 years, after experiencing verbal and physical abuse from his stepfather. Starting at the age of 12 years, Nick described being "angry all the time" with feelings of hopelessness toward his situation. He had problems with sleep, energy, and concentration and became more withdrawn and less interested in socializing or schoolwork. His appetite dropped significantly and he lost so much weight that friends wondered if he had an eating disorder. He also described frequent nightmares and flashbacks of the abuse and was hypervigilant, demonstrating an exaggerated startle response when he thought he saw his stepfather's car. From the age of 11 years, Nick also began having odd perceptual experiences, such as thinking that he heard his name being called when no one was there; or seeing shadows moving out of the corner of his eye. These experiences worsened along with his mood symptoms. Later, he began hearing voices calling him "stupid" or "dumb," and seeing shadowy figures and dead bodies on the wall. At the time of presentation, Nick confided to the doctor his belief that he had the ability to predict the future and read people's minds. There was no evidence of drug use. Nick was given the provisional diagnosis of major depression and posttraumatic stress disorder and was referred to the Early Diagnosis and Preventative Treatment of Psychotic Illnesses (EDAPT) clinic at University of California, Davis for evaluation of psychotic symptoms. After diagnostic interviews revealed that Nick had experienced his first psychotic break, the diagnosis and treatment of psychosis was discussed with Nick and his mother. They refused treatment because they believed that Nick's relatively good functioning precluded such a diagnosis. Over the next few months, however, mother reported significant decline. Nick continued to do poorly in school and was failing several classes. He stopped bathing and was becoming increasingly disheveled and malodorous. Finally, his mother became suspicious about one of Nick's friends, "Johnny," whom she had never met, but about whom Nick frequently talked. When the mother started receiving phone calls from other teenagers asking for Johnny, she began to suspect that this friend was not real. She revealed to the doctor her suspicion that Johnny was part of Nick's delusional system. Despite her efforts, Nick continued to refuse treatment because of paranoia about the medication. His condition quickly deteriorated and he was lost to follow-up.

The term "prodrome" indicates a period before the full manifestation of a psychotic illness, during which patients first experience changes in their emotions, cognition, or behavior that, although not meeting the threshold for the full disorder, indicate a deviation from the normal level of functioning. Much of the early research into prodromal symptoms is anecdotal, involving retrospective reports from first-break schizophrenia patients. Typical prodromal symptoms, in decreasing order of frequency, include: decreased concentration and attention, decreased motivation, depressed mood, sleep disturbance, anxiety, social withdrawal, suspiciousness, deterioration in role functioning, and irritability.[2] These retrospective reports indicate that although some patients experience few or no prodromal symptoms and transition directly into full psychotic illness,[3,4] others describe prodromal states lasting up to 20 years.[5,6] The prodrome is operationally defined as the period

---

[†] Vignettes are taken from actual patients seen in the Early Detection and Intervention for the Prevention of Psychosis Program (EDIPPP)/Early Diagnosis and Preventative Treatment of Psychotic Disorders (EDAPT) clinics at UC Davis. Names have been changed.

bridging the transition between the nonaffected state and the psychotic phase of illness.[2,7]

Cornblatt and colleagues[8] described two phases of the prodromal period: the early and late prodromal phases. The early prodromal phase typically occurs years before the onset of psychosis and consists of nonspecific symptoms, such as reduced concentration and motivation, irritability and depressed mood, anxiety, sleep disturbance, social withdrawal, suspiciousness, and impaired functioning. The late prodromal phase is believed to occur in the year before development of psychosis and is made up of symptoms that are closer to those experienced in the psychotic spectrum, but are considered subthreshold because they either occur transiently or are attenuated. Transient symptoms last at the most several days before subsiding spontaneously. Attenuated symptoms are those psychotic symptoms that the patient reports with less than full conviction. The patient questions the experience and expresses doubt as to the possibility of such symptoms and beliefs being true. Such subthreshold psychotic symptoms include paranoid ideation, unusual beliefs, magical thinking, thought disturbances, perceptual disturbances, ideas of reference, changes in thought and speech patterns, and atypical behavior and appearance. This progression has been referred to as the march of symptoms from the nonspecific and negative to more specific, positive psychotic symptoms.[9]

Retrospective data are limited in several ways, including recall bias and cognitive and emotional factors in the reporting patient and family members.[2] To obtain a truly accurate picture of this critical period of time before full expression of psychosis it is necessary to prospectively follow subjects who have not yet developed psychosis. This monitoring requires the development of an approach that allows us to identify individuals who are at substantial risk for developing a psychotic illness who can then be followed prospectively. The term "at-risk mental state" (ARMS) has been used to describe such populations who demonstrate clinical risk factors for subsequent psychosis.[10] Ultra high risk (UHR), clinical high risk, and ARMS are terms that are used interchangeably to describe these individuals, who are also functionally impaired and generally help-seeking. A detailed discussion of these clinical risk factors follows.

Phenomenological research of these risk factors done in Germany has expanded on work by Gerd Huber,[11] who described the symptoms that predate psychotic illness as basic because he believed that these symptoms were the basis or starting point for schizophrenia. Previously, behavioral observation of symptoms was emphasized. Huber, however, stressed the importance of a patient's subjective report of symptoms, proposing that patients were better reporters of early, more subtle changes in their cognitive, emotional, or physical status. These basic symptoms included subjective complaints of impaired energy, cognitive functioning, emotional functioning, motor functioning, bodily sensation, external perception, autonomic functioning, and tolerance to normal stress.[12] Huber also discussed the progression of symptoms from the nonspecific, which he called level 1 symptoms, to the more specific, or level 2 symptoms. In addition, he talked about outpost syndromes, which are clusters of symptoms and behaviors that resemble prodromes, but occur before the prodrome and resolve spontaneously without immediately progressing to psychosis.[2] Subsequent studies have shown that the presence of certain basic symptoms is in fact predictive of psychosis.[13,14] Huber acknowledged that these symptoms serve as potential harbingers of other mental disorders also.[12]

Over time, studies have shifted from examination of retrospective data of prodromal symptoms to prospective studies of at-risk patients. This shift has led to a worldwide increased focus on identification and characterization of individuals who are vulnerable to the development of psychosis. Consistent with this, research has increasingly focused on enhancing the accuracy of risk prediction to optimize the risk/benefit ratio of clinical interventions and on development of interventions aimed at reducing the impact of emerging psychotic illness.

At the PACE Clinic (Personal Assessment and Crisis Evaluation) in Melbourne, three distinct high-risk groups have been identified and followed prospectively to assess the rate of conversion to psychosis, the effectiveness of clinical interventions, and exploration of potential biological markers. Subjects in these studies met inclusion criteria for at least one of the following groups: (1) Attenuated Psychotic Symptoms Group, who experienced subthreshold, attenuated forms of positive psychotic symptoms during the past year; (2) Brief Limited Intermittent Psychotic Symptoms Group (BLIPS), who have experienced episodes of frank psychotic symptoms that have not lasted longer than a week and have spontaneously abated; or (3) Trait and State Risk Factor Group, who have a first-degree relative who has a psychotic illness or the identified client has a schizotypal personality disorder and they have experienced a significant decrease in functioning during the previous year.[9] Selection of these groups allowed the researchers the ability to focus on a group of individuals at higher risk for developing psychosis than the general population. By combining trait (genetic risk) and state (functional decline) risk factors, they have in essence closed in on individuals who are at higher risk for developing psychosis, thus enhancing the predictive power for psychosis conversion.[15]

HONING OUR DETECTION

The great number of our patients have shown for years before the break, clear signs of coming trouble. A number of them were brought to notice by the outcropping of behavior of a simple psychoneurotic sort. Anxiety conditions which deepen into schizophrenic panic occur in numbers.

—Henry Stack Sullivan, 1927[16]

As mentioned previously, the symptoms predating development of psychosis are often nonspecific and include inattention, irritability, and anxiety. In addition, the prodromal period often occurs in childhood and adolescence, when such symptoms may be seen in various psychiatric disorders. One method for improved detection of vulnerable individuals is to screen for attenuated or brief psychotic experiences in children who present with any behavioral changes or functional decline. In a prospective study of UHR individuals, Yung and colleagues[17] found that clinical symptoms that were highly predictive of later development of psychosis included: lower global assessment of functioning (GAF) at baseline, longer duration of prodromal symptoms, presence of low-grade psychotic symptoms, depression, and disorganization. Presence of at least four of these symptoms yielded accurate detection of individuals at high risk for development of psychosis.

KELLY

Kelly is a 16-year-old Asian female who initially presented because of complaints of sadness and anger that began 4 years prior when her older sister moved away for college.[1] She described the moods as occurring intermittently and accompanied by irritability, insomnia, and guilty ruminative thoughts. She had some thoughts of death, but denied suicidal intent or plan. Her family said that "on her good days" she would stand in front of the mirror admiring her hair and makeup and would act "hyper," but later would return to having low self-esteem. They denied decreased need for sleep or other manic symptoms and denied any psychotic symptoms. She was referred for psychotherapy, but failed to follow up. Two months later, she presented to the clinic at the urging of her family. Kelly reported experiencing two episodes lasting 4 days each during which she had decreased need for sleep and increased energy. During these periods, her behavior was highly erratic, including trying to involve others in outlandish schemes, such as driving 8 hours for lunch or stealing items from a garbage dump. She also spent excessive amounts of time on her hair and makeup. Her family reported that during these periods her speech was fast and difficult to follow, and that she was markedly irritable. Her family discovered writings by Kelly indicating that she thought of killing her sister because she believed that her sister was "out to get her." During the interview, Kelly admitted that she wrote this, but seemed perplexed by it. She remembered feeling that her sister was trying to kill her and that she needed to protect herself. Family reported that these 4-day periods were followed by a week of Kelly feeling lethargic and depressed. Kelly agreed and described feeling "hollow inside." In addition, she paid less attention to her appearance and described sleeping excessively and having an irritable mood and guilty ruminations.

Retrospective studies of first-break schizophrenic patients have consistently shown that mood and anxiety symptoms are some of the earliest seen in the prodromal period. Early symptoms have included depression, irritability, guilt, anhedonia, mood swings, suicidal ideation, anxiety, decreased motivation, fatigue, decreased concentration, restlessness, and appetite and sleep disturbance.[2] Prospective studies have also shown early presentation of mood and anxiety symptoms in the UHR populations. Meyer and colleagues[18] reported on their group of 24 adolescents who met criteria for one of the three UHR groups for a larger, prospective study. In this group of UHR teenagers, 50% received a diagnosis of major depression at baseline and 40% received a diagnosis of anxiety disorder, including (in decreasing order of frequency) anxiety disorder NOS, social phobia, generalized anxiety disorder, panic disorder, specific phobia, obsessive-compulsive disorder, and posttraumatic stress disorder. Svirskis and colleagues[19] also found that their subjects who met criteria for one of the three UHR groups had a high number of lifetime mood, anxiety, or somatization disorder diagnoses. Among these UHR subjects, researchers found that the odds ratio for receiving a lifetime mood disorder diagnosis was 3.28 compared with asymptomatic subjects and 6.34 for receiving an anxiety or somatization diagnosis. What becomes difficult to ascertain is whether these mood and anxiety symptoms represent comorbid conditions or are symptoms heralding a psychotic disorder. With further longitudinal studies, we can learn if those UHR patients who have mood and anxiety symptoms are more likely to develop an affective psychosis versus a nonaffective psychosis. It has been shown that recognition and treatment of depression in UHR patients is also important for the treatment of psychotic symptoms. In a study of nonpsychotic individuals experiencing "psychoticlike experiences," 40% were determined to have depression at baseline. Of those who had depression, 67.5% remitted by 6-month follow-up and those who had remitted also reported a decrease in psychoticlike experiences.[20]

MAX

Max was a 19-year-old white male who had been treated for depression with selective serotonin reuptake inhibitors for 3 years.[1] During these 3 years, Max became increasingly rebellious with parents and school authorities, listening to alternative music and getting caught vandalizing a public bathroom with friends. He was able to graduate high school and was accepted to a local university. There, he lived on his own and began using marijuana and cocaine heavily. After 6 months of drug use, Max had what he calls a "bad trip" with mushrooms, during which he ran into the street, babbling incoherently. During the next few months, Max continued living on his own and using drugs until his parents found him malnourished and incoherent. He was having difficulty finding words and was making odd movements with his eyes and mouth. He then moved back home and his parents monitored him closely to prevent drug use. In contrast to his previous oppositional behavior, he was now overly polite with family, yet remained somewhat aloof. His parents noticed that he lost interest in his previous hobbies of playing music and video games, but suddenly became interested in reading the Bible. Over the next few years, Max's condition worsened. He continued with intermittent drug use and his disorganized thinking worsened. He was hospitalized involuntarily several times, eventually leading to an extended admission in a residential treatment center where he remained off drugs during the year-long stay. His paranoia, hallucinations, and disorganized thinking continued in the absence of drug use and failed to respond to several medication trials. Max was eventually stabilized on clozapine and was discharged to live with his parents.

Although Max developed severe and debilitating psychotic symptoms that persisted despite cessation of drug use, in the early stages of illness there was confusion by various care providers as to how to reconcile his psychotic symptoms with his drug use. There is a great deal of evidence of an association between cannabis use and psychosis, including several prospective studies showing that cannabis use often occurs before the development of psychosis. A 15-year prospective study of 50,465 Swedish conscripts found that those who had tried cannabis by age 18 were 2.4 times as likely to later be diagnosed with schizophrenia than those who had not.[21] The risk for diagnosis increased with the frequency of cannabis use. After controlling for confounding variables, the risks were reduced, but still statistically significant. A later study of the same cohort also found a dose-response relationship between the frequency of cannabis use and risk for later diagnosis of schizophrenia.[22] These relationships persisted after controlling for the effects of other drug use and other confounders, including history of psychiatric symptoms at baseline. Other prospective studies revealed similar results, showing that cannabis use in adolescence was associated with later development of schizophrenia[23–26] and individuals who had any psychotic symptoms at baseline were more likely to develop schizophrenia or have continued psychotic symptoms if they used cannabis.[24,26] A recent meta-analysis of longitudinal studies looking at the relationship between cannabis use and psychosis found an increased risk for psychotic disorder with use of the drug.[27] Cannabis use is also associated with a younger age of onset of schizophrenia and increased likelihood for negative symptoms.[28] This evidence supports the classification of cannabis use as a risk factor for psychosis. An individual's risk for psychosis following cannabis use could be mediated by a functional polymorphism in the catechol-O-methyltransferase (COMT) gene, which encodes an enzyme that metabolizes dopamine in the frontal cortex. The homozygous val allele is associated with increased levels of dopamine in the midbrain and with a fivefold increased risk for developing psychotic symptoms with frequent cannabis use,[29] whereas the homozygous met allele did not have this increased risk. Those who had the intermediate val/met allele had double the risk.[30] This effect was only observed in those individuals who first used cannabis before the age of 18 years with no replication of results in individuals who first used after 18 years.

BENEFITS OF EARLY DETECTION

Investigations which we have carried on during the last two years into the newer therapeutic techniques used in schizophrenia have led to considerable preoccupation with patients in whom the disorder has shown much less progression than one finds in the usual schizophrenic individual dealt with routinely in hospital. From our experience and from reports of other workers in this field it appears that the therapeutic results to be obtained are considerably better in patients in whom there has been little progression toward chronicity. Indeed there is good reason to believe that with our therapeutic resources at their present level of development, their applicability to the state hospital situation will be considerably curtailed if we do not succeed in detecting cases earlier and insuring their being brought promptly under treatment.

—D. Ewen Cameron, 1938[3]

In their review of the prodromal psychosis, Yung and McGorry[2] illustrated the path of events that can occur with patients experiencing prodromal symptoms of psychosis (**Fig. 1**). This path is a hypothetical course for patients, with the y-axis representing the severity of symptoms and the x-axis the time scale. The first arrow indicates the point when the patient first notices some change in him or herself. These changes are not yet noticeable to family and friends, however. These changes may be vague and nonspecific, but are not psychotic. The second arrow indicates when these nonpsychotic but notable symptoms are also observed by family and friends, who may pick up on mood or behavioral changes. The third arrow indicates when the patient first notices psychotic symptoms in him or herself, which are not yet noticeable to others. The fourth arrow indicates when family and friends first notice psychotic symptoms in the patient and the fifth arrow indicates the point of first psychiatric intervention.

The first attempts to improve clinical outcome focused on reducing the time between the fourth and fifth arrows, that is, to reduce the time that an individual experiences psychotic symptoms before receiving care. One meta-analysis looking at the relationship between duration of untreated psychosis (DUP) and outcome revealed

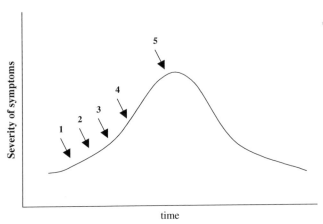

Arrow Points: 1 = patient fist notices some change in self, 2 = family or friends first notice some change in patient, 3 = patient first notices psychotic symptoms in self, 4 = family or friends first notice psychotic symptoms in patient, 5 = first psychiatric intervention.
From Yung and McGorry, 1996

Fig. 1. Development of psychosis over time, with arrows indicating points of change noted by the patient or informants. (*From* Yung AR, McGorry PD. The prodromal phase of first-episode psychosis: past and current conceptualizations. Schizophr Bull 1996;22(2):353–70; with permission.)

that shorter DUP was associated with greater response to antipsychotic treatment,[31] whereas another meta-analysis revealed that patients who had a longer DUP were more likely to have depression and anxiety at baseline and at 6- and 12-month follow-up and were more likely to experience more positive and negative symptoms and to have poorer overall functioning at 6- and 12-month follow-up.[32]

The Norwegian TIPS study looked at the initiation of an early detection (ED) program to reduce duration of untreated psychosis. Patients in this ED area were compared with those from a parallel area that did not have such an intervention and both areas were indistinguishable in sociodemographic and treatment service variables. The ED-area patients were detected earlier in their illness than the control group (5-week median duration of illness for the ED area, as compared with 16 weeks for control group).[33] At baseline, the patients from the ED area were in better clinical condition and had fewer negative symptoms and less risk for suicide.[34,35] Both groups received the same treatment, but the ED-area group demonstrated fewer negative symptoms at 1- and 2-year follow-up and improved mood and cognitive scores.[33,36]

Other early intervention studies were based on providing assertive, specialized care and comparing it to control groups who were assigned to standard care. The OPUS trial in Denmark involved 547 patients randomly assigned to either standard of care (at community mental health centers in large cities) or to an integrated treatment program. The latter involved an intense and assertive approach, including family involvement, social skills training, community involvement, and lower patient-to-clinician ratios. The intervention lasted 2 years and demonstrated improved clinical and functional outcomes for the integrated treatment group at 1- and 2-year follow-up.[37,38] A 5-year follow-up study revealed that the previously seen clinical effects were not maintained after the program had ended. They did find that the patients from the experimental group were living more independently, spending fewer days in the hospital, and using less supported housing, although these findings did not persist with further statistical analysis.[39]

Another study involving assertive treatment was the Lambeth Early Onset Team, based in England. This intervention compared residents in the Lambeth borough of London, who were randomly assigned to either an intensive outreach group with extended hours of service and specialized training in the management of early psychosis, or to standard of care, which was delivered by nonspecialized community mental health teams. At 18-month follow-up, the patients in the specialized care group were less likely to have hospital readmissions and less likely to drop out of care.[40]

Although such intensive programs may seem to be cost prohibitive, data from similar projects in Sweden and Australia have shown reduced costs for the patients in the intervention groups because of the focus on treatment in the community and subsequently reduced inpatient costs.[41,42]

These early intervention strategies, which are focused on initiating treatment with newly psychotic patients as quickly as possible to improve clinical outcome, are considered secondary prevention. To be considered primary prevention, the intervention should occur before the first presentation of psychosis, with hopes to prevent, delay, or reduce the onset of full illness. As we discussed previously, the prepsychotic symptoms are often nonspecific, so to improve efficacy of such interventions, groups have closed in on populations who had multiple risk factors and therefore were more likely to develop psychosis.[15] Researchers have been intervening with these UHR groups, while monitoring the conversions to full psychotic illness. Going back to the hypothetical symptom course in **Fig. 1**, these groups are attempting to improve overall outcome by addressing the left-hand side of the symptom curve; by giving more services to patients at the first or second arrow, they hope to reduce the height of the overall curve.

The first step in this process is accurate identification of the target population. The Structured Interview for Prodromal Syndromes (SIPS) is a structured diagnostic interview, somewhat analogous to the Structured Clinical Interview for DSM-IV (SCID), and is used to identify patients in the three UHR groups. The interview is made up of various components, including the Scale of Prodromal Symptoms (SOPS),[43–46] the Schizotypal Personality Disorder Checklist,[45] a family history questionnaire,[47] and a GAF scale.[48] The SIPS has established predictive validity, and groups can attain excellent interrater reliability after brief training.[49]

After identifying patients as UHR, groups like the PACE clinic offer various intensive services, including case management, supportive counseling, and antidepressant medication, if needed.[50] Intervening before presentation of illness raises concern of treatment being provided to false positives, meaning patients who would never have gone on to develop psychosis. Researchers have been mindful of this concern, only offering antipsychotic medications when the patient is clearly experiencing psychotic symptoms. Sensitivity is required when talking to the patients and families about their potential risk for psychosis, understanding the anxiety and stigma that such discussions can bring.

The rate of conversion from UHR to psychosis in these groups has ranged from 30% to 50%,[17,51–55] which is much greater than the rates of first-episode psychosis in the general population or the short-term rates of symptom development in individuals at high genetic risk (eg, siblings) in whom the lifetime risk is about 10%. This higher conversion rate indicates that the groups studied have been accurately identified as having increased vulnerability for psychosis. In some follow-up studies researchers have noted a reduction in the rate of conversion to psychosis over the years, which they acknowledge could be because of a dilution effect from enrolling patients who were false positives. The increased emphasis on early detection and attention to individuals who have nonspecific symptoms may be resulting in the selection of individuals who would never have gone on to develop psychosis. Instead of developing psychosis, these false-positive individuals could have resolution of symptoms or could go on to develop nonpsychotic disorders. The decreased conversion rate could also be attributable to patients becoming false false-positives, meaning that their trajectory was toward psychotic illness, but they were prevented from psychosis conversion by the interventions provided.[55] At this point, it is not possible to accurately distinguish between these possibilities.

TREATMENT/MANAGEMENT

The treatment goals in the UHR population are twofold: to treat the patient's current symptoms as the presenting disease and to improve immediate functioning, along with treating the current symptoms as risk markers for future disease. This process means monitoring the patient for worsening illness while using available interventions to minimize symptoms and improve patient's functioning. Groups working with the UHR population have attempted to engage patients in various psychosocial interventions using a recovery model of treatment. These interventions include case management; individual therapy, including psychoeducation and cognitive-behavioral therapy (CBT); multifamily support groups; and supported education and employment.

Studies have shown that CBT in UHR patients has resulted in decreased positive symptoms of psychosis[56] and reduced likelihood of being prescribed an antipsychotic.[57] There was evidence that those treated with CBT demonstrated decreased progression to psychosis compared with controls when baseline cognitive factors were controlled.[57]

Treatment trials with medications are limited. An open study with aripiprazole in UHR subjects demonstrated improvements in prodromal symptoms without significant adverse events.[58] A trial comparing needs-focused intervention (NFI) to NFI plus amisulpride revealed improved functioning with the combined group.[59] There is also evidence to suggest that treatment with antidepressants can improve the outcome in these patients.[8,60] A double-blind, placebo-controlled trial of olanzapine failed to show a significant effect of the drug. The low power of this study could have affected the outcome; the subjects in the placebo group had 2.5 times the rate of conversion to psychosis as the medication group.[61]

To improve the risk/benefit ratio for treatment, we must improve our ability to accurately identify individuals at high risk for developing psychosis. Cannon and colleagues[62] detected certain clinical factors that improved the positive predictive value in detecting individuals at risk for psychosis. The risk factors that predicted a high risk for conversion to psychosis included a genetic risk for schizophrenia with recent deterioration in functioning, higher levels of unusual thought content, higher levels of suspicion/paranoia, greater social impairment, and a history of substance abuse. Positive predictive power increased dramatically (68%–80%) when two to three of the variables were combined in prediction algorithms.

Prospective studies following UHR patients and controls have shown that the UHR patients who later became psychotic demonstrated declines in visual memory and attentional set-shifting before becoming psychotic.[63] Similarly, prospective MRI studies have shown a decrease in baseline thickness of anterior cingulate cortex (ACC) gray matter in UHR individuals who later become psychotic compared with UHR individuals who do not.[64,65] Fornito and colleagues[66] also demonstrated reduced ACC gray matter in UHR subjects who subsequently became psychotic as compared with healthy controls and UHR subjects who did not become psychotic. In this study, baseline ACC differences between the two high-risk groups predicted time to psychosis onset, with every 1-mm decrease in ACC thickness being associated with a 20% increase in risk for psychosis. Waltergang and colleagues[67] found that UHR subjects who later become psychotic had baseline thickening of the anterior genu of the callosum that was predictive of an individual's risk for conversion to psychosis. When baseline and repeat MRIs were done in UHR subjects, reductions in the gray matter volume of the hippocampus were seen after subjects developed psychosis.[64]

FUTURE DIRECTIONS

The limited data regarding treatment of UHR patients underscores the need for further research in this population and the importance of referring these patients to specialists. The Robert Wood Johnson Foundation launched a national program, the Early Detection and Intervention for the Prevention of Psychosis Program (EDIPPP), based on previous work done at the Portland Identification and Early Referral (PIER) program in Portland, Maine. This group, based at the Maine Medical Center, has used extensive community outreach and support to identify youth at risk for psychosis. The patients in the active treatment group were provided evidence-based psychosocial support and psychoeducation, and multifamily support group and medication treatment when needed. Patients at lower risk for psychosis were put into a comparison group that met with a case manager for monitoring, support, and referrals for additional treatment as needed but did not receive intensive services. The success of this program has been seen in the lower-than-expected rate of psychosis in the intensive services group at 1-year follow-up. Fourteen percent of the at-risk patients who enrolled in PIER experienced a full psychotic episode, which is lower than expected based on the conversion rates mentioned earlier (personal communication).

In hopes of replicating these findings, the Robert Wood Johnson Foundation has funded four other sites across the country to develop similar models: The Mid-Valley Behavioral Care Network in Salem, Oregon; the Washtenaw Community Health Organization in Ypsilanti, Michigan; the University of California, Davis in Sacramento, California; and the Zucker Hillside Hospital in Glen Oaks, New York. In addition to the clinical interventions mentioned earlier, the at-risk youth will be monitored from a neuropsychiatric perspective to search for potential biological markers of psychotic illness. Participation in research of this kind is crucial in improving our treatment of psychotic illness and preventing the typically devastating course that these patients often experience.

Research in this UHR population presents an avenue of hope for patients and families struggling to cope with the debilitating effects of schizophrenia. As clinicians, we must be vigilant for individuals who present with the aforementioned risk factors and then carefully screen for unusual thought content, suspiciousness, grandiosity, perceptual disturbances, or disorganized communication. By referring these patients to specialty clinics that provide increased support and services, there is the potential that we can change the trajectory of their illness. Further research and funding is required to increase availability of such services and to reduce the time it takes patients to access care once ill. It is anticipated that this shift toward early intervention and prevention of illness will change the nature of psychiatric treatment in individuals who have psychotic illness and improve functional outcomes and quality of life for affected individuals.

REFERENCES

1. Meares A. The diagnosis of prepsychotic schizophrenia. Lancet 1959;1:55–8.
2. Yung AR, McGorry PD. The prodromal phase of first-episode psychosis: past and current conceptualizations. Schizophr Bull 1996;22(2):353–70.
3. Cameron ED. Early schizophrenia. Am J Psychiatry 1938;95:567–78.
4. Varsamis J, Adamson JD. Early schizophrenia. Can Psychiatr Assoc J 1971;16: 487–97.
5. Conrad K, editor. Die beginnende schizophrenie. Stuttgart, Germany: Georg Thieme Verlag; 1958.
6. Beiser M, Erickson D, Fleming JAE, et al. Establishing the onset of psychotic illness. Am J Psychiatry 1993;150:1349–54.
7. Cornblatt BA, Lencz T, Obuchowski M, et al. The schizophrenia prodrome: treatment and high-risk perspectives. Schizophr Res 2002;54:177–86.
8. Cornblatt BA, Lencz T, Smith CW, et al. The schizophrenia prodrome revisited: a neurodevelopmental perspective. Schizophr Bull 2003;29:633–51.
9. Phillips LJ, Yung AR, Yuen HP, et al. Prediction and prevention of transition to psychosis in young people at incipient risk for schizophrenia. Am J Med Genet 2002; 114:929–37.
10. McGorry PD, Singh BS. Schizophrenia: risk and possibility. In: Raphael B, Burrows GD, editors. Handbook of studies on preventive psychiatry. Amsterdam: Elsevier; 1995. p. 491–514.
11. Gross G. The onset of schizophrenia. Schizophr Res 1997;28:187–98.
12. Koehler K, Sauer H. Huber's basic symptoms: another approach to negative psychopathology in schizophrenia. Compr Psychiatry 1984;25(2):174–82.

13. Klosterkotter J, Ebel H, Schultze-Lutter F, et al. Diagnostic validity of basic symptoms. Eur Arch Psychiatry Clin Neurosci 1996;246:147–54.
14. Klosterkotter J, Hellmich M, Steinmeyer EM, et al. Diagnosing schizophrenia in the initial prodromal phase. Arch Gen Psychiatry 2001;58:158–64.
15. Bell RQ. Multiple-risk cohorts and segmenting risk as solutions to the problem of false positives in risk for the major psychoses. Psychiatry 1992;55:370–81.
16. Sullivan HS. The onset of schizophrenia. Am J Psychiatry 1927;6:105–34.
17. Yung AR, Phillips LJ, Yuen HP, et al. Psychosis prediction: 12-month follow up of a high-risk ("prodromal") group. Schizophr Res 2003;60:21–32.
18. Meyer SK, Bearden CE, Lux SR, et al. The psychosis prodrome in adolescent patients viewed through the lens of DSM-IV. J Child Adolesc Psychopharmacol 2005;15(3):434–51.
19. Svirskis T, Korkeila J, Heinimaa M, et al. Axis-I disorders and vulnerability to psychosis. Schizophr Res 2005;75:439–46.
20. Yung AR, Buckby JA, Cosgrave EM, et al. Association between psychotic experiences and depression in a clinical sample over 6 months. Schizophr Res 2007; 91:246–53.
21. Andreasson S, Allebeck P, Engstrom A, et al. Cannabis and schizophrenia. A longitudinal study of Swedish conscripts. Lancet 1987;2:1483–6.
22. Zammit S, ALlebeck P, Andreasson S, et al. Self reported cannabis use as a risk factor for schizophrenia in Swedish conscripts of 1969: historical cohort study. Br Med J 2002;325:1199–203.
23. Arseneault L, Cannon M, Poulton R, et al. Cannabis use in adolescence and risk for adult psychosis: longitudinal prospective study. Br Med J 2002;325: 1212–3.
24. Van Os J, Bak M, Hanssen M, et al. Cannabis use and psychosis: a longitudinal population-based study. Am J Epidemiol 2002;156:319–27.
25. Fergusson DM, Horwood JL, Swain-Campbell NR. Cannabis dependence and psychotic symptoms in young people. Psychol Med 2003;33:15–21.
26. Henquet C, Krabbendam L, Spauwen J, et al. Prospective cohort study of cannabis use, predisposition for psychosis, and psychotic symptoms in young people. BMJ 2005;330:11–6.
27. Moore THM, Zammit S, Lingford-Hughes A, et al. Cannabis use and risk of psychotic or affective mental health outcomes: a systematic review. Lancet 2007; 370:319–28.
28. Veen ND, Selten JP, Van der Tweel I, et al. Cannabis use and age at onset of schizophrenia. Am J Psychiatry 2004;161:501–6.
29. Meyer-Lindenberg A, Nichols T, Callicott JH, et al. Impact of complex genetic variation in COMT on human brain function. Mol Psychiatry 2006;11:867–77.
30. Caspi A, Moffitt TE, Cannon M, et al. Moderation of the effect of adolescent-onset cannabis use on adult psychosis by a functional polymorphism in the catechol-O-methyltransferase gene: longitudinal evidence of a gene x environment interaction. Biol Psychiatry 2005;57:1117–27.
31. Perkins DO, Gu H, Boteva K, et al. Relationship between duration of untreated psychosis and outcome in first-episode schizophrenia: a critical review and meta-analysis. Am J Psychiatry 2005;162(10):1785–804.
32. Marshall M, Lewis S, Lockwood A, et al. Association between duration of untreated psychosis and outcome in cohorts of first-episode patients. Arch Gen Psychiatry 2005;62:975–83.
33. Larsen TK, Melle I, Auestad B, et al. Early detection of first-episode psychosis: the effect on 1-year outcome. Schizophr Bull 2006;32(4):758–64.

34. Melle I, Larsen TK, Haahr U, et al. Reducing the duration of untreated first-episode psychosis: effects on clinical presentation. Arch Gen Psychiatry 2004;61: 143–50.
35. Melle I, Johannesen JO, Friis S, et al. Early detection of the first episode of schizophrenia and suicidal behavior. Am J Psychiatry 2006;163(5):800–4.
36. Melle I, Larsen TK, Haahr U, et al. Prevention of negative symptom psychopathologies in first-episode schizophrenia. Arch Gen Psychiatry 2008;65(6):634–40.
37. Thorup A, Petersen L, Jeppesen P, et al. Integrated treatment ameliorates negative symptoms in first episode psychosis—results from the Danish OPUS trial. Schizophr Res 2005;79:95–105.
38. Petersen L, Nordentoft M, Jeppesen P, et al. Improving 1-year outcome in first-episode psychosis. Br J Psychiatry 2005;187(48):s98–103.
39. Bertelsen M, Jeppesen P, Petersen L, et al. Five-year follow-up of a randomized multicenter trial of intensive early intervention vs standard treatment for patients with a first episode of psychotic illness. Arch Gen Psychiatry 2008;65(7):762–71.
40. Craig TKJ, Garety P, Power P, et al. The Lambeth early onset (LEO) team: randomized controlled trial of the effectiveness of specialized care for early psychosis. Br Med J 2004;329(7474):1067.
41. Mihalopoulos C, McGorry PD, Carter RC. Is phase-specific, community-oriented treatment of early psychosis an economically viable method of improving outcome? Acta Psychiatr Scand 1999;100(1):47–55.
42. Culberg J, Mattsson M, Levander S, et al. Treatment costs and clinical outcome for first episode schizophrenia patients: a 3-year follow-up of the Swedish "parachute project" and two comparison groups. Acta Psychiatr Scand 2006;114(4): 274–81.
43. Miller TJ, McGlashan TH, Woods SW, et al. Symptom assessment in schizophrenic prodromal states. Psychiatr Q 1999;70:273–87.
44. McGlashan TH, Miller TJ, Woods SW, et al. A scale for the assessment of prodromal symptoms and states. In: Miller TJ, Mednick SA, McGlashan TH, et al, editors. Early intervention in psychotic disorders. Dordrecht, The Netherlands: Kluwer Academic Publishers; 2001. p. 135–49.
45. Hawkins KA, Quinlan D, Miller TJ, et al. Factorial structure of the scale of prodromal symptoms. Schizophr Res 2004;68(2–3):339–47.
46. American Psychiatric Association. DSM-IV: diagnostic and statistical manual of mental disorders. 4th edition. Washington, DC: APA; 1994.
47. Andreasen NC, Endicott J, Spitzer RL, et al. The family history method using diagnostic criteria: reliability and validity. Arch Gen Psychiatry 1977;34:1229–35.
48. Hall R. Global assessment of functioning: a modified scale. Psychosomatics 1995;36:267–75.
49. Miller TJ, McGlashan TH, Rosen JL, et al. Prodromal assessment with the structured interview for prodromal syndromes and the scale of prodromal symptoms: predictive validity, interrater reliability, and training to reliability. Schizophr Bull 2003;29(4):703–15.
50. Yung AR, McGorry PD, Francey SM, et al. PACE: a specialized service for young people at risk of psychotic disorders. Med J Aust 2007;187(7):s43–6.
51. Yung AR, Phillips LJ, Yuen HP, et al. Risk factors for psychosis in an ultra high-risk group: psychopathology and clinical features. Schizophr Res 2004;67:131–42.
52. Miller TJ, McGlashan TH, Rosen JL, et al. Prospective diagnosis of the initial prodrome for schizophrenia based on the structured interview for prodromal syndromes: preliminary evidence of interrater reliability and predictive validity. Am J Psychiatry 2002;159:863–5.

53. Mason O, Startup M, Halpin S, et al. State and trait predictors of transition to first episode psychosis among individuals with at risk mental states. Schizophr Res 2004;71:227–37.

54. Larsen TK. The transition from premorbid period to psychosis: how can it be described? Acta Psychiatr Scand 2002;106:s10–1.

55. Yung AR, Yuen HP, Berger G, et al. Declining transition rate in ultra high risk (prodromal) services: dilution or reduction of risk. Schizophr Bull 2007;33(3):673–81.

56. French P, Shryane N, Bentall RP, et al. Effects of cognitive therapy on the longitudinal development of psychotic experiences in people at high risk of developing psychosis. Br J Psychiatry 2007;191:s82–7.

57. Morrison AP, French P, Parker S, et al. Three-year follow-up of a randomized controlled trial of cognitive therapy for the prevention of psychosis in people at ultra-high risk. Schizophr Bull 2007;33(3):682–7.

58. Woods SW, Tully EM, Walsh BC, et al. Aripiprazole in the treatment of the psychosis prodrome. Br J Psychiatry 2007;191:s96–101.

59. Ruhrmann S, Bechdolf A, Kuhn K-U, et al. Acute effects of treatment for prodromal symptoms for people putatively in a late initial prodromal state of psychosis. Br J Psychiatry 2007;191:s88–95.

60. Cornblatt BA, Lencz T, Smith CW, et al. Can antidepressants be used to treat the schizophrenia prodrome? Results of a prospective, naturalistic treatment study of adolescents. J Clin Psychiatry 2007;68:546–57.

61. McGlashan TH, Zipursky RB, Perkins D, et al. Randomized, double-blind trial of olanzapine versus placebo in patients prodromally symptomatic for psychosis. Am J Psychiatry 2006;163:790–9.

62. Cannon TD, Cadenhead K, Cornblatt B, et al. Prediction of psychosis in youth at high clinical risk. Arch Gen Psychiatry 2008;65(1):28–37.

63. Wood SJ, Brewer WJ, Koutsouradis P, et al. Cognitive decline following psychosis onset. Br J Psychiatry 2007;191:s52–7.

64. Pantelis C, Velakoulis D, McGorry PD, et al. Neuroanatomical abnormalities before and after onset of psychosis: a cross-sectional and longitudinal MRI comparison. Lancet 2003;361:281–8.

65. Borgwardt SJ, Riecher-Rossler A, Dazzan P, et al. Regional gray matter volume abnormalities in the at risk mental state. Biol Psychiatry 2007;61:1148–56.

66. Fornito A, Yung AR, Wood SJ, et al. Anatomic abnormalities of the anterior cingulate cortex before psychosis onset: an MRI study of ultra-high-risk individuals. Biol Psychiatry 2008;64(9):758–65.

67. Waterfang M, Yung AR, Wood AG, et al. Corpus callosum shape alterations in individuals prior to the onset of psychosis. Schizophr Res 2008;103(1–3):1–10.

Cognitive-Behavioral Therapy and Dialectical Behavior Therapy; Adaptations Required to Treat Adolescents

Laurence Y. Katz, MD[a],*, Sarah A. Fotti, MD[a], Lara Postl, MD[b]

KEYWORDS

- Cognitive-behavioral therapy • Dialectical behavior therapy
- Adolescents • Anxiety • Depression

Psychotherapy with children and adolescents presents a set of challenges for the therapist that is qualitatively different from the challenges of psychotherapy with adults. Children and adolescents are not "little adults" and thus require a developmental approach to psychotherapy and modification of the treatment. Cognitive behavioral therapy (CBT) and dialectical behavior therapy (DBT) are two types of psychotherapy used in the treatment of children and adolescents. CBT is a psychotherapeutic model that posits that individuals with, for example mood and anxiety disorders, have cognitive distortions and behavioral deficits that can be targeted for change in therapy resulting in improvements in emotional, cognitive, and behavioral functioning.[1] DBT is a principle-based psychotherapy developed by Linehan that blends standard cognitive-behavioral therapy with Eastern philosophy and meditation practices and shares elements with psychodynamic, client-centered, gestalt, paradoxical, and strategic approaches.[2] However, DBT is not used with children and CBT with children is a subspecialty practice, so this article will focus on the developmental approach to the use of these treatments with adolescents as may be applicable to the practice of a general psychiatrist. Manuals and texts describing the details of these treatments are available elsewhere (eg, Roblek and Piacentini,[3] Lewinsohn and colleagues,[4] Brent and colleagues,[5] Rohde and colleagues,[6] and Wood and colleagues).[7] Thus, this chapter will provide a brief review of the research on the use of these treatments but primarily will focus on the clinical differences between conducting these treatments with

[a] Department of Psychiatry, PsycHealth Centre, PZ-162 771 Bannatyne Avenue, University of Manitoba, Winnipeg, MB R3E 3N4, Canada
[b] Faculty of Medicine, PsycHealth Centre, PZ-162 771 Bannatyne Avenue, University of Manitoba, Winnipeg, MB R3E 3N4, Canada
* Corresponding author.
E-mail address: lkatz@hsc.mb.ca (L.Y. Katz).

Psychiatr Clin N Am 32 (2009) 95–109
doi:10.1016/j.psc.2008.10.005
0193-953X/08/$ – see front matter © 2009 Elsevier Inc. All rights reserved.

adolescents as compared with adults. Anxiety disorders and depressive disorders are the most common indications for these treatments and thus will be the focus of the discussion of CBT. DBT as used with suicidal adolescents is also described. Finally, a brief review of controlled studies in children and adolescents with other diagnoses is provided.

RESEARCH ON COGNITIVE BEHAVIORAL THERAPY AND ANXIETY IN ADOLESCENCE

Anxiety disorders are among the most common psychiatric disorders in children and adolescents.[8] However, the evidence base for treatment of anxiety in youths is relatively limited.[9] Initial studies of CBT for anxiety showed positive results.[10,11] More recently there have been several randomized controlled trials (RCTs) that have examined CBT in various formats including individual child,[10,12] family focused,[11,13] and group.[14] A number of these studies have demonstrated a significant effect of CBT compared with controls and alternate treatments.[15]

Recent systematic reviews of CBT for the treatment of anxiety disorders in youth appear to demonstrate benefit of CBT in comparison with waiting list or no-treatment controls. Cartwright and colleagues[16] performed a meta-analysis of several studies that compared CBT with waiting list and found there to be a significant remission rate of diagnosed anxiety disorders in the CBT group compared with control. In addition, a more recent meta-analysis by James and colleagues[9] found similar results showing that just over half of subjects respond to CBT compared with a natural response rate of one third.

Although CBT for anxiety disorders appears to be effective when compared with wait list and attention controls, two trials that compared CBT with educational support found no greater benefit to CBT.[17,18] Muris and colleagues[19] compared CBT with emotional disclosure and no treatment controls and found CBT to be superior to emotional disclosure; however, neither was significantly more effective than no treatment.

In a comparison of CBT literature, CBT for symptoms of anxiety appears to yield greater effect sizes than those for depression across studies. Chu and Harrison[15] conducted a comprehensive review of RCTs that tested CBT for anxiety and depression. Their findings suggest that CBT for anxious youth consistently yields moderate to large effects across variables in comparison with CBT for depression, which showed consistent but small effects. CBT appeared to produce comparatively greater behavioral and coping changes in anxiety samples, which supports the possibility that different processes may mediate CBT for anxious and depressed youth.

The CBT and anxiety literature for children and adolescents has generally considered anxiety disorders such as social anxiety disorder, generalized anxiety disorder, and overanxious disorder as a single group.[9] However, there have been several studies that have examined other anxiety disorders such as posttraumatic stress disorder (PTSD) and obsessive compulsive disorder (OCD) specifically. To date, there are no rigorous RCTs in children and adolescents with either phobias or panic disorder.

Although CBT is a well-documented intervention for adults with OCD, its effectiveness has not been extensively studied in youth populations. A recent comprehensive RCT[20] by the Pediatric OCD Treatment Study Team (POTS) comparing CBT and sertraline found the combination of treatments to be slightly more effective than CBT alone. Sertraline alone was proven to be significantly superior to placebo; however, the effect size of CBT alone was larger than sertraline alone. This led the authors to the conclusion that children and adolescents with OCD should begin treatment with CBT alone or with CBT plus a selective serotonin reuptake inhibitor (SSRI). Further RCTs and reviews have found similar results suggesting that CBT appears to be a promising treatment for OCD in children and adolescents.[21,22] Similarly, studies examining abuse-related PTSD in children and adolescents found trauma-focused CBT to be effective in not only reducing PTSD-related symptoms but also in reducing parallel depression and abuse-related shame when compared with child-centered therapy.[23,24]

In general the reviewed studies have shown benefit for CBT in the treatment of anxiety disorders; however, there have been several methodological shortfalls identified. The most significant of which appears to be difficulties in the process of randomization as well as limited active control comparison groups. In addition, study samples generally included children and adolescents with mild to moderate symptoms of anxiety mostly recruited from community and outpatient populations and did not include severe cases. Therefore, additional studies would be useful to further clarify the efficacy and effectiveness of CBT in treating child and adolescent anxiety disorders.

IMPLEMENTATION OF COGNITIVE BEHAVIORAL THERAPY FOR ANXIETY DISORDERS IN ADOLESCENTS

Anxiety disorders are associated with significant impairment in peer relationships, and family and school functioning. There is also an association with suicidal behaviors and comorbid psychiatric disorders such as depression and substance abuse.[9,16] CBT for adolescents is an empirically supported treatment, as described earlier. In this discussion, differences between CBT for adults and adolescents with anxiety disorders will be highlighted.

Before describing specific techniques, a composite case example of an adolescent with generalized anxiety disorder will be presented. This is the most common anxiety disorder in adolescents, affecting between 3% and 5%.[25]

The patient is a 16-year-old female who lives with her parents and younger brother. She is in grade 10. She has a longstanding history of anxiety. She has many worries ranging from the safety of her parents to her school performance. She has always been an A student but continues to worry that she will fail. She is unable to control the worry, has difficulty concentrating, and difficulty falling asleep. She also describes feeling "on edge" a lot of the time. She often misses school because she is too worried about making mistakes in class and has been unable to get a part-time job because of her worry that she will not be successful. She currently has no symptoms of depression and no other anxiety disorder symptoms. Her parents are very supportive but are becoming frustrated and don't know how to help her.

CBT for adolescents with anxiety can be conducted individually or in groups. The most commonly used treatment manual was developed by Kendall and is called the "Coping Cat Program."[3] This program typically involves 16 to 20 sessions, which begin with skills training followed by exposure exercises. An acronym used in this program is FEAR (Feeling frightened, Expecting bad things to happen, Actions/attitudes that will help, Review and reward). The adolescent is taught to recognize anxious feelings and bodily sensations, identify and challenge cognitive distortions, develop a coping plan, and, finally, evaluate coping responses and reward themselves appropriately.

There are some important developmental differences that may influence the manner in which CBT is performed in teenagers.[3] First, their ability to recognize and process emotions is still developing, along with their ability to think in an abstract way. Using role-playing, stories and metaphors may be helpful in demonstrating some of the abstract CBT concepts given these developmental limitations. Adolescents also tend to be focused on the present and may have a difficult time envisioning how working on current difficulties will improve their future, especially when doing challenging exposure exercises. In the context of these considerations there are three distinct aspects of using CBT with adolescents that will be discussed in more detail: alliance, role of parents, and homework/compliance.

Creating an alliance with adolescents is a different endeavor than with adults for a few reasons. First, adolescents are not usually the ones to initiate treatment. Parents or other outside influences are usually the initiators of treatment. Adolescents are also at a stage in their development in which they are struggling with autonomy and individuation. This may makes it challenging to connect with an adult therapist, who may be seen as another authority figure in their lives. Thus, collaboration in therapy is emphasized (consistent with the collaborative empiricism inherent in CBT) in addition to highlighting confidentiality to improve the likelihood of creating a successful alliance. Furthermore, it has been found that active participation by the teen and using his or her suggestions in session has been associated with positive treatment outcomes.[26] Being too forceful in pushing a teen to talk about anxiety when he or she is not ready to has been shown to negatively affect the treatment alliance.[26]

Parents/caregivers have an influential role in the lives of most teens; therefore, they also have an important role in CBT. The literature is mixed with regard to outcome studies involving parents because it depends on the item of interest being measured.[13,27] Given that genetics and environmental modeling of anxiety have been well studied, involving parents may be valuable. They may help with the learning of coping skills, be "coaches" in exposure exercises, and help develop a behavioral rewards system to motivate the teen to work on anxiety and to remove any reinforcement of the teen's anxious behavior. In addition, parents may be valuable co-therapists who continue facilitating treatment gains when CBT is terminated.[13,27]

Homework is a key component of CBT. It is well known that teens do not generally love homework, so it is challenging to design homework assignments that they will think worth their while. CBT homework creates opportunities to practice skills to build mastery and enhance capabilities. It also allows the therapist to assess whether the teen understands the material, as most will be reluctant to confess if they are having trouble. To increase the likelihood that homework is completed, it is vital to begin with easily achievable assignments that have successful outcomes. In addition, having a reward system that is meaningful to the teen is imperative.[28] The first step in dealing with noncompliance is to determine the reason, which may range from forgetting and avoidance, to the assignment being too difficult. The next step is to work on the homework together in session and strategize various ways for the homework to get done. It is important to keep in mind that although completing homework is essential, the teen should not be made to feel guilty or inadequate as the probability of homework being completed will drastically decrease.

To highlight some of the above principles, the following is a brief excerpt from the treatment of the previously described 16-year-old female with generalized anxiety disorder and school refusal:

T (Therapist): So, I hear that it was difficult to get to school this week.

P (Patient): Yeah, I was too tired and I wasn't feeling well so I didn't go, I read a book and watched TV instead.

C (Caregivers/parents): She gets really anxious and says she is too sick to go to school and then she seems fine at home after that. We know that school is important and try to get her to go, but the more we push she gets mad so we let her stay home. It is very frustrating because she seems fine the rest of the day and even goes out with friends sometimes when she misses school.

T: What do you worry will happen if you go to school?

P: I always feel sick and anxious at school and feel better when I stay at home. I also worry that something bad might happen to my parents if I go to school.

T: As we have talked about in previous sessions, we know that when you miss school your "annoying anxiety" is acting up again. We also know that one of the best ways to beat it is to go to school anyways. This way you will show the anxiety that you are in charge and it will back off as you start attending school regularly. When you are at school you can use some of the relaxation we have talked about and also your anxiety coping thoughts. What do you think about that?

P: I don't know, it sounds really hard. It has worked before, but I think my "annoying anxiety" is getting worse.

T: What do you think about getting your parents involved as coaches again? Their job will be to make sure you go to school no matter what and coach you to use the skills you already know. I would like you to write them down again today to take home with you.

P: I guess I can try that, but I would like to work toward doing it by myself, without my parents' help.

This brief dialog from a CBT session illustrates externalizing the anxiety by giving it another name and involving the parents in therapy.

The above principles can be applied to generalized anxiety disorder, social anxiety disorder, and, to some extent, specific phobia. In working with teens with panic disorder many of the same techniques may be used. However, one important caveat is that there are usually more somatic symptoms in panic disorder with adolescents.[3] These may take the form of the classic cardiopulmonary symptoms, gastrointestinal symptoms, or neuromuscular symptoms such as trembling, numbness, and tingling. Therefore, it is essential to target these symptoms in CBT by doing relaxation exercises, cognitive restructuring, panic induction, and exposure therapy.[29]

Using CBT in the treatment of OCD and PTSD is more specialized than treating the above-mentioned disorders. There are a lot of similarities in treating adults and teens, including the importance of exposure with response prevention, but some of the developmental considerations mentioned earlier will come into play. Specifically, with OCD it is vital to recognize, re-label, and externalize intrusive thoughts as OCD, and develop strategies to cope with anxiety other than with compulsive behaviors. It is helpful to come up with a separate name for the OCD so that the teen can develop skills to conquer or manage the disorder so that it is not experienced as a part of the teen's identity.[22,30] CBT for PTSD in adolescents is similar to adults, with a few adaptations. It is important to take into account parental reactions and their coping strategies. Modifying both the adolescents' and parents' unhelpful trauma-related appraisals is vital.[31] With younger teens, using projective drawing and telling stories that reference the trauma may provide an opportunity to begin talking about the trauma.[32]

RESEARCH ON COGNITIVE BEHAVIORAL THERAPY AND DEPRESSION IN ADOLESCENCE

CBT is the most studied nonpharmacologic intervention for the treatment of depression in youth.[1] Initial meta-analyses conducted throughout the late 1990s may have overestimated the effect sizes for CBT on measures of depression,[1] as recent meta-analyses have shown more modest effects. However, CBT for youth depression continues to be a promising intervention and appropriate treatment choice.

Initial studies found that CBT reliably outperformed wait list control and attention placebo conditions[33] and early meta-analyses found CBT outcomes to yield medium to large effect sizes.[34] In addition, Brent and colleagues[5] compared CBT to family therapy and a supportive therapy control and found that significantly more adolescents who received CBT than supportive therapy no longer met criteria for major depression. Their data favored CBT over family and supportive therapy in reducing remission rates. Similarly, Wood and colleagues[7] found a brief CBT program to be superior to relaxation therapy alone, across multiple indices. Meta-analyses that pooled findings across early clinical trials documented consistent significant effect sizes for CBT.[33–35]

More recent investigations have brought into question the relative strength of CBT for the treatment of youth depression. The success of antidepressant medications in comparative clinical trials as well as the decreased effect sizes found in recent meta-analyses suggests that treatment effects may be more modest in clinical settings than previously thought. The publication of the Treatment for Adolescent Depression study (TADS) in 2004[36] showed outcomes for CBT that were less encouraging. However, there was evidence that CBT may be beneficial in buffering youth against negative life stressors and suicidal thinking.[1] This led to the recommendation that the combination of fluoxetine and CBT for adolescent depression is the best treatment option and that CBT should be readily available as part of a comprehensive treatment strategy.[36] In contrast to the TADS study, a randomized controlled trial done by Goodyer and colleagues[37] looked at the effects of fluoxetine treatment alone and in combination with CBT in a population of moderately to severely depressed adolescents receiving routine clinical care and found that there was no evidence to support the combination treatment over fluoxetine alone. In addition, Weisz and colleagues[38] recently published the most comprehensive meta-analysis for CBT and depression in youth to date and found that the overall effects of psychotherapy treatment including CBT do not surpass and may actually lag significantly behind treatments for other youth conditions.

Differences in methodological characteristics have likely contributed to the discrepancies in efficacy seen between earlier and more recent studies of CBT for adolescent depression.[39] Adolescents who appear to have had more severe illness and more significant comorbidities that may in part account for the differences seen in effects characterized samples used in recent investigations of CBT. Finally, differences in design factors may have contributed to the conflicting results seen in the literature. CBT generally performs well when compared with the passage of time or attention conditions, however when compared with alternate treatments or active controls the effects are not as significant.[1]

Although CBT for the treatment of adolescent depression appears to have a more modest effect in the valid treatment population than initially thought, the effect has been shown to be significantly greater than zero across studies. All things considered, the results indicate that CBT for youth depression is a reasonable treatment option and should be available as part of a comprehensive treatment plan for depressed adolescents.

IMPLEMENTATION OF COGNITIVE BEHAVIORAL THERAPY FOR DEPRESSIVE DISORDERS IN ADOLESCENTS

As has been previously described, there are significant differences in the application of CBT for adolescents as compared with adults. The developmental considerations and the strategies for modifying the treatment approach described above for the use of CBT with anxiety disorders largely apply to the use of CBT with depression. Detailed reviews of the various CBT models available for adolescents with depression are available elsewhere (eg, Weersing and Brent[1] and Rohde and colleagues).[6] This discussion will focus on the differences in conducting CBT with adolescents as opposed to adults, considering the factors relevant to depression that were not discussed in the section on anxiety disorders.

As described by Weersing and Brent[1] a review of the research on CBT for adolescents finds that there are four commonly studied models. The coping with depression for adolescents model (CWD-A) is the most studied,[4] whereas the Pittsburgh cognitive therapy model,[5] the brief cognitive therapy model used in the United Kingdom,[7,40,41] and the TADS model[6] are also commonly found in the literature. CWD-A is a group therapy course that includes psychoeducation, pleasant activity scheduling, social skills training, and cognitive restructuring. In the Pittsburgh cognitive therapy model, the treatment was individual therapy driven by cognitive case conceptualization, with no preset exercises or homework and the content focused largely on cognitive restructuring, behavioral activation, and problem-solving skills. In the TADS model, the treatment was individual therapy with both required and optional family sessions. It blended elements of CWD-A, the Pittsburgh cognitive therapy manual, and the investigators' own expertise. Finally, in the brief cognitive therapy model, common CBT techniques were used but the interventions were low dose.[1] All of these models are based on fundamental CBT principles found in CBT models for adults. However, what is common to all of these models for adolescents is consideration of the developmental factors described above in the discussion of CBT for anxiety disorders. Consideration of these factors leads to modifications of the application of CBT appropriate to the stage of development of the patient. A case description will be provided and then discussion of some of the necessary modifications and strategies will follow.

The patient is a 15-year-old female who lives with her biological parents and siblings. She attends high school but has had significant problems over the past few months with her grades dropping substantially. Her major concern is that she notices that she is incredibly irritable. She has had longstanding squabbles with her parents but now cannot tolerate them at all and is constantly arguing with them. Of particular concern to her is that she now finds that she cannot be around her friends either as they are now "annoying." Thus, she withdraws to her room and isolates herself from others. She spends a lot of time crying and lonely. These symptoms have been steadily worsening over the past few months. She has had thoughts of suicide but has never attempted and states she would not do that. She has also cut herself on two occasions when particularly distressed but is not currently planning on harming herself. She has experimented with alcohol and marijuana but does not use regularly. She has longstanding sleep problems that have worsened during this episode. She eats erratically and notices that she often does not eat partly out of lack of appetite and partly out of some concern about her weight. She is of normal body weight.

This composite case description highlights common symptomatology of depressed adolescents. It also illustrates one of the biggest challenges in conducting CBT with adolescents. As described in DSM-IV,[42] irritability is a common symptom of depression in adolescents. Establishing an alliance with an irritable, emotionally dysregulated adolescent is a challenge that may impact the outcome of therapy.[43] It often requires that the therapist have a "thick skin" and be able to tolerate not only intense emotion in the room but often hostility. Irritable depressed teenagers will often devalue therapy and the therapist in moments of distress. The ability of the therapist to tolerate the distress and assist the adolescent in re-regulating himself or herself can profoundly enhance the alliance. Working with depressed adolescents requires this tolerance.

A nonjudgmental stance is another key factor in developing rapport with adolescents. Depressed adolescents often experience their environment and in particular adults as judgmental. A therapist who adopts a nonjudgmental, accurately empathic, genuine, and tolerant stance will be able to establish a working alliance with a diverse range of adolescents and their families.[6]

In the CBT models described above there are modifications for use with adolescents. However, working with a 13-year-old and working with a 17-year-old can be quite different. Furthermore, chronological age does not determine capability and thus the developmental capacity of each adolescent must be determined in an ongoing manner. Many of the models described above use techniques to enhance learning and engagement in the therapy. For example, the use of cartoon strips to assist in the identification of negative cognitions.[44] However, the use of such a technique must be appropriately developmentally targeted, as some late adolescents will find such a technique irritating and in fact damaging to the alliance. In addition, each CBT model puts varying degrees of emphasis on cognitive versus behavioral components of the treatment. In adolescents, assessment of the capacity of the adolescent to use cognitive constructs given their still-developing cognitive and abstraction capabilities is critical. Some adolescents will require greater emphasis on the behavioral strategies because of an inability to use the cognitive procedures.

Like CBT for anxiety disorders, CBT for depression models also recognize the role of family in the life of the adolescent. Most models either directly include or allow for family involvement in the treatment. Unfortunately, in studies conducted thus far, including families in the treatment has not been shown to add to the treatment gains that occur with CBT alone.[4,45]

As described above, CBT is often used in conjunction with antidepressant medication as part of a comprehensive treatment plan for a moderately to severely depressed adolescent. In the composite case described above, the initial sessions would be focused on building a therapeutic alliance around the comprehensive treatment plan.

Therapist (T): Based on what you've been telling me, depression seems to be really interfering in your life.

Patient (P): Well duh!

T: You've described a bunch of really difficult things happening that make it understandable that you would feel this way but I also wonder if sometimes your thoughts and what you do also cause you troubles. What do you think?

P: What do you mean?

T: Well sometimes something happens that upsets us and then when I'm upset I start to think in ways that make me more upset and then sometimes I do things that make the situation worse.

P: Oh yeah, when I get pissed off with my friends its like everything they do annoys me and then I start to get so annoyed with them I think about all the stuff they're doing to piss me off and then I start yelling at them and it just gets worse and worse.

T: Exactly, so what we are talking about is using medication to try and help with how you feel but then also working to see if thoughts are affecting how you feel and also looking at whether what you are doing is impacting on how you feel. Then we would help you to learn new ways of thinking that do not intensify your feelings and help you to act in ways that improve your mood. Hopefully the combination of all these things will get you relief from how you've been feeling.

P: All right, I'll give it a try but I doubt that it is going to work.

T: That would be one of those thoughts that I was talking about.

RESEARCH ON DIALECTICAL BEHAVIOR THERAPY WITH SUICIDAL ADOLESCENTS

Dialectical behavior therapy (DBT) is an empirically supported treatment[46,47] developed by Linehan[48] for adult women with borderline personality disorder who have chronic suicidal and nonsuicidal self-injurious behavior. To date, there are no published RCTs of dialectical behavior therapy for adolescents. However, there are two promising controlled studies of DBT modified for suicidal adolescents that have been published.[49,50] In the Rathus and Miller study,[49] 111 adolescent outpatients referred to an adolescent depression and suicide program received either 12 weeks of DBT or treatment as usual. It is not a randomized trial and adolescents with more severe symptomatology were referred for DBT. DBT was shown to reduce inpatient psychiatric days and treatment dropouts as compared with treatment as usual. Notably, there were no suicide attempts in the DBT group during the study. In the Katz and colleagues[50] study, 62 adolescent inpatients received 2 weeks of either DBT or treatment as usual. DBT as compared with treatment as usual was found to reduce behavioral incidents during the hospitalization. There was also a 100% retention rate in the DBT program. In the 1-year follow-up, both treatments were found to reduce depression and suicidal ideation. Given the promising data generated by these studies, an RCT of 16 weeks of DBT for suicidal adolescent outpatients as compared with treatment as usual is currently under way in Norway.

IMPLEMENTATION OF DIALECTICAL BEHAVIOR THERAPY FOR SUICIDAL ADOLESCENTS

As mentioned above, DBT has been modified for use with adolescents. Miller and colleagues[2] have described the modifications for suicidal adolescent outpatients in detail and Katz and Cox[51] have described the modifications for acute-care inpatients. In DBT, the treatment is always provided by a treatment team and not by an individual in isolation. The following discussion will provide a brief description of the differences between adult and adolescent DBT models.

Shorter Duration

Standard adult DBT is of 1-year duration. Although this duration of treatment may be used with adolescents, many programs have modified the duration of treatment. In their text, Miller and colleagues[2] describe a 16-week DBT program. The rationale for the shortening of treatment includes that adolescents may find it difficult to commit to 1 year of treatment. Service demands may also factor in to the decision making on duration of treatment and currently there are no data in adolescents as to what is appropriate treatment duration. In many programs that do offer shorter length of treatment, the opportunity to either repeat the cycle of treatment or to "graduate" into a "graduate group" is available.

Multifamily Skills Training

In DBT for suicidal adolescents, modifications have been made to the delivery of skills training groups. Given that adolescents reside with caregivers who play a significant role in their emotional experience, the caregivers participate in the skills training groups. The principle is that the caregivers will require skills to effectively assist the adolescent in becoming skillful. The caregivers participate fully in the group in that they are there to learn the same skills as the adolescents and do the homework. The involvement of caregivers in the groups allows the skills trainers to observe the interactions between caregiver and adolescent and provide in vivo skills coaching. In standard DBT, individual therapists take phone calls from their patients to provide in vivo coaching on the use of skills during a crisis. In DBT for suicidal adolescents, this is also true but in addition the skills trainers take crisis calls from caregivers participating in the skills groups to provide the caregivers with in vivo coaching on applying the skills to their parenting.

Modification of the Wording of the Skills Manual

There is not currently a skills training manual for DBT for suicidal adolescents. Thus, the manual for skills training and the associated handouts are taken from the adult manual developed by Linehan.[52] Many programs have modified the wording of the handouts to make them more "adolescent friendly."[2] However, there are no data on the use of any modifications to the skills manual.

Walking the Middle Path

In standard DBT there are four skills training modules: core mindfulness, distress tolerance, emotion regulation, and interpersonal effectiveness. In the course of their work with adolescents, Miller and colleagues[2] found that the adolescent and his or her family had significant deficits that went beyond those that were addressed by the four existing modules in standard DBT. Miller and colleagues[2] identified a set of behavioral patterns that exist in the family constellations of suicidal adolescents and that parents, patients, and even therapists vacillate and become polarized along the three dimensions. Parents and therapists can become polarized along the dimension of excessive leniency versus authoritarian control, fostering dependence versus forcing autonomy and pathologizing normative behaviors versus normalizing pathological behaviors. The identification of these patterns led Miller and colleagues[2] to develop a fifth skills module for adolescents called "walking the middle path" to provide the skills necessary for adolescents and their caregivers to change these behavioral patterns. In this skills module the adolescent and his or her caregiver are taught basic behavioral principles, validation strategies, and how to think and act dialectically.

As-Needed Family Sessions

Finally, in addition to including the caregiver in the skills-training group as described above, it is recognized that the adolescent is still residing in an environment that will be establishing contingencies for his or her behavior. As such, it is often necessary to meet with the adolescent and his or her family/caregiver for as-needed family therapy sessions.

In DBT for suicidal adolescents, the therapist uses a variety of strategies to help the adolescent understand his or her emotional experiences while at the same time working to get the adolescent to commit to change. The therapist uses behavioral chain analysis to elicit an understanding of the events of the day and allow for determination of what strategies might have been used to change the course of the events and allow for a more adaptive outcome. The dialog below is an example of a small part of a chain analysis at the point where the adolescent has described the events of the day and the therapist is clarifying and ensuring understanding of the events.

T: So what did you want to have happen when you took the pills?

P: At that time, I wanted to die.

T: So let me make sure I've got this. You'd had a really tough time for the last few days and were sad, frustrated, and angry with your mom because she wouldn't let you go out to hang out with your friends, which you thought would help with how you were feeling. When you couldn't persuade her you thought of dying and went and impulsively took the pills.

P: Yeah, that's right.

T: Just to clarify, when you took the pills were you thinking about your mom?

P: Not really, I was really upset and just didn't want to have to deal with all this any more.

T: Okay, so I've got one question.

P: What's that?

T: You're saying that you were upset that your mom wouldn't let you hang out with your friends, which I get, but you didn't go ballistic on your mom you took pills to try to die. Do your friends like to hang out with dead people?

P: Well, no.

T: Do you see what I am getting at? We have got to find a way to help you achieve your goals and not just escape from pain. I understand wanting to hang out with your friends and I think we can help you to achieve that. Maybe not at any hour of the night, but if you use your interpersonal skills I think we can get this worked out. We are going to have to look at how we can get you to be able to think to use those skills at those crunch times. I also want you to remember that you have the option of paging me if you think that I can be helpful to you in how to use your skills with your mom at that moment. Are you willing to work on a plan for how to use your skills?

RESEARCH ON COGNITIVE BEHAVIORAL THERAPY FOR SOMATOFORM AND EATING DISORDERS

Few studies have been conducted on the subject of CBT and somatoform illness in children and adolescents. Pain complaints, including recurrent abdominal pain in particular, are a common presentation in school-aged children and adolescents. However, there has been discrepancy as to effective management techniques.[53] Several recent studies have suggested the effectiveness of CBT intervention in reducing chronic pain syndromes in youth. Research by Sanders and colleagues[54] has shown that cognitive-behavioral intervention for recurrent abdominal pain was more effective than wait list intervention. In addition, CBT helped with reduction of pain symptoms more quickly, thoroughly, and for longer periods of time when compared with standard medical care.[55] Further RCTs by Duarte and colleagues[56] and Robins and colleagues[53] compared cognitive-behavioral family intervention with standard medical care to a control group that included patients receiving standard medical care alone. Both studies found a reduction in the amount of abdominal pain and the frequency of pain crises in the groups receiving cognitive-behavioral family therapy. Robins and colleagues reported reductions in both child and parent reported pain and somatization. Sanders and colleagues reported the positive effects to be maintained at 6- and 12-month follow-up.[54] Duarte and colleagues[56] found that the CBT intervention was better for predicting and terminating pain episodes but not for dampening crises once started. Limitations of these studies included small sample sizes and selection bias in randomization. In addition, the CBT techniques used in treatment were not standardized across studies. Nonetheless, the results appear promising and suggest that combined medical and behavioral health intervention is effective in reducing perceived pain and somatization in children and adolescents. Related empiric studies examining CBT for other commonly occurring pediatric pain disorders, including recurrent pediatric headache, have also yielded positive results demonstrating significant reductions in pain with CBT treatments.[57,58]

Similarly, few studies have focused on the area of CBT treatment for childhood and adolescent eating disorders. Family-based models have proven to be effective in the treatment of adolescents with anorexia nervosa and bulimia nervosa[59]; however CBT remains largely unstudied as a treatment option in youth populations. CBT is the treatment of choice for adults with bulimia nervosa[59] and therefore may prove to be a useful intervention for bulimia in adolescents. A recent RCT by Schmidt and colleagues[60] compared the efficacy of family therapy and CBT-guided self-care in adolescents with bulimia nervosa or eating disorder not otherwise specified. Their findings suggest that CBT-guided self-care resulted in earlier reduction in binge eating than family therapy and that CBT had an advantage in terms of outcome and acceptability. Further research is required to further delineate the effectiveness and benefit of CBT for the treatment of eating disorders in children and adolescents.

SUMMARY

Although the benefits of CBT for anxiety and depressive disorders may not be as effective as once believed, it is nevertheless still an effective treatment and important part of the therapeutic armamentarium. To use CBT with adolescents, the therapist must factor in developmental considerations and use treatment models designed with these considerations in mind. The effectiveness of DBT for suicidal adolescents remains unknown despite promising preliminary studies. However, there is no well-established, empirically supported treatment for suicidal adolescents and thus DBT has been widely implemented around the world. DBT for suicidal adolescents also is a modification of the adult approach factoring in developmental considerations. For the general psychiatrist who is treating adolescents, these treatments can have great utility in achieving desired outcomes but require familiarity with the principles described in this article.

REFERENCES

1. Weersing R, Brent D. Cognitive behavioral therapy for depression in youth. Child Adolesc Psychiatr Clin N Am 2006;15:939–57.
2. Miller AL, Rathus JH, Linehan MM. Dialectical behavior therapy with suicidal adolescents. New York: Guilford Press; 2007.
3. Roblek T, Piacentini J. Cognitive-behavior therapy for childhood anxiety disorders. Child Adolesc Psychiatr Clin N Am 2005;14:863–76.
4. Lewinsohn PM, Clarke GN, Hops H, et al. Cognitive-behavioral treatment for depressed adolescents. Behav Ther 1990;21:385–401.
5. Brent D, Holder D, Kolko D, et al. A clinical psychotherapy trial for adolescent depression comparing cognitive, family, and supportive treatments. Arch Gen Psychiatry 1997;54:877–85.
6. Rohde P, Feeny NC, Robins M. Characteristics and components of the TADS CBT approach. Cogn Behav Pract 2005;12:186–97.
7. Wood A, Harrington R, Moore A. Controlled trial of a brief cognitive-behavioral intervention in adolescent patients with depressive disorders. J Child Psychol Psychiatry 1996;37:737–46.
8. Costello E, Egger H, Angold A. Prevalence and comorbidity. Child Adolesc Psychiatr Clin N Am 2005;14:631–48.
9. James A, Soler A, Weatherall R. Cognitive behavioral therapy for anxiety disorders in children and adolescents. Cochrane Database Syst Rev 2005;Oct19(4): CD004690.
10. Kendall P, Flannery-Schroeder E, Panichelli-Mindel S, et al. Treating anxiety disorders in youth: a second randomized clinical trial. J Consult Clin Psychol 1997; 65:366–80.
11. Barret P, Dadds M, Rapee R. Family treatment of childhood anxiety: a controlled trial. J Consult Clin Psychol 1996;64:333–42.
12. Kendall P. Treating anxiety disorders in youth: results of a randomized clinical trial. J Consult Clin Psychol 1994;62:100–10.

13. Wood J, Piacentini J, Southam-Gerow M, et al. Family cognitive behavioral therapy for child and anxiety disorders. J Am Acad Child Adolesc Psychiatry 2006; 45:314–21.
14. Flannery-Schroeder E, Kendall P. Group and individual cognitive-behavioral treatments for youth with anxiety disorders: a randomized clinical trial. Cognit Ther Res 2000;24:251–78.
15. Chu B, Harrison T. Disorder-specific effects of CBT for anxious and depressed youth: a meta-analysis of candidate mediators of change. Clin Child Fam Psychol Rev 2007;10:352–72.
16. Cartwright-Huttons S, Roberts C, Chitsabesan P, et al. Systematic review of the efficacy of cognitive-behaviour therapies for childhood and adolescent anxiety disorders. Br J Clin Psychol 2004;43:421–36.
17. Last C, Hansen C, Franco N. Cognitive-behavioral treatment of school phobia. J Am Acad Child Adolesc Psychiatry 1998;37:404–11.
18. Silverman W, Kurtines W, Ginsburg G, et al. Contingency management, self control, and education support in the treatment of childhood phobic disorders: a randomized clinical trial. J Consult Clin Psychol 1999;67:675–87.
19. Muris P, Meesters C, Gobel M. Cognitive coping versus emotional disclosure in the treatment of anxious children: a pilot-study. Cogn Behav Ther 2002;31:59–67.
20. The Pediatric OCD Treatment Study (POTS) Team. Cognitive-behavior therapy, sertraline, and their combination for children and adolescents with obsessive-compulsive disorder: the pediatric OCD treatment study (POTS) randomized controlled trial. JAMA 2004;292(16):1969–76.
21. O'Kearney R, Anstey K, von Sanden C. Behavioral and cognitive behavioral therapy for obsessive compulsive disorder in children and adolescents. [review]. Cochrane Database Syst Rev 2006;Oct18(4):CD004856.
22. Watson H, Rees C. Meta-analysis of randomized, controlled treatment trials for pediatric obsessive-compulsive disorder. J Child Psychol Psychiatry 2008; 49(5):489–98.
23. Cohen J, Deblinger E, Mannarino A, et al. A multi-site, randomized controlled trial for children with abuse-related PTSD symptoms. J Am Acad Child Adolesc Psychiatry 2004;43(4):393–402.
24. Deblinger E, Mannarino A, Cohen J, et al. A follow-up study of a multisite, randomized, controlled trial for children with sexual abuse-related PTSD symptoms. J Am Acad Child Adolesc Psychiatry 2006;45(12):1474–84.
25. Brookman RR, Sood AA. Disorders of mood and anxiety in adolescents. Adolesc Med 2006;17:79–95.
26. Creed TA, Kendall PC. Therapist alliance-building behavior within a cognitive-behavioral treatment for anxiety in youth. J Consult Clin Psychol 2005;73(3): 498–505.
27. Barmish AJ, Kendall PC. Should parents be co-clients in cognitive-behavioral therapy for anxious youth? J Clin Child Adolesc Psychol 2005;34(3):569–81.
28. Hudson JL, Kendall PC. Showing you can do it: homework in therapy for children and adolescents with anxiety disorders. J Clin Psychol 2002;58(5):525–34.
29. Hannesdottir DK, Ollendick TH. The role of emotion regulation in the treatment of child anxiety disorders. Clin Child Fam Psychol Rev 2007;10:275–93.
30. Piacentini J, Langley AK. Cognitive-behavioral therapy for children who have obsessive-compulsive disorder. J Clin Psychol 2004;60(11):1181–94.
31. Smith P, Yule W, Perrin S, et al. Cognitive-behavioral therapy for PTSD in children and adolescents: a preliminary randomized controlled trial. J Am Acad Child Adolesc Psychiatry 2007;46(8):1051–61.

32. Shooshtary MH, Panaghi L, Moghadam JA. Outcome of cognitive behavioral therapy in adolescents after natural disaster. J Adolesc Health 2008;42:466–72.

33. Lewinsohn P, Clarke G. Psychosocial treatments for adolescent depression. Clin Psychol Rev 1999;19:329–42.

34. Reinecke M, Ryan N, Dubois D. Cognitive-behavioral therapy of depression and depressive symptoms during adolescence: a review and meta-analysis. J Am Acad Child Adolesc Psychiatry 1998;37:26–34.

35. Michael K, Crowley S. How effective are treatments for child and adolescent depression? A meta-analytic review. Clin Psychol Rev 2002;22:247–69.

36. Treatment for Adolescents with Depression Study Team (TADS). Fluoxetine, cognitive-behavioral therapy, and their combination for adolescents with depression: treatment for adolescents with depression study (TADS) randomized controlled trial. JAMA 2004;292(7):807–20.

37. Goodyer I, Dubicka B, Wilkinson P, et al. Selective serotonin reuptake inhibitors and routine specialist care with and without cognitive behavioral therapy in adolescents with major depression: randomized controlled trial. BMJ 2007; 335(7611):142.

38. Weisz J, McCarty C, Valeri S. Effects of psychotherapy for depression in children and adolescents: a meta-analysis. Psychol Bull 2006;132(1):132–49.

39. Klein J, Jacobs R, Reinecke M. Cognitive-behavioral therapy for adolescent depression: a meta-analytic investigation of changes in effect-size estimates. J Am Acad Child Adolesc Psychiatry 2007;46(11):1403–13.

40. Vostanis P, Feehan C, Grattan E, et al. A randomized controlled outpatient trial of cognitive-behavioral treatment for children and adolescents with depression: 9-month follow-up. J Affect Disord 1996;40:105–16.

41. Kerfoot M, Harrington R, Harrington V, et al. A step too far? Randomized trial of cognitive-behavior therapy delivered by social workers to depressed adolescents. Eur Child Adolesc Psychiatry 2004;13(2):92–9.

42. American Psychiatric Association. Diagnostic and statistical manual. (4th edition). Washington (DC): American Psychiatric Association; 1994.

43. Shirk SR, Gudmundsen G, Kaplinski HC, et al. Alliance and outcome in cognitive-behavioral therapy for adolescent depression. J Clin Child Adolesc Psychol 2008;37(3):631–9.

44. Clarke GN, Hornbrook M, Lynch F, et al. A randomized trial of a group cognitive intervention for preventing depression in adolescent offspring of depressed parents. Arch Gen Psychiatry 2001;85:1127–34.

45. Clarke GN, Rohde P, Lewinsohn PM, et al. Cognitive-behavioral treatment of adolescent depression: efficacy of acute group treatment and booster sessions. J Am Acad Child Adolesc Psychiatry 1999;38:272–9.

46. Linehan MM, Comtois KA, Murray AM, et al. Two year randomized trial and follow-up of dialectical behavior therapy vs. therapy by experts for suicidal behaviors and borderline personality disorder. Arch Gen Psychiatry 2006;63:757–66.

47. Verheul R, van den Bosch LM, Koeter MW, et al. Dialectical behavior therapy for women with borderline personality disorder: 12 month randomized clinical trial in the Netherlands. Br J Psychiatry 2003;182:135–40.

48. Linehan MM. Cognitive-behavioral treatment of borderline personality disorder. New York: Guilford Press; 1993.

49. Rathus JH, Miller AL. Dialectical behavior therapy adapted for suicidal adolescents. Suicide Life Threat Behav 2002;32:146–57.

50. Katz LY, Gunasekara S, Cox BJ, et al. Feasibility of dialectical behavior therapy for parasuicidal adolescent inpatients. J Am Acad Child Adolesc Psychiatry 2004;43:276–82.

51. Katz LY, Cox BJ. Dialectical behavior therapy for suicidal adolescent inpatients: a case study. Clin Case Stud 2002;1:81–92.
52. Linehan MM. Skills training manual for treating borderline personality disorder. New York: Guilford Press; 1993.
53. Robins P, Smith S, Glutting J, et al. A randomized-controlled trial of a cognitive-behavioral family intervention for pediatric recurrent abdominal pain. J Pediatr Psychol 2005;30(5):397–408.
54. Sanders M, Rebgetz M, Morrison M, et al. Cognitive-behavioral treatment of recurrent nonspecific abdominal pain in children: an analysis of generalization, maintenance and side effects. J Consult Clin Psychol 1989;57:294–300.
55. Sanders M, Shepherd R, Cleghorn G, et al. The treatment of recurrent abdominal pain in children: a controlled comparison of cognitive-behavioral family intervention and standard pediatric care. J Consult Clin Psychol 1994;62:306–14.
56. Duarte M, Penna F, Andrade E, et al. Treatment of nonorganic recurrent abdominal pain: cognitive-behavioral family intervention. J Pediatr Gastroenterol Nutr 2006;43:59–64.
57. Holden E, Deichmann M, Levy J. Empirically supported treatments in pediatric psychology: recurrent pediatric headache. J Pediatr Psychol 1999;24:91–109.
58. Beames L, Sanders M, Bor W. The role of parent training in the cognitive behavioral treatment of children's headaches. Behav Psychother 1989;20:167–80.
59. National Collaborating Centre for Mental Health. Eating disorders: core interventions in the treatment and management of anorexia nervosa, bulimia nervosa, and related eating disorders. London: National Institute for Clinical Excellence; 2004.
60. Schmidt U, Lee S, Beecham J, et al. A randomized controlled trial of family therapy and cognitive behavior therapy guided self-care for adolescents with bulimia nervosa and related disorders. Am J Psychiatry 2007;164:591–8.

Child and Adolescent Psychopharmacology Update

Molly McVoy, MD[a],*, Robert Findling, MD[b]

KEYWORDS

- Pediatric • Medication • Treatment • Psychopharmacology
- Mood disorder • Anxiety • Autism

Understanding pediatric psychopharmacology is often an important part of the practice of a general psychiatrist. A substantial number of children and adolescents are affected by a major psychiatric illness.[1,2] For many of these youths, medication management may be an important treatment option.[2] In addition, access to child and adolescent psychiatrists may be limited because child and adolescent psychiatry is an underserved medical subspecialty.[3] Considering that many pediatricians and family practitioners may feel treating these ill children is outside of their scope of practice, many of them are brought to general psychiatrists for treatment.[3]

There are some key issues for a general psychiatrist to consider before he or she begins prescribing psychotropic medications to children and adolescents. The most important is that agents that are effective in adults may not be effective in youths.[2] Similarly, medications that are well tolerated in adults may be associated with accentuated or additional risks when prescribed to young people. Thus, simply translating the practice of adult psychiatry to the pediatric population is not advisable.[2]

Historically, there has been a paucity of methodologically stringent data about the psychopharmacologic treatment of neuropsychiatric disorders in the pediatric population (with attention deficit hyperactivity disorder being a significant exception).[4] Fortunately, there has recently been a significant increase in research dedicated to the medication therapy of the pediatric population.[4] This article is an effort to summarize those recent advances and bring the general psychiatrist up to date on the evidence-based psychopharmacologic treatment of children and adolescents.

[a] Child and Adolescent Psychiatry, University Hospitals Case Medical Center, Walker Building, 1st floor, 10524 Euclid Avenue, Cleveland, Ohio 44106, USA
[b] Child and Adolescent Psychiatry, University Hospitals Case Medical Center, Case Western Reserve University School of Medicine, 10524 Euclid Avenue, Cleveland, Ohio 44106, USA
* Corresponding author.
E-mail address: molly.mcvoy@uhhospitals.org (M. McVoy).

Psychiatr Clin N Am 32 (2009) 111–133
doi:10.1016/j.psc.2008.11.002
0193-953X/08/$ – see front matter © 2009 Elsevier Inc. All rights reserved.

ATTENTION DEFICIT HYPERACTIVITY DISORDER

Attention deficit hyperactivity disorder (ADHD) is one of the most common and well-studied neuropsychiatric disorders in children and adolescents. It affects approximately 5% of children in the United States.[5] The gold standard of psychopharmacology for ADHD management has historically been psychostimulants.[4] Stimulant treatment of ADHD has been studied for more than 70 years, longer even than antibiotics.[4] Currently, stimulants can be conceptualized as falling into two fundamental groups: methylphenidate-based and amphetamine-based medications. In numerous randomized controlled trials, both classes of treatments have been shown to be generally well tolerated and superior to placebo, with a consistently large effect size.[6] No major differences in efficacy and tolerability have been found between methylphenidate- and amphetamine-based medications in the multiple studies comparing the two.[6] To date, no consistent patient profile has been established that preferentially identifies responders to methylphenidate- versus amphetamine-based stimulants.

Originally, marketed stimulants were immediate-release formulations that required multiple daily dosing, often during the school day, a result of the stimulants' short half-lives. In order to address the shortcomings associated with the need for frequent dosing, long-acting formulations were developed. The benchmark stimulants used to treat ADHD, methylphenidate and dextroamphetamine, have been available in long-acting preparations since the 1980s. Ritalin SR and Dexedrine Spansules were the earliest long-acting formulations of methylphenidate and amphetamine, respectively. Although there were data that these early preparations were superior to placebo, clinical practice and further research found that these early long-acting formulations had significant variability in terms of both efficacy and duration of action.[7,8] Overall, they did not appear to offer substantial improvements over the original, immediate-release formulations.[7-9]

Because the first-generation formulations did not effectively achieve once-daily dosing, newer once-daily formulations of both methylphenidate and dextroamphetamine were developed. Several oral versions of long-acting methylphenidate have been available for almost a decade (Concerta, Metadate, Ritalin LA) as have amphetamine-based treatments (Dexedrine ER and Adderall XR). In multiple, randomized controlled trials, these long acting formulations have been found to be therapeutically superior to placebo and generally well tolerated.[4-6] Differences between the medications remain primarily related to duration and onset of action.[4-6]

Aside from the preparations described above, a transdermal formulation of methylphenidate has recently been developed: the methylphenidate-transdermal system (Daytrana). Methylphenidate transdermal consists of a mixture of methylphenidate contained in a polymer-based adhesive.[10] The medication diffuses out of the patch into the skin continuously over the recommended 9-hour wear time.[10] In a double-blind, placebo-controlled trial, the methylphenidate-transdermal system was well tolerated and significantly better than placebo.[10] It should be noted that the length of time the patch is worn can be adjusted to less than the standard 9-hour wear time in order to fit the schedule and demands of the individual child.[11]

In the past, all methylphenidate treatments have consisted of a racemic mixture of two enantiomers, d-threo and l-threo methylphenidate.[12] Recently, formulations that consist only of d-threo methylphenidate have been released onto the market (Focalin and Focalin XR). These compounds were developed because of reports that the d-isomer may be the therapeutically active form of the agent.[12] Several studies have compared the efficacy of d,l-methylphenidate with pure d-methylphenidate (dexmethylphenidate). To date, no significant difference in the efficacy and safety of the two formulations has been reported.[12,13]

Recent data suggest that there may be a difference in the onset and duration of action of d,l-methylphenidate versus d-methylphenidate.[12,13] One study reported that dexmethylphenidate may have a faster onset of action than d,l-methylphenidate.[12,13] However, conflicting reports exist as to the duration of action of the two formulations: one study has found d,l-methylphenidate to have a longer duration of action while another found that dexmethylphenidate lasted longer.[12,13] In short, despite potential differences in onset and duration of action, the two preparations appear to provide overall comparable symptom relief and tolerability.[12,13]

In addition to methylphenidate, as noted above, several long-acting formulations of amphetamine-based medications exist. Lisdexamfetamine (Vyvanse) has most recently entered the market. Lisdexamfetamine is a compound consisting of a pro-drug of dextroamphetamine.[6,14] This inactive formulation is metabolized into the active drug after ingestion and allows for once-daily dosing. Several placebo-controlled studies have found it to be effective and safe in children.[6,14] No studies currently exist that compare the efficacy of lisdexamfetamine with other long-acting formulations of amphetamine treatments.[6]

Stimulant treatment in children and adolescents has raised questions regarding adverse cardiac events, in the past.[3,5] The rate of adverse cardiac events, including sudden death, in children treated with stimulant medication does not currently appear to exceed that of the general pediatric population.[3,5] At present, several guidelines do not recommend routine cardiac evaluation prior to stimulant treatment. A careful history for significant cardiac disease or symptoms and family history, looking particularly for sudden cardiac death, is recommended.[3,5] Consultation with a cardiologist for children with pre-existing cardiac disease or a concerning history is also recommended if considering stimulant treatment.[3,5]

Aside from stimulant treatment, there is one other Food and Drug Administration (FDA)-approved treatment for ADHD: a norepinephrine reuptake inhibitor, atomoxetine (Strattera). This has been shown to be generally safe and effective for the treatment of children, adolescents, and adults with ADHD.[6] Because of the larger effect size of stimulants when compared to atomoxetine, several treatment guidelines recommend atomoxetine as a second-line agent for the general ADHD population. For those children who cannot tolerate stimulant treatment, whether because of underlying medical conditions, anxiety disorders, tic disorders, substance abuse problems, or intolerable side effects, these guidelines recommend atomoxetine as a first-line agent.[6]

Finally, α-adrenoceptor agonists, such as clonidine and guanfacine, have been prescribed off-label as alternatives or adjuvants to stimulant treatment. α-adrenoceptor agonists have robust evidence for the treatment of tics.[15–17] However, there are also data to suggest α-agonists may be generally safe and effective in treating ADHD and ADHD comorbid with tics.[18,19] In addition, some clinicians have used α-adrenoceptor agonists for sleep induction in children, although there is limited evidence to support this practice.[20]

Similar to stimulant treatment, previous formulations of α-agonists have required multiple daily dosing for the treatment of ADHD. In order to improve the utility of these medications, new long-acting formulations of both guanfacine and clonidine are being developed. Furthest along in development is a long-acting formulation of guanfacine, a selective $\alpha2$-agonist. Guanfacine ER (Intuniv) was studied in a randomized, placebo-controlled trial and found to be both safe and superior to placebo in children ages 6 to 17.[19] It has received an FDA-approvable letter for use in ADHD treatment.[21] In addition, a sustained-release formulation of clonidine (Clonicel) is being studied as part of the drug-development process.[22] Studies comparing the long-acting versus short-acting formulations of α-agonists have not yet been performed.

DISRUPTIVE BEHAVIOR DISORDERS

Disruptive behavior disorders (DBD), including oppositional defiant disorder and conduct disorder, are common diagnoses psychiatrists encounter when treating youth.[23,24] Aggression and aggressive behaviors are symptoms frequently targeted with pharmacotherapy.[23,24] When evaluating these children, characterizing the type of aggression they are displaying can be helpful in order to inform treatment decisions. Aggression in DBDs can be thought of as falling somewhere on a continuum between predatory aggression and impulsive/affective aggression.[25,26] Predatory aggression involves planning and control while impulsive/affective aggression is characterized by reactivity, lack of planning, and minimal control.[25,26] This second, impulsive type of aggression is the type of aggression that appears to respond most robustly to pharmacotherapy.[25,26]

Recent data suggest that treating the impulsive/affective type of aggression associated with DBDs may reduce the many negative long-term consequences of DBDs.[26,27] It should be emphasized, however, that psychosocial interventions, such as family- and school-based interventions, as well as psychotherapy are recommended in many treatment guidelines as first-line interventions for DBDs.[27,28] Nevertheless, as part of a comprehensive treatment strategy, pharmacologic interventions are often considered and employed for affective/impulsive aggression, particularly when psychosocial interventions have been unsuccessful.[27,28]

When evaluating and treating a child with aggression as a potential target symptom for pharmacotherapy, it is recommended that a clinician first perform a meticulous assessment and diagnosis. Aggression is a nonspecific group of behaviors that may occur both in normal development and as part of many pediatric psychiatric diagnoses.[25,27] The first step in treatment planning is to understand and treat the underlying diagnosis that is resulting in the aggressive behaviors.[25,27] That is, aggression stemming from a primary mood disorder would be treated differently than one stemming from an anxiety disorder.[27] It is important to note that the treatment studies discussed below describe the treatment of youths with disruptive behavior disorders alone or comorbid with ADHD, generally free from other comorbid Axis I disorders. That is to say, the studies below do not discuss the treatment of aggression, per se, but impulsive aggression associated with DBDs.

In targeting this impulsive aggression associated with DBDs, clinicians have prescribed mood stabilizers, typical antipsychotics, and atypical antipsychotics off-label.[27] However, to date, there are no FDA-approved treatments for children and adolescents with DBDs.[21]

Historically, the typical antipsychotics and mood stabilizers were the mainstays of treatment for aggression in youth stemming from DBDs.[29,30] Haloperidol, in several studies, was found to be effective in reducing aggression in youth, particularly in those with irritability.[31] However, these studies found that the pediatric population appears to be significantly more vulnerable to extrapyramidal side effects of typical antipsychotics than the adult population.[32] Consequently, this side-effect profile appears to have significantly limited typical antipsychotics' clinical utility in treating DBD-associated aggression in children and adolescents.

Among mood stabilizers, lithium and divalproic acid formulations (DVPX) have the most extensive literature supporting the treatment of DBDs in youth.[26,27,31,32] Both lithium and DVPX have been found to be more effective than placebo in treating aggressive symptoms in youth with DBDs.[26,27,31,32] However, the need for therapeutic drug monitoring and their side-effect profiles may limit their clinical use in youth with DBDs.[26,32]

The atypical antipsychotics appear to have become the most commonly prescribed medications in this patient population.[27,29] Risperidone, quetiapine, olanzapine, and aripiprazole all have been studied in DBDs.[28] Among the atypical antipsychotics, risperidone has the most robust data supporting its use in children and adolescents.[33,34] Studies have found that risperidone may be beneficial both in the short-term and long-term treatment of aggressive behaviors associated with DBDs.[33,34]

There are less data on the use of other atypical antipsychotics in the treatment of DBDs in youths.[28] However, olanzapine, quetiapine, and aripiprazole have been studied in this population.[28] Olanzapine has been reported to effectively treat aggressive symptoms in youth with the combination of DBD and low IQ in retrospective and open-label trials.[35,36] However, side effects, especially weight gain, were noted as significant problems for the study participants.[37,38] Similar to olanzapine, research on quetiapine in DBDs has shown some promise.[28] Several open-label studies have found that quetiapine is beneficial in DBDs and relatively well tolerated.[29–41] Aripiprazole, in one open label trial, has shown evidence of both safety and efficacy in treating children and adolescents with DBDs and aggressive symptoms.[42]

In summary, treating aggression associated with DBDs first involves careful evaluation and diagnosis to rule out other causes of the aggressive behavior. For impulsive/affective aggression stemming from DBDs and targeted with pharmacotherapy, typical antipsychotics, mood stabilizers, and atypical antipsychotics have been used. Side effects have limited the use of typical antipsychotics and mood stabilizers and it appears atypical antipsychotics, risperidone, in particular, have become a mainstay of treatment supported by evidenced-based data.

MAJOR DEPRESSIVE DISORDER

A key example of the pitfalls associated with extrapolating adult therapeutic data to children and adolescents is evident when one considers the pharmacologic treatment of major depressive disorder (MDD). Research into psychopharmacologic interventions for youth with MDD has identified significant differences in both efficacy and safety of antidepressants as compared to adults.[43]

Historically, tricyclic antidepressants (TCAs) have been a mainstay in the treatment of adult MDD. In spite of the development of selective serotonin reuptake inhibitors (SSRIs), they continue to have a role in the treatment of adult depression.[44] Prior to the 1980s, TCAs were also a primary treatment of pediatric depression.[45] However, once outcomes with tricyclics were studied in the pediatric population, no significant difference between TCAs and placebo was found.[45] There have been multiple negative randomized, controlled trials of TCAs in pediatric depression.[45–47] In addition, concerns regarding a narrow therapeutic index, anticholinergic side effects, ECG changes, and sudden death have been raised in children and adolescents treated with TCAs.[48] Consequently, TCAs are not generally recommended as treatment for youth with MDD.[43]

Over the last 10 years, there has been a significant increase in the number of randomized, controlled trials related to the pharmacologic treatment of pediatric depression.[2] Currently, the only FDA-approved antidepressant for youth suffering from MDD is fluoxetine.[43] Several randomized, controlled trials have found fluoxetine to be significantly more effective than placebo in treating depression in the pediatric population.[49,50] In addition to being effective for the acute treatment of MDD, a recent study found that fluoxetine was effective in delaying the onset of relapse of depression in children and adolescents.[51]

Other SSRIs have been studied in children and adolescents with depression but the majority have not found active treatment with an antidepressant to be statistically different than placebo.[43] Several theories for the reasons behind this have been proposed, including the large placebo response in this population, methodologic shortcomings regarding both the design and implementation of the trials, and true differences in efficacy between the individual SSRIs.[43]

Although this article focuses primarily on psychopharmacologic treatment of children and adolescents, psychotherapeutic treatment is worth mentioning here regarding the treatment of pediatric MDD. There is methodologically stringent literature regarding the combination of medication and psychotherapy in this patient population. The Treatment for Adolescents with Depression Study was a multicenter, randomized clinical trial designed to study fluoxetine alone, cognitive behavior therapy (CBT) alone, the combination of the two, and placebo in the treatment of adolescent depression.[52–54] This National Institute of Mental Health (NIMH)-funded study found that fluoxetine was superior to both placebo and CBT, but that the combination of CBT and fluoxetine was superior to the medication treatment alone.[53] In addition, it was found that the addition of CBT to fluoxetine offered some protection against the emergence of suicidal events.[53]

Beyond the acute treatment of pediatric depression, there is very limited evidence regarding the treatment of refractory depression in youth. An NIMH-funded study, the Treatment of SSRI-Resistant Depression in Adolescents trial examined four different interventions in adolescents whose depression did not respond to treatment by an SSRI. They compared switching this group to another SSRI, venlafaxine, SSRI plus CBT, or venlafaxine plus CBT.[55] At the end of 12 weeks, they found no difference in clinical response between the venlafaxine group and the SSRI group. The addition of CBT did make a significant difference, however. The investigators found that adding CBT to either an SSRI or venlafaxine in this group was significantly better, in clinical response, than switching the medication alone.[55]

In addition to significant differences in efficacy between children and adults, there are important safety issues that are particular to the treatment of children and adolescents with MDD. In the forefront of the concerns has been the report of an associated increase in suicidal events in children and adolescents treated with SSRIs. In 2003, the FDA began looking into the effects of antidepressants on spontaneously reported suicidality (suicidal adverse events, suicidal ideation, and suicidal attempts).[56] The FDA evaluated the results of 24 randomized, controlled trials involving the treatment of youth with antidepressants and found a small but statistically significant increase in the occurrence of "suicidal adverse events" when compared to placebo. However, no completed suicides were reported throughout the studies.[57] A second meta-analysis found a similar small increase in the relative risk for self-reported suicidality.[43] A black-box warning was placed on all antidepressants in 2004, regarding the risk of suicide in children and adolescents.[56] Overall, these studies have found an approximately 2% increase in the risk of suicidal ideation in youth who were treated with antidepressants versus those who were not.[43]

Although there have been recent concerns, as stated above, about the possibility of antidepressants increasing suicidality, pharmacoepidemiologic studies have not borne this out.[43,57,58] These studies show a decline in child and adolescent suicide with increased use of antidepressants in the treatment of pediatric MDD.[57] Because of all of the above, multiple treatment guidelines conclude that the overall risk/benefit ratio favors treating moderate or severe pediatric depression with medication, primarily SSRIs.[43,58]

However, these guidelines also recognize the risk associated with antidepressant pharmacotherapy and stress the importance of close monitoring during medication treatment. Currently, the FDA recommends monitoring patients weekly for first 4 weeks after initiation of an antidepressant, then every other week for the next 8 weeks.[21] After 12 weeks, the FDA recommends monitoring "as clinically indicated."[21] In addition, as stated above, the combination of CBT with medication appears to both add benefit and reduce the risk of suicidality in adolescents.[53] Treating moderate-to-severe depression in adolescents with both medication and CBT may, therefore, help to achieve the most rapid response with the smallest amount of risk.[53] Similar data concerning younger children's response to medication alone versus medication and psychotherapy do not exist at this time.

In addition to the concern regarding suicidality, treating children and adolescents with antidepressants raises concerns regarding the risk of pediatric bipolar disorder for several reasons. A child treated with an antidepressant because of a presentation consistent with MDD may develop manic or hypomanic symptoms after initiation of treatment.[59] This may be because of a latent bipolar disorder that was not evident on initial presentation.[59,60] Additionally, subclinical hypomanic symptoms may have been present prior to the presentation of MDD that were not elicited by the clinician.[59,60] Finally, a child may present with irritability and insomnia that is treated presumptively as MDD, but in fact represents a mixed episode. Treating such children with antidepressants risks producing more rapid cycling or worsening of manic and mixed symptoms.[60] Consequently, it is recommended that clinicians monitor children and adolescents beginning antidepressant treatment for the emergence of manic or hypomanic symptoms.[43] In addition, a meticulous clinical history with attention to the possibility of past manic or hypomanic symptoms and an examination of the family history for a history of bipolar disorder is recommended.[60]

BIPOLAR DISORDER

Pediatric bipolar disorder is a chronic and disabling condition.[60] Controversy has surrounded what constitutes the spectrum of pediatric bipolar disorder.[59–61] The issues involved in this controversy and the particulars of the diagnostic process are beyond the scope of this article (see Horst, of this issue). However, less controversial is the diagnosis of bipolar I disorder in children.[59,60] The treatment for youth diagnosed with this serious condition is the focus of this section.

Historically, there has been a dearth of research with methodologic rigor on the treatment of bipolar disorder in children and adolescents.[60,61] However, in recent years there has been a significant increase in the data available for treatment of these youth.[60,61] These studies of bipolar disorder primarily focus on youth in manic or mixed states.[60,61] Consequently, little is known still about the management of pediatric bipolar depression, the maintenance treatment of pediatric bipolar disorder, and the pharmacotherapy of major depression in youth with family histories of bipolar disorder.[60,61] At this point, there are three medication treatments approved by the FDA for the psychopharmacologic management of pediatric bipolar disorder: lithium for children aged 12 and up, and aripiprazole and risperidone for youth aged 10 to 17 in manic or mixed states.[60,61]

Lithium was one of the first medications used for the treatment of bipolar disorder in adults and remains an important mood stabilizer in that population.[62–65] In children and adolescents, there are prospective studies, several open label trials, and one randomized controlled trial supporting its use in pediatric bipolar disorder.[63–65] Many of these studies have lacked methodologic rigor and FDA approval of lithium in youth appears to be based primarily on data from adult studies.[63–65] More definitive research on lithium in children is currently being conducted with National Institute of Child Health and Human Development support.[62,66] However, until more definitive data become available, it appears that lithium may be a relatively safe and effective treatment for adolescents in acute manic or mixed states.[63–65]

In addition to lithium, medications originally used to treat epilepsy, the anticonvulsants, have been used to treat bipolar disorder in both children and adults. Divalproic acid-based preparations, carbamazepine, topiramate, and oxcarbazepine are the best studied of the anticonvulsants in the treatment of bipolar disorder.[60,61] Early research on DVPX consisted of open label trials and generally reported DVPX as effective in reducing mixed and manic symptoms in adolescents.[60,61] However, two recent randomized, controlled trials have provided contradictory results.[67,68] One three-site, National Institutes of Health (NIH)-sponsored study found DVPX superior to placebo in treating manic symptoms in youth.[67] However, a larger, industry-supported, multisite study found no difference between DVPX and placebo.[68] Differences in study design and implementation may account for the discrepant results and more data on valproate's efficacy in comparison with placebo are still needed. Several studies have found that divalproate had efficacy equal to lithium in the acute treatment of pediatric bipolar disorder.[69,70]

Carbamazepine outcome data in youth is restricted to case reports. Currently, no controlled data are available to confirm or refute its use in children and adolescents.[61,71] Placebo-controlled data supporting its use in adults, however, may warrant further methodologically rigorous investigations into its use in the pediatric population.[72] Oxcarbazepine was studied in one randomized, controlled trial in youth with bipolar disorder.[73] This study found no statistically significant difference in efficacy between oxcarbazepine and placebo.[73]

Finally, among the anticonvulsants, one randomized controlled trial comparing topiramate to placebo in youths was discontinued early because of consistently negative results in the adult population. However, after this study was terminated, results of the trial suggested that topiramate was well tolerated in youth and provided some benefit when compared to placebo.[74] Again, because of the appearance of potential benefits, further research into topiramate's use is indicated.[74]

In recent years, much of the research on pediatric bipolar disorder has focused on the atypical antipsychotics.[75-80] As stated previously, risperidone and aripiprazole have FDA approval for the treatment of mixed and manic states in youth aged 10 to 17. Risperidone, olanzapine, quetiapine, aripiprazole, and ziprasidone have all been studied in placebo-controlled clinical trials involving young people with bipolar disorder.[75-80] To date, all have been positive studies, that is, they have found that these atypical antipsychotics are more effective in the acute treatment of manic or mixed states in children than placebo (Table 1).[75-80]

Most studies have been three-arm studies; they have looked at placebo, a supposed minimal-effective dose of the medication, and a higher dose.[75-80] In these three-arm studies (see Table 1), results indicate that both active-treatment arms were therapeutically superior to placebo and found no difference in treatment efficacy between the two doses of medication.[75-79] Although the higher doses showed no additional benefit, they did show an increase in side effects.[75-79]

In summary, three medication treatments are currently approved by the FDA for the treatment of youth in manic and mixed states: lithium for children ages 12 and up, and aripiprazole and risperidone for youths aged 10 to 17. Although the data are somewhat limited, lithium appears generally safe and effective in youth in manic or mixed states. In addition, since their advent, much of the research has focused on the atypical antipsychotics and, to date, all placebo-controlled trials have found the atypical antipsychotics more effective in treating manic or mixed states than placebo. The presumed minimally effective doses that have been studied in these trials have been found to be as therapeutically effective as the higher dosages and with lower side effects.

ANXIETY DISORDERS

Anxiety symptoms and anxiety disorders are a common occurrence in childhood, with a diagnosable anxiety disorder occurring in 10% to 20% of children.[81,82] Among

Table 1
A typical antipsychotics in the treatment of pediatric mania and/or mixed mania

Medication	Author	Sample Size	Dosing	Findings
Aripiprazole	Chang et al, 2008	296	10 mg/day 30 mg/day	Both doses of aripiprazole were significantly more effective than placebo; no significant treatment or tolerability differences were noted between medication doses
Olanzapine	Tohen et al, 2007	161	2.5 mg/day–20 mg/day (avg. 10.7 mg/day)	Olanzapine was more effective for reducing manic symptoms than placebo; also had significant increase in side effects (SE) (weight gain, elevated glucose, and cholesterol, sedation)
Quetiapine	DelBellow et al, 2008	283	400 mg/day 600 mg/day	Both doses of quetiapine were significantly more effective than placebo; no significant treatment differences were noted between medication doses; more SE (somnolence, sedation, dizziness) were reported with higher dose
Risperidone	Pandina et al, 2008	137	0.5 mg/day–2.5 mg/day 3 mg/day–6 mg/day	Both dosage ranges of risperidone were significantly more effective than placebo; no significant treatment differences were noted between medication doses; more SE (somnolence, HA, fatigue) were reported with higher dose
Ziprasidone	DelBellow et al, 2008	150	80 mg/day–160 mg/day	Ziprasidone was significantly more effective in reducing manic symptoms than placebo but also had significant increase in SE (sedation, somnolence, nausea)

medications, SSRIs have the most evidence supporting their use in youth with anxiety, although several medication groups have been studied.[81,82] Although the psychopharmacologic treatment of children and adolescents is the focus of this article, psychotherapeutic treatment deserves a special mention, especially in the treatment of anxiety disorders.[81,82] In children with anxiety disorders, CBT has substantial evidence supporting its use and is often recommended in combination with medication therapy.[81,82]

In order to understand the research surrounding the pharmacologic treatment of pediatric anxiety disorders, it is helpful to think of them as falling in four basic categories: (1) broad anxiety disorders, which include generalized anxiety disorder, social phobia, and separation anxiety disorder; (2) obsessive-compulsive disorder (OCD); (3) posttraumatic stress disorder (PTSD); and (4) panic disorder.

Research concerning the pharmacologic treatment of the broad anxiety disorders has primarily focused on the use of SSRIs.[81–88] Sertraline, fluoxetine, paroxetine, and fluvoxamine all have placebo-controlled data that indicate treatment superiority for acute management of anxiety in comparison with placebo in both children and adolescents.[81–88] In addition to these SSRIs, venlafaxine also has several recent randomized, controlled trials that indicate it may be more effective than placebo in reducing anxiety symptoms in youth with generalized anxiety disorder and social phobia.[89,90] However, there are currently no FDA-approved medications for the treatment of these disorders in children and adolescents.

As stated above, in addition to medications, cognitive behavior therapy is often recommended in the treatment of these disorders.[81,82] However, there are limited data comparing the relative benefits of CBT and medications in this population.[81,82] The NIMH is currently supporting a study (Child Adolescent Anxiety Multimodal Treatment Study) that is designed to compare sertraline treatment alone, CBT alone, and their combination in comparison with placebo in the treatment of social phobia and generalized anxiety disorder.[91]

In contrast to the broad anxiety disorders, there are several FDA-approved medications for the treatment of OCD in youth. To date, sertraline has FDA approval in children ages 6 and up, fluoxetine ages 7 and older, fluvoxamine ages 8 and up, and clomipramine for youth aged 10 and older. As with the broad anxiety disorders, SSRIs have the most robust research supporting their use in this population.[92–95] Sertraline, fluoxetine, fluvoxamine, and paroxetine all have positive randomized trials supporting their therapeutic superiority to placebo.[92–95]

Again, in contrast to the broad anxiety disorders, there is evidence comparing CBT with medication management in OCD. In the Pediatric OCD Treatment Study, CBT alone, sertraline alone, and CBT plus sertraline were compared with placebo in youth aged 7 to 17 with OCD.[96] Data suggest that the combination of CBT plus sertraline was the most effective treatment and that both CBT alone and sertraline alone were more effective than placebo.[96] In addition, the results indicated that CBT alone was a more effective treatment than sertraline alone in treating children with OCD.[96] In early-onset OCD, defined as OCD beginning before puberty, it has been found that family-based CBT is effective in reducing both obsessions and compulsions in pre-adolescent patients.[97]

The pharmacologic treatment of pediatric posttraumatic stress disorder has very limited evidence, and there are no medications currently approved by the FDA for this indication.[98] Several medications have been studied in open trials and case series.[98] Open-label trials of citalopram show contradictory results: one in 2001 demonstrated benefit while another in 2002 did not.[99] There are several case studies on both in-patients and out-patients with PTSD reporting a reduction in anxiety symptoms with the use of clonidine.[100–102] In addition, quetiapine has been reportedly used with success in youth with PTSD in detention centers.[103] One controlled study exists that suggested propranolol was effective in reducing the symptoms of PTSD in the study population.[104]

In pediatric panic disorder, no controlled data exist regarding its pharmacologic treatment.[105] A pilot study of SSRI treatment in a small number of children indicated efficacy in reducing panic symptoms, but suggested the need for a benzodiazepine during treatment initiation.[106] Overall, however, there is a dearth of data on the pharmacologic treatment of children with panic disorder. More methodologically stringent studies are warranted.[105]

In summary, anxiety disorders are common, disabling conditions affecting youth, but there is limited evidence regarding the pharmacotherapeutic interventions used to treat them. The broad anxiety disorders have evidence supporting the use of SSRIs to reduce symptoms in children and adolescents. Similarly, SSRI management of OCD has significant data behind it. In contrast, there is limited research on the psychopharmacologic management of pediatric PTSD and panic disorder. Multiple medication classes have been clinically used in this population, including SSRIs, α-agonists, and atypical antipsychotics, although there are no FDA-approved medications for anxiety disorders in youth.

AUTISM AND PERVASIVE DEVELOPMENTAL DISORDERS

Autism is the prototypic pervasive developmental disorder. It is characterized by dysfunction in socialization, language, and repetitive behaviors.[107,108] In addition to these core features, patients diagnosed with this disorder often struggle with other behaviors that impair their ability to function in daily life.[107,108] These include symptoms of inattention, hyperactivity, mood instability, and aggression.[107,108] As part of a comprehensive treatment plan, including school support, occupational and physical therapy, and social skills training, pharmacotherapy may be utilized to help youth manage the symptoms described above.[108]

One of the core features of autism is the presence of repetitive, stereotyped behaviors and compulsions. As in patients with OCD, several antidepressants have data supporting their use in reducing compulsions in autistic youth.[109] Fluoxetine has placebo-controlled data that indicate it may be more effective than placebo in reducing stereotyped behavior in autism, and may be generally well tolerated.[110,111] Citalopram, escitalopram, and sertraline all have open-trial data that indicate possible benefit in reducing compulsive behavior in these children.[112–115] Although benefit is suggested for these SSRIs, several studies found a significant occurrence of what some others have termed, "behavioral-activating side effects" with SSRI treatment in autistic youth, including aggression, agitation, and hyperactivity.[109–115] Aside from SSRIs, clomipramine, a tricyclic antidepressant, has been studied in this population.[116,117] Although clomipramine showed superior clinical efficacy to placebo, significant side effects were experienced by many of the patients, including urinary retention, worsening behavior, and sedation.[116,117]

Patients with autism often suffer from symptoms of inattention and hyperactivity. As with patients diagnosed with ADHD, psychostimulants are the most well-studied medications for ADHD symptoms associated with autism.[118–120] A recent double-blind, placebo-controlled, crossover study was conducted investigating methylphenidate in youth with pervasive developmental disorders.[120] Methylphenidate was superior to placebo in reducing inattention and hyperactivity symptoms in this population, but at a significantly lower response rate than in typically developing children with ADHD.[120] In addition, children in this study appeared to have a relatively high incidence of adverse events.[120] Amphetamine-based stimulants have very limited data in youth with autism, with the most recent data from the 1970s.[121–123] These data suggest poor tolerability for amphetamines in children with autistic spectrum disorders.[121–123] However, definitive studies with current methodologies are not yet available.

Data regarding α-agonists in the treatment of inattention and hyperactivity associated with autism is limited.[124–127] Two placebo-controlled trials of clonidine demonstrate significant reduction in hyperactive behavior in youth with autism.[124,125] Open-label data also indicate that guanfacine may be effective in reducing inattentive and hyperactive symptoms in these youth.[126,127] However, as with stimulant treatment, patients appeared to have significant adverse effects with alpha agonists, including sleep disruption, fatigue, and changes in appetite.[124–127]

Aggression and self-injurious behaviors can be disabling for children with autism and have been the focus of many types of pharmacotherapy.[107] Currently, risperidone is the only FDA-approved medication to treat the irritability sometimes associated with pervasive developmental disorders.[107,128–130] Risperidone has several placebo-controlled trials that indicate it is efficacious in reducing aggression, tantrums, and self-injurious behaviors in the short- and long-term, and is generally well tolerated.[128–130] Quetiapine has also been studied, but has been found to have more modest benefit and more problematic side effects than risperidone in this population.[131,132] In addition, although olanzapine has been reported to have moderate efficacy in reducing aggressive symptoms, weight gain has been significantly problematic in the study populations.[133–135] Ziprasidone and aripiprazole have very limited data in this patient group.[136–140] Further research may be warranted.

In addition to atypical antipsychotics, mood stabilizers have been used clinically to treat irritability and aggression in children with autism.[107,141,142] One placebo-controlled trial showed significant benefit of divalproex sodium in reducing aggressiveness and mood lability.[141]

Finally, for the core dysfunction of autism, impairment in social functioning, effective or FDA-approved pharmacotherapeutic interventions have not been identified at this point.[142,143] D-cycloserine, a glutamate agonist, which has shown limited success in the negative symptoms of schizophrenia, has been studied with mixed results in children with autism.[142,143] In addition, tetrahydrobiopterin, a compound involved in catecholamine synthesis, was found to have modest benefit in socialization in a small study of children with autism.[143]

In summary, many pharmacologic interventions have been used clinically for behavior dysfunctions related to pervasive developmental disorders. Unfortunately, treatment with respect to the core social dysfunction remains elusive. Medication treatment of associated behaviors involves identifying specific behaviors and targeting with medication appropriately. However, it should be noted that patients suffering from pervasive developmental disorders often display therapeutic and adverse reactions that differ significantly from those in the general pediatric population. As existing research is somewhat limited in this area, further methodologically stringent clinical trials are needed.

PSYCHOTIC DISORDERS

Early-onset schizophrenia and schizoaffective disorder are severe and chronic diseases.[144–146] Up to 33% of individuals with schizophrenia report having symptom onset before the age of 18.[144–146] Those patients who do have psychotic symptoms in their youth often have a less favorable prognosis than those with adult-onset psychotic disorders.[144–146] Effective treatment, therefore, is important, in this severely ill population. Since their advent, atypical antipsychotics appear to be, clinically, the most commonly used medications for pediatric psychotic disorders. However, recent research has suggested that first-generation antipsychotics may be equally effective acutely.[144,147] Definitive data and recommendations on which specific antipsychotic should be considered first line in children and adolescents with schizophrenia and schizoaffective disorder are not available. Currently, FDA-approved treatments include aripiprazole and risperidone for the treatment of adolescents aged 13 to 17 with schizophrenia.

Early studies on pediatric psychotic disorders focused on the first-generation antipsychotics, including haloperidol, thiothixene, thioridazine, and loxapine.[148–150] Haloperidol and loxapine have both been studied in comparison to placebo in adolescents and both were reported to be therapeutically superior to placebo.[148,149] However, both loxapine and haloperidol were associated with substantial rates of extra-pyramidal symptoms (EPS) and sedation in comparison to placebo.[148,149] Thiothixene and thioridazine were compared in a similar study population and were found to reduce psychotic symptoms, but were associated with dose-limiting sedation.[150]

Because of concerns regarding the side effects of typical antipsychotics in juveniles, particularly EPS, the atypical antipsychotics have become much more commonly prescribed. Risperidone, olanzapine, and aripiprazole have been studied in comparison with placebo in the acute treatment of early-onset schizophrenia.[151–159] In addition, clozapine, in spite of its side-effect profile, has evidence to support its use in the treatment of refractory schizophrenia in youth.[160–163]

Risperidone was studied in a three-arm, placebo-controlled trial. The data suggest that both active treatments (1 mg/day–3 mg/day and 4 mg/day–6 mg/day) were superior to placebo in reducing psychotic symptoms. However, the higher dose treatment group had significantly greater extrapyramidal side effects than the lower dose group, with a similar degree of symptom reduction.[158] Olanzapine was studied in a blinded, 6-week, placebo-controlled, flexible dosing study in adolescents.[159] Treatment with olanzapine resulted in significantly greater reduction in symptoms than placebo. However, considerable weight gain (average of 4.3 kg), in addition to sedation and liver enzyme elevation, were noted with olanzapine treatment.[159] Recent data were published of a three-arm, placebo-controlled trial of aripiprazole in adolescents with schizophrenia.[157] In this study, both doses of aripiprazole (10 mg or 30 mg/day) were statistically superior to placebo in reducing psychotic symptoms, with no significant difference between the treatment arms. Significantly more EPS was noted in the aripiprazole-treatment groups with mild degrees of weight gain in comparison to placebo.[157]

Until recently, there were very little data available to compare one antipsychotic with another, in particular first-generation versus second-generation antipsychotics in youth.[147] In the Treatment of Early-Onset Schizophrenia Spectrum Disorders Study, risperidone, olanzapine, and molindone were compared over 8 weeks.[147] No differences were found between the treatment groups in regard to therapeutic effects. Olanzapine was associated with such significant weight gain, however, that randomization to this treatment group was ended early.[147] In addition, more akathisia was reported with molindone treatment. No differences in other reports of EPS between the three treatment groups were noted, however.[147]

With respect to treatment-resistant schizophrenia, clozapine remains the treatment of choice for adults.[160–163] The data in children are less robust, but consistently indicate that clozapine is superior to other typical and atypical antipsychotics for youths who have failed treatment with at least two previous antipsychotics.[160–163] Several open trials indicate clozapine is effective in reducing psychotic symptoms in youth with treatment-refractory schizophrenia.[160] In addition, clozapine has been compared to both haloperidol and high-dose olanzapine in double-blind comparison studies for treatment-resistant early-onset schizophrenia.[161–163] Clozapine was shown to be therapeutically superior in both studies. However, side effects, including seizures and neutropenia, remain a concern for patients treated with clozapine.[160–163]

In summary, although beneficial, antipsychotic treatment of early-onset psychotic disorders continue to have substantial shortcomings, including EPS, metabolic dysfunction, and overall increased side effects when compared with the adult population. These illnesses are chronic and severe, and youth with schizophrenia are often more susceptible to side effects than adults. Among first-generation anitpsychotics, haloperidol, molindone, thiothixene, thioridazine, and loxapine have been studied and found to be generally effective in reducing psychotic symptoms. However, concerns regarding EPS and tardive dyskinesia remain serious. Olanzapine, risperidone, and aripiprazole have been shown to be therapeutically superior to placebo in psychotic youth. However, weight gain continues to be a major consideration with atypical antipsychotics and, in particular, with olanzapine. Clozapine appears to remain the treatment of choice for refractory early-onset schizophrenia, although the data are limited.

SUMMARY

There has been a significant increase in the number of methodologically rigorous studies concerning the psychopharmacologic treatment of children and adolescents in recent years. This has allowed clinicians to make better informed and more evidenced-based decisions when evaluating and treating youth. Although the research has increased in volume and rigor of late, further research is still needed. Studies evaluating the long-term safety of medication treatment in children and adolescents remain limited. In addition, data on head-to-head comparisons of medications are necessary. Comparisons of medication, psychotherapy, and the combination have begun, but further investigations are warranted. Finally, research into predictors of response and tolerability may aid in determining the optimal medication choices for particular patients. In conclusion, the consideration of pharmacologic treatment continues to be important for many children and adolescents with psychiatric illness.

REFERENCES

1. Kessler RC, Wang PS. The descriptive epidemiology of commonly occurring mental disorders in the United States. Annu Rev Public Health 2008;29:115–29.
2. Vitiello B. Research in child and adolescent psychopharmacology: recent accomplishments and new challenges. Psychopharmacology 2007;191:5–13.
3. Hoagwood K, Kelleher K, Feil M, et al. Treatment services for children with ADHD: a national perspective. J Am Acad Child Adolesc Psychiatry 2000; 39(2):198–206.
4. McClellan JM, Werry JS. Evidence-based treatments in child and adolescent psychiatry: an inventory. J Am Acad Child Adolesc Psychiatry 2003;42(12): 1388–400.
5. Pliska S, AACAP Work Group on Quality Issues. Practice parameter for the assessment and treatment of children and adolescents with attention-deficit/hyperactivity disorder. J. Am Acad Child Adolesc Psychiatry 2007;46(7):894–921.
6. Findling R. Evolution of the treatment of attention-deficit/hyperactivity disorder in children: a review. Clin Ther 2008;30(5):942–57.
7. Swanson J, Wigal S, Wigal T, et al. A comparison of once-daily extended-release methylphenidate formulations in children with attention-deficit/hyperactivity

disorder in the laboratory school (The COMACS study). Pediatrics 2004;113(3): 206–16.

8. Pelham W, Sturges J, Hoza J, et al. Sustained release and standard methylphenidate effects on cognitive and social behavior in children with attention deficit disorder. Pediatrics 1987;80(4):491–501.

9. Brown G, Ebert M, Mikkelse E, et al. Behavior and motor activity response in hyperactive children and plasma amphetamine levels following a sustained release preparation. J Am Acad Child Psychiatry 1980;19:225–39.

10. Findling R, Bukstein O, Melmed R, et al. A randomized, double-blind, placebo-controlled, parallel-group study of methylphenidate transdermal system in pediatric patients with attention-deficit/hyperactivity disorder. J Clin Psychiatry 2008; 69:149–59.

11. Wilens T, Boellner S, Lopez F, et al. Varying the wear time of the methylphenidate transdermal system in children with attention-deficit/hyperactivity disorder. J Am Acad Child Adolesc Psychiatry 2008;47(6):700–8.

12. Wigal S, Swanson J, Fiefel D, et al. A double-blind, placebo-controlled trial of dexmethylphenidate hydrochloride and d,l-threo-methylphenidate hydrochloride in children with attention-deficit/hyperactivity disorder. J Am Acad Child Adolesc Psychiatry 2004;43(11):1406–14.

13. Muniz R, Brams M, Mao A, et al. Efficacy and safety of extended-release dexmethylphenidate compared with d,l-methylphenidate and placebo in the treatment of children with attention-deficit/hyperactivity disorder: a 12-hour laboratory classroom study. J Child Adolesc Psychopharmacol 2008;15(3): 248–56.

14. Biederman J, Boellner S, Childress A, et al. Lisdexamfetamine dimesylate and mixed amphetamine salts extended-release in children with ADHD: a double-blind, placebo-controlled, crossover analog classroom study. Biol Psychiatry 2007;62:970–6.

15. Du Y, Li F, Vance A, et al. Randomized double-blind multicentre placebo-controlled clinical trial of the clonidine adhesive patch for the treatment of tic disorders. Aust N Z J Psychiatry 2008;42(9):807–13.

16. Gaffney G, Perry P, Lund B, et al. Risperidone versus clonidine in the treatment of children and adolescents with Tourette's syndrome. J. Am Acad Child Adolesc Psychiatry 2002;41(3):330–6.

17. Cummings D, Singer H, Krieger M, et al. Neuropsychiatric effects of guanfacine in children with mild Tourette syndrome: a pilot study. Clin Neuropharmacol 2002;25(6):325–32.

18. Kurlan R, Goetz C, McDermott M, et al. Treatment of ADHD in children with tics: a randomized controlled trial. Neurology 2002;58:527–36.

19. Biederman J, Melmed R, Patel A, et al. A randomized, double-blind, placebo-controlled study of guanfacine extended release in children and adolescents with attention-deficit/hyperactivity disorder. Pediatrics 2008;121(1):73–84.

20. Carskadon M, Cavall A, Rosekind M, et al. Sleepiness and nap sleep following a morning dose of clonidine. Sleep 1989;12(4):338–44.

21. Available at: www.fda.gov.

22. Available at: www.addrenex.com/lead_product.html.

23. Bambauer K, Connor D. Characteristics of aggression in clinically referred children. CNS Spectr 2005;10(9):709–18.

24. Nock M, Kaxdin A, Hiripi E, et al. Prevalence, subtypes, and correlates of DSM-IV conduct disorder in the National Comorbidity Survey replication. Psychol Med 2006;36(5):699–710.

25. Findling R. Atypical antipsychotic treatment of disruptive behavior disorders in children and adolescents. J Clin Psychiatry 2008;69(Suppl 4):9–14.
26. Pappadopulos E, MacIntyre J, Crismon M, et al. Treatment recommendations for the use of antipsychotics for aggressive youth. J Am Acad Child Adolesc Psychiatry 2003;42(2).
27. Steiner H, Remsin L. Practice parameter for the assessment and treatment of children and adolescents with oppositional defiant disorder. J Am Acad Child Adolesc Psychiatry 2007;46(1):126–41.
28. Findling R, Steiner H, Weller E, et al. Use of antipsychotics in children and adolescents. J Clin Psychiatry 2005;66(Suppl 7):29–40.
29. Campbell M, Rapoport J, Simpson G, et al. Antipsychotics in children and adolescents. J Am Acad Child Adolesc Psychiatry 1999;38(5):537–45.
30. Ruths S, Steiner H. Psychopharmacologic treatment of aggression in children and adolescents. Pediatr Ann 2004;33(5):319–27.
31. Campbell M, Small A, Green W, et al. Behavioral efficacy of haloperidol and lithium carbonate. A comparison in hospitalized aggressive children with conduct disorder. Arch Gen Psychiatry 1984;41(7):650–6.
32. Malone R, Delaney M, Luebbert J, et al. A double-blind placebo-controlled study of lithium in hospitalized aggressive children and adolescents with conduct disorder. Arch Gen Psychiatry 2000;57:649–54.
33. Reyes M, Buitelaar J, Toren P, et al. A randomized, double-blind, placebo-controlled study of risperidone maintenance treatment in children and adolescents with disruptive behavior disorders. Am J Psychiatry 2006;163(3):402–10.
34. Turgay A, Binder C, Snyder R, et al. Long-term safety and efficacy of risperidone for the treatment of disruptive behavior disorders in children with subaverage IQs. Pediatrics 2002;110(3):1–12.
35. Connor D, Fletcher K, Wood J, et al. Neuroleptic-related dyskinesias in children and adolescents. J Clin Psychiatry 2001;62(12):967–74.
36. Biederman J, Mick E, Faraone S, et al. risperidone for the treatment of affective symptoms in children with disruptive behavior disorder: a Post hoc analysis of data from a 6-week, multicenter, randomized, double-blind, parallel-arm study. Clin Therap 2006;28(5):794–800.
37. Handen B, Hardan A. Open-label, prospective trial of olanzapine in adolescents with subaverage intelligence and disruptive behavior disorders. J Am Acad Child Adolesc Psychiatry 2006;45(8):928–35.
38. Masi G, Milone A, Canepa G, et al. Olanzapine treatment in adolescents with severe conduct disorder. Eur Psychiatry 2006;21:51–7.
39. Kronenberger W, Giauque A, Lafata D, et al. Quetiapine addition in methylphenidate treatment-resistant adolescents with comorbid attention-deficit/hyperactivity disorder, conduct/oppositional-defiant disorder, and aggression: a prospective, open-label study. J Child Adolesc Psychopharmacol 2007;17(3):334–47.
40. Findling R, Reed M, O'Riordan M, et al. A 26-week open-label study of quetiapine in children with conduct disorder. J Child and Adolesc Psychopharmacol 2007;17(1):1–9.
41. Findling R, Reed M, O'Riordan M, et al. Effectiveness, safety, and pharmacokinetics of quetiapine in aggressive children with conduct disorder. J Am Acad Child Adolesc Psychiatry 2006;45(7):792–800.
42. Findling R, Blumer J, Kauffmann R, et al. Pharmacokinetic effects of aripiprazole in children and adolescents with conduct disorder. Presented at the XXIVth Collegium Internationale Neuro-Psychopharmacologicum Congress. 2004.

43. Birmaher B, Brent D, et al. Practice parameter for the assessment and treatment of children and adolescents with depressive disorders. J Am Acad Child Adolesc Psychiatry 2007;46(11):1503–26.
44. Thase M, Nelson J, Papakostas G, et al. Augmentation strategies in the treatment of major depressive disorder. CNS Spectr 2007;12(12 Suppl 22):3–5.
45. Geller B, Reisling D, Leonard H, et al. Critical review of tricyclic antidepressant use in children and adolescents. J Am Acad Child Adolesc Psychiatry 1999; 38(5):513–6.
46. Geller B, Cooper T, Graham D, et al. Pharmacokinetically designed double-blind placebo-controlled study of nortriptyline in 6- to 12-year-olds with major depressive disorder. J Am Acad Child Adolesc Psychiatry 1992;31(1):34–44.
47. Birmaher B, Waterman S, Ryan N, et al. Randomized, controlled trial of amitriptyline versus placebo for adolescents with "treatment-resistant" major depression. J Am Acad Child Adolesc Psychiatry 1998;37(5):527–35.
48. Wilens T, Biederman J, Baldessarini R, et al. Cardiovascular effects of therapeutic doses of tricyclic antidepressants in children and adolescents. J Am Acad Child Adolesc Psychiatry 1996;35(11):1491–501.
49. Emslie G, Heiligenstein J, Wagner K, et al. Fluoxetine for acute treatment of depression in children and adolescents: a placebo-controlled, randomized clinical trial. J Am Acad Child Adolesc Psychiatry 2002;41(10):1205–15.
50. Emslie G, Rush A, Weinberg W, et al. A double-blind, randomized, placebo-controlled trial of fluoxetine in children and adolescents with depression. Arch Gen Psychiatry 1997;54(11):1031–7.
51. Emslie G, Heiligenstein J, Hoog S, et al. Fluoxetine treatment for prevention of relapse of depression in children and adolescents: a double-blind, placebo-controlled study. J Am Acad Child Adolesc Psychiatry 2004;43(11):1397–405.
52. March J, Silva S, Vitiello B, et al. The treatment study for adolescents with depression study (tads): methods and message at 12 weeks. J Am Acad Child Adolesc Psychiatry 2006;45(12):1393–403.
53. March J, Silva S, Petrycki S, et al. Fluoxetine, cognitive-behavioral therapy, and their combination for adolescents with depression: treatment for adolescents with depression study (TADS) randomized controlled trial. JAMA 2004;292(7):807–20.
54. March J, Silva S, Petrycki S, et al. The treatment for adolescents with depression study (TADS). Arch Gen Psychiatry 2007;64(10):1132–44.
55. Brent D, Emslie G, Clarke G, et al. Switching to another SSRI or to venlafaxine with or without cognitive behavioral therapy for adolescents with SSRI-resistant depression: the TORDIA randomized controlled trial. JAMA 2008;299(23): 901–13.
56. Libby A, Brent D, Morrato E, et al. Decline in treatment of pediatric depression after FDA advisory on risk of suicidality with SSRIs. Am J Psychiatry 2007;164(6):884–91.
57. Brent D. Antidepressants and pediatric depression—the risk of doing nothing. N Engl J Med 2004;351(16):1598–601.
58. Cheung A, Zuckerbrot R, Jensen P, et al. Guidelines for adolescent depression in primary care (GLAD-PC): II. Treatment and ongoing management. Pediatrics 2007;120(5):1313–26.
59. McClellan J, Kowatch R, Findling R, et al. Practice parameter for the assessment and treatment of children and adolescents with bipolar disorder. J Am Acad Child Adolesc Psychiatry 2007;46(1):107–25.
60. Findling R, Gracious B, McNamara N, et al. Rapid, continuous cycling and psychiatric co-morbidity in pediatric bipolar 1 disorder. Bipolar Disord 2001;3: 202–10.

61. Smarty S, Findling R. Psychopharmacology of pediatric bipolar disorder: a review. Psychopharmacology 2007;191:39–54.

62. Findling R, Frazier J, Kafantaris V, et al. The collaborative lithium trials (CoLT): specific aims, methods, and implementation. Child Adolesc Psychiatry Ment Health. 2008;2(21).

63. Kafantaris V, Coletti D, Dicker R, et al. Lithium treatment of acute mania in adolescents: a placebo-controlled discontinuation study. J Am Acad Child Adolesc Psychiatry 2004;43(8):984–93.

64. Kafantaris V, Coletti D, Dicker R, et al. Lithium treatment of acute mania in adolescents: a large open trial. J Am Acad Child Adolesc Psychiatry 2003;42(9): 1038–45.

65. Patel N, DelBello M, Bryan H, et al. Open-label lithium for the treatment of adolescents with bipolar depression. J Am Acad Child Adolesc Psychiatry 2006; 45(3):289–97.

66. Available at: http://bpca.nichd.nih.gov/clinical/studies/index.cfm.

67. Kowatch R, Findling, R, Schefer R, et al. Pediatric bipolar collaborative mood stabilizer trial.

68. Wagner K, Redden L, Kowatch R, et al. Safety and efficacy of Divalproex ER in youth with mania. AACAP; 2007.

69. Findling R, McNamara N, Youngstrom E, et al. Double-blind 18-month trial of lithium versus divalproex maintenance treatment in pediatric bipolar disorder. J Am Acad Child Adolesc Psychiatry 2005;44(5):409–17.

70. Ginsberg L. Carbamazepine extended-release capsules: a retrospective review of its use in children and adolescents. Ann Clin Psychiatry 2006;18(1): 3–7.

71. Weisler R, Kalali A, Ketter T, et al. A multicenter, randomized, double-blind, placebo-controlled trial of extended-release carbamazepine capsules as monotherapy for bipolar disorder patients with manic or mixed episodes. J Clin Psychiatry 2004;65:478–84.

72. Vieta E, Cruz N, Garcia J, et al. A double-blind, randomized, placebo-controlled prophylaxis trial of oxcarbazepine as adjunctive treatment to lithium in the long-term treatment of bipolar I and II disorder. Int J Neuropsychopharmacology 2008;11(4):445–52.

73. Wagner K, Kowatch R, Emslie G, et al. A double-blind, randomized, placebo-controlled trial of oxcarbazepine in the treatment of bipolar disorder in children and adolescents. Am J Psychiatry 2006;163(7):1179–86.

74. Delbello M, Findling R, Kushner S, et al. A pilot controlled trial of topiramate for mania in children and adolescents with bipolar disorder. J Am Acad Child Adolesc Psychiatry 2005;44(6):539–47.

75. Wagner K, Nyilas M, Johnson B, et al. Long-term efficacy of aripiprazole in children (10–17 years old) with mania. AACAP; 2007.

76. Correll C, Auran C, Johsnon B, et al. Safety and tolerability of aripiprazole in children (10–17) with mania. AACAP; 2007.

77. DelBello M, Findling R, Earley W, et al. Efficacy of quetiapie in children and adolescents with bipolar mania: a 3-week, double-blind, randomized, placebo-controlled trial.

78. Pandina G, DelBello M, Kushner S, et al. Risperidone for the treatment of acute mania in bipolar youth. AACAP; 2007.

79. DelBello M, Findling R, Wang P, et al. Efficacy and safety of ziprasidone in pediatric bipolar disorder. APA Annual Meeting, 2008.

80. Tohen M, Kryzhanovskaya L, Carlson G, et al. Olanzapine versus placebo in the treatment of adolescents with bipolar mania. Am J Psychiatry 2007;164(10):1547–56.
81. Williams T, Miller B. Pharmacologic management of anxiety disorders in children and adolescents. Curr Opin Pediatr 2003;15:483–90.
82. Connoly S, Bernstein G, Work Group on Quality Issues. Practice parameter for the assessment and treatment of children and adolescents with anxiety disorders. J Am Acad Child Adolesc Psychiatry 2007;46(2):267–83.
83. Birmaher B, Axelson D, Monk K, et al. Fluoxetine for the treatment of childhood anxiety disorders. J Am Acad Child Adolesc Psychiatry 2003;42(4):415–23.
84. Clark D, Birmaher B, Axelson D, et al. Fluoxetine for the treatment of childhood anxiety disorders: open-label, long-term extension to a controlled trial. J Am Acad Child Adolesc Psychiatry 2005;44(12):1263–70.
85. Cheer S, Figgit D. Spotlight on fluvoxamine in anxiety disorders in children and adolescents. Paediatr Drugs 2001;3(10):763–81.
86. Research Unit on Pediatric Psychopharmacology Anxiety Study Group (RUPP). Fluvoxamine for the treatment of anxiety disorders in children and adolescents. N Engl J Med 2001;344(17):1279–85.
87. Rynn M, Siqueland L, Rickels K, et al. Placebo-controlled trial of sertraline in the treatment of children with generalized anxiety disorder. Am J Psychiatry 2001; 158(12):2008–14.
88. Wagner K, Berard R, Stein M, et al. A multicenter, randomized, double-blind, placebo-controlled trial of paroxetine in children and adolescents with social anxiety disorder. Arch Gen Psychiatry 2004;61:1153–62.
89. March J, Entusah R, Rynn M, et al. A randomized controlled trial of venlafaxine ER versus placebo in pediatric social anxiety disorder. Biol Psychiatry 2007;62: 1149–54.
90. Rynn M, Riddle M, Yeung P, et al. Efficacy and safety of extended-release venlafaxine in the treatment of generalized anxiety disorder in children and adolescents: two placebo-controlled trials. Am J Psychiatry 2007;164:290–300.
91. ClinicalTrials.gov.
92. Riddle M, Reeve E, Yaryura-Tobias J, et al. Fluvoxamine for children and adolescents with obsessive-compulsive disorder: a randomized, controlled, multicenter trial. J Am Acad Child Adolesc Psychiatry 2001;40(2):222–9.
93. Geller D, Wagner K, Emslie G, et al. Paroxetine treatment in children and adolescents with obsessive-compulsive disorder: a randomized, multicenter, double-blind, placebo-controlled trial. J Am Acad Child Adolesc Psychiatry 2004;43(11):1387–96.
94. Cook E, Wagner K, March J, et al. Long-term sertraline treatment of children and adolescents with obsessive-compulsive disorder. J Am Acad Child Adolesc Psychiatry 2001;40(10):1175–81.
95. March J, Biederman J, Wolkow R, et al. Sertraline in children and adolescents with obsessive-compulsive disorder: a multicenter randomized controlled trial. JAMA 1998;280(20):1752–6.
96. March J, Foa E, Gammon P, et al. Cognitive-behavior therapy, sertraline, and their combination for children and adolescents with obsessive-compulsive disorder; the pediatric OCD treatment study (POTS) randomized controlled trial. JAMA 2004;292(16):1969–76.
97. Freeman J, Garcia A, Fucci C, et al. Family-based treatment of early-onset obsessive-compulsive disorder. J Child Adolesc Psychopharmacol 2003; 13(Suppl 1):571–80.

98. Perrin S, Smith P, Yule W, et al. Practitioner review: the assessment and treatment of post-traumatic stress disorder in children and adolescents. J Child Psychol Psychiatry 2000;41(3):277–89.

99. Seedat S, Stein D, Ziervogel C, et al. Comparison of response to a selective serotonin reuptake inhibitor in children, adolescents, and adults with posttraumatic stress disorder. J Child Adolesc Psychopharm 2002;12(1):37–46.

100. Porter D, Bell D. The use of clonidine in post-traumatic stress disorder. J Natl Med Assoc. 1999;91(8):475–7.

101. Harmon R, Riggs P. Clonidine for posttraumatic stress disorder in preschool children. J Am Acad Child Adolesc Psychiatry 1996;35(9):1247–9.

102. Lustig S, Botelho C, Lynch L, et al. Implementing a randomized clinical trial on a pediatric psychiatric inpatient unit at a children's hospital: the case of clonidine for post-traumatic stress. Gen Hosp Psychiatry 2002;24:422–9.

103. Stathis S, Martin G, McKenna J, et al. A preliminary case series on the use of quetiapine for posttraumatic stress disorder in juveniles within a youth detention center. J Clin Psychopharmacol 2005;25(6):539–44.

104. Famular R, Kinscherff R, Fenton T, et al. Propanolol treatment for childhood posttraumatic stress disorder, acute type. A pilot study. Am J Dis Child 1988; 142(11):1244–7.

105. Diler R. Panic disorder in children and adolescents. Yonsei Med J 2003;44(1): 174–9.

106. Renaud J, Birmaher B, Wassick S, et al. Use of selective serotonin reuptake inhibitors for the treatment of childhood panic disorder: a pilot study. J Child Adolesc Psychopharm 1999;9(2):73–83.

107. Leskovec T, Rowles B, Findling R, et al. Pharmacological treatment options for autism spectrum disorders in children and adolescents. Harv Rev Psychiatry 2008;16(2):97–112.

108. Aman M. Treatment planning for patients with autism spectrum disorders. J Clin Psychiatry 2005;66(Suppl 10):38–45.

109. McDougle C, Kresch L, Posey D, et al. Repetitive thoughts and behaviors in pervasive developmental disorders: treatment with serotonin reuptake inhibitors. J Autism Dev Disord 2000;30(5):427–35.

110. Cook E, Rowlett R, Jaselskis C, et al. Fluoxetine treatment of children and adults with autistic disorder and mental retardation. J Am Acad Child Adolesc Psychiatry 1992;31(4):739–45.

111. Hollander E, Phillips A, Chaplin W, et al. A placebo controlled crossover trial of liquid fluoxetine on repetitive behaviors in childhood and adolescent autism. Neuropsychopharm 2005;30:582–9.

112. Steingard R, Zimnitzky B, DeMaso D, et al. Sertraline treatment of transition-associated anxiety and agitation in children with autistic disorder. J Child Adolesc Psychopharm Springfielder 1997;7(1):9–15.

113. Hellings J, Kelley L, Gabrielli W, et al. Sertraline response in adults with mental retardation and autistic disorder. J Clin Psychiatry 1996;57(8):333–6.

114. Owley T, Walton L, Sat J, et al. An open-label trial of escitalopram in pervasive developmental disorders. J Am Acad Child Adolesc Psychiatry 2005;44(4): 343–8.

115. Namerow L, Thomas P, Bostic J, et al. Use of citalopram in pervasive developmental disorders. J Dev Behav Pediatr 2003;24(2):104–8.

116. Reminton G, Sloman L, Konstantareas M, et al. Clomipramine versus haloperidol in the treatment of autistic disorder: a double-blind, placebo-controlled, crossover study. J Clin Psychopharm 2001;21(4):440–4.

117. Sanches L, Campbell M, Small A, et al. A pilot study of clomipramine in young autistic children. J Am Acad Child Adolesc Psychiatry 1996;35(4):537–44.
118. DiMartino A, Melis G, Ciancehetti C, et al. Methylphenidate for pervasive developmental disorders: safety and efficacy of acute single dose test and ongoing therapy: an open-pilot study. J Child Adolesc Psychopharm 2004;14(2):207–18.
119. Handen B, Johnson C, Lubetsky M, et al. Efficacy of methylphenidate among children with autism and symptoms of attention-deficit hyperactivity disorder. J Autism Dev Disord 2000;30(3):245–55.
120. Research Units on Pediatric Psychopharmacology (RUPP). Randomized, Controlled, Crossover Trial of Methylphenidate in Pervasive Developmental Disorders with Hyperactivity.
121. Volkmar F, Cohen D, Hoshino Y, et al. Phenomenology and classification of the childhood psychoses. Psychol Med 1988;18(1):191–201.
122. Campbell M, Fish B, David R, et al. Response to triiodothyronine and dextroamphetamine: a study of preschool schizophrenic children. J Autism Child Schizophr 1972;2(4):343–58.
123. Campbell M, Small A, Collins P, et al. Levodopa and levoamphetamine: a crossover study in young schizophrenic children. Curr Ther Res Clin Exp 1976;19(1):70–86.
124. Fankhauser M, Karumanchi V, German M, et al. A double-blind, placebo-controlled study of the efficacy of transdermal clonidine in children. J Clin Psychiatry 1992;53(3):77–82.
125. Jaselskis C, Cook E, Fletcher K, et al. Clonidine treatment of hyperactive and impulsive children with autistic disorder. J Clin Psychopharmacol 1992;12(5):322–7.
126. Posey D, Puntney J, Sasher T, et al. Guanfacine treatment of hyperactivity and inattention in pervasive developmental disorders: a retrospective analysis of 80 cases. J Child Adolesc Psychopharm 2004;14(2):233–41.
127. Scahill L, Aman M, McDougle C, et al. A prospective open trial of guanfacine in children with pervasive developmental disorders. J Child Adolesc Psychopharm 2006;16(5):589–98.
128. Research Units on Pediatric Psychopharmacology Autism Network (RUPP). Risperidone treatment of autistic disorder: longer-term benefits and blinded discontinuation after 6 months. Am J Psychiatry 2005;162(7):1361–9.
129. McDougle C, Scahill L, Aman M, et al. Risperidone for the core symptom domains of autism: results from the study by the autism network of the research units on pediatric psychopharmacology. Am J Psychiatry 2005;162(6):1142–8.
130. Aman M, Arnold E, McDougle C, et al. Acute and long-term safety and tolerability of risperidone in children with autism. J Child Adolesc Psychopharm 2005;15(6):869–84.
131. Findling R, McNamara N, Gracious B, et al. Quetiapine in nine youths with autistic disorder. J Child Adolesc Psychopharm 2004;14(2):287–94.
132. Martin A, Koenig K, Scahill L, et al. Open-label quetiapine in the treatment of children and adolescents with autistic disorder. J Child Adolesc Psychopharm 1999;9(2):99–107.
133. Hollander E, Wasserman S, Swanson E, et al. A double-blind placebo-controlled pilot study of olanzapine in childhood/adolescent pervasive developmental disorder. J Child Adolesc Psychopharm 2006;16(5):541–8.
134. Kemner C, Willemsen S, deJonge M, et al. Open-label study of olanzapine in children with pervasive developmental disorder. J Clin Psychopharm 2002;22(5):455–60.

135. Malone R, Cater J, Sheikh R, et al. Olanzapine versus haloperidol in children with autistic disorder: an open pilot study. J Am Acad Child Adolesc Psychiatry 2001;40(8):887–94.

136. Duggal H. Ziprasidone for maladaptive behavior and attention-deficit/hyperactivity disorder symptoms in autistic disorder. J Child Adolesc Psychopharm 2007;17(2):261–3.

137. Cohen S, Fitzgerald B, Khan S, et al. The effect of a switch to ziprasidone in an adult population with autistic disorder: chart review of naturalistic, open-label treatment. J Clin Psychiatry 2004;65:110–3.

138. McDougle C, Kem D, Posey D, et al. Case series: use of ziprasidone for maladaptive symptoms in youths with autism. J Am Acad Child Adolesc Psychiatry 2002;41(8):921–7.

139. Valicenti M, Demb H. Clinical effects and adverse reactions of off-label use of aripiprazole in children and adolescents with developmental disabilities. J Child Adolesc Psychopharm 2006;16(5):549–60.

140. Shastri M, Alla L, Sabaratnam M, et al. Aripiprazole use in individuals with intellectual disability and psychotic or behavioral disorders: a case series. J Psychopharm 2006;20(6):863–7.

141. Hardan A, Jou R, Handen B, et al. A retrospective assessment of topiramate in children and adolescents with pervasive developmental disorders. J Child and Adolesc Psychopharm 2004;14(3):426–32.

142. Posey D, Kern D, Swiezy N, et al. A pilot study of D-cycloserine in subjects with autistic disorder. Am J Psychiatry 2004;161(11):2115–7.

143. Danfors T, von Knorring A, Hartvig P, et al. Tetrahydrobiopterin in the treatment of children with autistic disorder. J Clin Psychopharm 2005;25(5):485–9.

144. Kumra S, Oberstar J, Sikich L, et al. Efficacy and tolerability of second-generation antipsychotics in children and adolescents with schizophrenia. Schizophrenia Bulletin 2008;34(1):60–71.

145. Correll C. Assessing and maximizing the safety and tolerability of antipsychotics used in the treatment of children and adolescents. J Clin Psychiatry 2008; 69(Suppl 4):26–36.

146. Thomas L, Woods S. The schizophrenia prodrome: a developmentally informed review and update for psychopharmacologic treatment. Child Adolesc Psychiatr Clin N Am 2006;15:109–33.

147. Sikich L, Frazier J, McLellan J, et al. Double-blind comparison of first- and second-generation antipsychotics in early-onset schizophrenia and schizoaffective disorder: findings from the treatment of early-onset schizophrenia spectrum disorders (TEOSS) study. Am J Psychiatry 2008;AiA:1–13.

148. Spencer E, Kafantaris V, Padron-Gayol M, et al. Haloperidol in schizophrenic children: early findings from a study in progress. Psychopharmacol Bull 1992; 28(2):183–6.

149. Pool D, Bloom W, Mielki D, et al. A controlled evaluation of loxitane in seventy-five adolescent schizophrenic patients. Curr Ther Res Clin Exp 1976;19(1):99–104.

150. Realmuto G, Erickson W, Yellin A, et al. Clinical comparison of thiothixene and thioridazine in schizophrenic adolescents. Am J Psychiatry 1984;141(3):440–2.

151. Bishop J, Pavuluri M. Review of risperidone for the treatment of pediatric and adolescent bipolar disorder and schizophrenia. Neuropsychiatr Dis Treat 2008;4(1):55–68.

152. Armenteros J, Whitaker A, Welikson M, et al. Risperidone in adolescents with schizophrenia: an open pilot study. Am J Acad Child Adolesc Psychiatry 1997;36(5):694–700.

153. Mozes T, Ebert T, Michal S, et al. An open-label comparison of olanzapine versus risperidone in the treatment of childhood-onset schizophrenia. J Child Adolesc Psychopharmacol 2006;16(4):393–403.
154. Zalsman G, Carmon E, Martin A, et al. Effectiveness, safety, and tolerability of risperidone in adolescents with schizophrenia: an open-label study. J Child Adolesc Psychopharmacol 2003;13(3):319–27.
155. Gothelf D, Apter A, Reidman J, et al. Olanzapine, risperidone, and haloperidol in the treatment of adolescent patients with schizophrenia. J Neural Transm 2003; 110(5):545–60.
156. van Bruggen J, Tijseen J, Dingemans P, et al. Symptom response and side-effects of olanzapine and risperidone in young adults with recent onset schizophrenia. Int Clin Psychopharmacol 2003;18(6):341–6.
157. Findling R, Robb A, Nyilas M, et al. A multiple-center, randomized, double-blind, placebo-controlled study of oral aripiprazole for treatment of adolescents with schizophrenia. Am J Psychiatry 2008;AiA:1–10.
158. Kushner S, Unis A, Copenhaver M, et al. Acute and continuous efficacy and safety of risperidone in adolescents with schizophrenia. AACAP; 2007.
159. Kryzhanovskaya L, Schulz C, McDougle C, et al. Efficacy and safety of olanzapine in adolescents with schizophrenia: results from a double-blind, placebo-controlled trial. Presented at the 44th College of Neuropsychopharmacology.
160. Kranzler H, Kester H, Gerbino-Rosen G, et al. Treatment-refractory schizophrenia in children and adolescents: an update on clozapine and other pharmacologic interventions. Child Adolesc Psychiatr Clin N Am 2006;15:135–59.
161. Kumra S, Kranzler H, Gerbino-Rosen G, et al. Clozapine and "high-dose" olanzapine in refractory early-onset schizophrenia: a 12-week randomized and double blind comparison. Biol Psychiatry 2008;63(5):524–9.
162. Kumra S, Frazier J, Jacobsen L, et al. Childhood onset schizophrenia. A double-blind clozapine-haloperidol comparison. Arch Gen Psychiatry 1996;53(12): 1090–7.
163. Shaw P, Sporn A, Gogtay N, et al. Childhood Onset Schizophrenia. A double-blind clozapine-olanzapine comparison. Arch Gen Psychiatry 2006;63:721–30.

The Wraparound Approach in Systems of Care

Nancy C. Winters, MD[a],*, W. Peter Metz, MD[b]

KEYWORDS

- Wraparound • Systems of care • Family-driven care
- Youth-guided care • Strengths-based planning

Child and adolescent psychiatrists and general psychiatrists who serve children and adolescents with complex mental health needs, generally find themselves interfacing with multiple child-serving systems, including mental health, child welfare, juvenile justice, developmental disabilities, addictions services, and primary health care. In these systems of care, psychiatrists will likely encounter the term "wraparound," which describes a key intervention ushered in with the system-of-care model of service delivery. To effectively integrate and coordinate psychiatric interventions with other services provided in the system of care, psychiatrists should become familiar with the wraparound approach. This article describes wraparound's historical context, philosophy, procedures, and the evidence supporting its effectiveness.

HISTORICAL CONTEXT

To understand the wraparound approach, it is helpful to review the context in which it was created and continues to flourish. Over the past 25 years there has been a major paradigm shift in the philosophy and organization of services for the estimated 4.5 to 6.3 million children and adolescents in the United States with serious emotional and behavioral disorders and their families.[1] In the 1960s through the 1980s, several reports documented a disorganized and fragmented system that was grossly failing these children.[2,3] Services in their communities were largely unavailable, resulting in frequent placement in out-of-state residential facilities. In response to these reports, the federal government established the Child and Adolescent Service System Program (CASSP) under the auspices of the National Institutes of Mental Health. CASSP articulated core values and guiding principles for a system of care for children and adolescents with severe emotional disturbance. These principles have served as

[a] Department of Psychiatry, Oregon Health & Science University, 3181 SW Sam Jackson Park Road OP02, Portland, OR 97239-3098, USA
[b] Division of Child and Adolescent Psychiatry, University of Massachusetts Medical Center, 55 Lake Avenue North, Worcester, MA 01655, USA
* Corresponding author.
E-mail address: winterna@ohsu.edu (N.C. Winters).

Psychiatr Clin N Am 32 (2009) 135–151
doi:10.1016/j.psc.2008.11.007
0193-953X/08/$ – see front matter © 2009 Published by Elsevier Inc.

psych.theclinics.com

a template for the evolution of child-serving systems across the nation targeting this population. The system-of-care framework developed by CASSP is defined as a comprehensive spectrum of mental health and other services and supports organized into a coordinated network to meet the diverse and changing needs of children and adolescents with severe emotional disorders and their families.[4] The major emphases of the CASSP principles are: (1) individualized care that recognizes strengths in the child, family and community and is tailored to the individual needs and preferences of the child and family; (2) family inclusion at every level of the clinical process and system development; (3) collaboration and coordination between different child-serving agencies and integration of services across agencies; (4) provision of culturally competent services; and (5) serving youth in their communities, or the least-restrictive setting that meets their clinical needs, using natural supports in the community whenever possible.

In 1992 the federal Center for Mental Health Services (CMHS), part of the Substance Abuse and Mental Health Services Administration (SAMHSA), made the largest investment to date in children's mental health services when they established the Comprehensive Community Services for Children and Youth and Their Families. Through this initiative, CMHS has funded over 100 6-year demonstration projects in diverse communities in all 50 states, as well as Native American tribes and United States territories, to implement systems-of-care programs, which must include a wraparound approach to service planning for children and adolescents with serious emotional disturbance and their families. The goals of these programs have been to implement CASSP values, provide a broad array of individualized, family-centered, and community-based services, and ensure the full involvement of families in the care of their children and development of local services. Specific performance measures defined by CMHS for the system-of-care grants, include: (1) increased interagency collaboration as measured by referrals from nonmental health agencies; (2) decreased use of in-patient or residential treatment by 20%; (3) improved child outcomes in areas such as school attendance and law-enforcement contacts; (4) decreased overall functional impairment of youth; (5) increased family satisfaction with services; (6) increased stability of living arrangements; and (7) decreased levels of family stress.[5]

Extensive data from the nationwide outcomes evaluation of this CMHS initiative indicates that system-of-care programs have reduced the number of hospital and out-of-home residential placements, improved school performance, improved youths' behavioral and emotional functioning, reduced violations of the law, and provided more services to children and families who need them.[6] These outcomes have supported continually increasing congressional appropriations for the program, from an initial appropriation of $5 million to the current appropriation of over $100 million.

Implementation of system-of-care values and principles has also been promoted in several states by class action law suits that were settled with consent decrees or, most recently in Massachusetts, with a judgment requiring availability of intensive home and community-based services, including the wraparound approach, to eligible children and their families, with support from federal Medicaid funding. However, the experience in many of these states is that without enactment of legislation mandating these services, the systems of care developed by these states reverted to a pre-suit level once federal court oversight ended.

Implicit within its public health orientation, system-of-care methodology has a place in preventive efforts, especially for young at-risk children. Nevertheless, the primary target population continues to be children and adolescents with "serious emotional disturbance." The CMHS definition of serious emotional disturbance (SED) stipulates that the child or adolescent has a mental or emotional disturbance listed in the

Diagnostic and Statistical manual of Mental Disorders,[7] which must be associated with significant functional impairments interfering with major life domains, such as home, school, and community. Children with SED who are served in systems of care generally require the services of two or more child-serving agencies, such as mental health, education, juvenile justice, child welfare, or developmental disabilities. Therefore, coordination among different providers is critically important.

The goal of serving these youth more effectively in their communities and allowing them to maintain their relationships with families, schools, and neighbors is a central goal of systems of care. To that end, community-based treatment and supports are provided to the child or youth and family, often in the home, to enable the youth to stay at home. These include an array of individualized services, such as respite, mobile crisis services, crisis shelter care, intensive home-based services, skills-building, and mentoring, among others (**Box 1**).

The move away from out-of-home residential treatment toward community-based services has received support from a number of sources, including the limited effectiveness of hospital and residential treatment,[9] advocacy from family organizations such as the Federation of Families for Children's Mental Health (FFCMH),[10] and promising outcomes of home- and community-based interventions.[11,12] Additionally, it

---

Box 1
The range of community-based services that may be included in a system of care[8]

Case management (service coordination)

Community-based in-patient psychiatric care

Counseling (individual, group, and youth)

Crisis residential care

Crisis outreach teams

Day treatment

Education/special education services

Family support

Health services

Independent living supports

Intensive family-based counseling (in the home)

Legal services

Protection and advocacy

Psychiatric consultation

Recreation therapy

Residential treatment

Respite care

Self-help or support groups

Small therapeutic group care

Therapeutic foster care

Transportation

Tutoring

Vocational counseling

stands to reason that separating young people from their families to receive treatment makes it unlikely that problems in the home context will be addressed adequately, with the result that they may resurface after discharge.[13]

The system-of-care model places the child and family at the center of the clinical process and as full partners at all levels of system planning.[14,15] Through federal support and technical assistance to family advocacy organizations, such as the FFCMH and National Association for the Mentally Ill, the concept of "family-driven care" was developed and it is now a cornerstone of systems of care. Family-driven, as defined by the FFCMH,[16] means that families have a primary decision-making role in the care of their own children, as well as the policies and procedures governing care for all children in their community, state, tribe, territory, and nation. Family-driven care has had a significant influence on national policy for both child and adult mental health[9] and was embraced by the President's New Freedom Commission, which has as one of its six major goals that mental health care is consumer and family-driven.[17]

The concept of consumer- and family-driven care has been expanded to include youth-guided care, which allows youth to provide meaningful guidance to mental health professionals based on their own experience as recipients of services.[18] "Youth-guided," as defined by SAMHSA,[19] means that youth have the right to be empowered, educated, and given a decision-making role in the care of their own lives, as well as the policies and procedures governing the care of all youth in the community, state, and nation. Youth voice is being developed by a national organization Youth M.O.V.E. (Motivating Others through Voices of Experience). Youth M.O.V.E.[20] was organized with the support of CMHS to improve services that support positive growth and development by uniting the voices of youth and young adults who have lived experience in various systems, including mental health, juvenile justice, education, and child welfare. Guidelines for family-driven and youth-guided care guidelines call for families and youth to be given complete information and included in all decision-making about their care.

WHAT IS "WRAPAROUND"?

"Wraparound," coined in North Carolina,[21] is an approach that incorporates the guiding principles and values of CASSP and has evolved into a well-described and widely applied intervention. Wraparound is a definable planning process that results in a unique set of community services and natural supports that are individualized for a child and family to achieve a positive set of outcomes.[22] Services are "wrapped around" the child and family in their natural environments. The wraparound planning process is child- and family-centered, builds on child and family strengths, is community-based (using a balance of formal and informal supports), is culturally relevant, flexible, and coordinated across agencies; it is outcome driven, and provides unconditional care.[23] The term "wraparound" has intuitive appeal and has entered the lexicon of most child-serving clinicians and agencies. There is sometimes confusion about whether wraparound refers to the services themselves or the planning process, but over the years wraparound has been operationalized as a planning process with core elements. An emerging consensus on wraparound includes the following ten essential elements:[22,23,24,25]

> Efforts are based in the community.
> Wraparound must be a team-driven process involving the family, child, natural supports, agencies, and community services working together to develop, implement, and evaluate the individualized plan.

Families must be full and active partners at every level of the wraparound process.

Services and supports must be individualized, built on strengths, and meet the needs of children and families across life domains to promote success, safety, and permanence in home, school, and community.

The process must be culturally competent, building on unique values, preferences, and strengths of children and families, and their communities.

Wraparound child and family teams must have flexible approaches and adequate flexible funding.

Wraparound plans must include a balance of formal services and informal community and family supports.

There must be an unconditional commitment to serve children and their families.

The plans should be developed and implemented based on an interagency, community-based, collaborative process.

Outcomes must be determined and measured for the individual child, for the program, and for the system.

How Wraparound Works

The wraparound process is a specific model of an individualized, family-driven and youth-guided team planning process. Through the team process, the child and family drive care planning by determining an overall vision of how the family will know when things are better; the composition of the team (unless custody lies with child welfare, in which case child welfare must have a place on the team); goals and desired outcomes of services regarding specific needs; evaluating the effectiveness of services; and having a meaningful role in all decisions, including those that impact funding of services. Empowering families and youth as drivers of the team process provides them an experience of "voice and choice," in which their goals, preferences, needs, and strengths guide all efforts. The personal expertise the family has about itself and its community is viewed as equally important to the expertise that professionals on the team have about their respective disciplines and agencies. Full inclusion of the youth and family as partners in the team process is expressed by the core concept "nothing about us without us."[26] It means that no decisions are made about care plans without parent or caregiver participation, but does not preclude communications between team members that do not include the family.

While the child and family are the driving forces of the team in that care plans generated by the team ultimately must be approved by the family, the generation of options to meet identified needs and the implementation of options selected in the child's care plan occurs through the team process. The team is facilitated by a care coordinator or care manager, and frequently there is also a paid family partner or family support specialist, who helps support family engagement and voice in the planning process. The family partner is a person who has experience raising a youth with SED and often is a person who comes from a similar cultural background as the family. The care coordinator and family partner have a primary responsibility to support a "no shame, no blame" atmosphere in the team meetings, in which mutual respect is actively modeled and recrimination and disrespect between team members is actively discouraged.

The team process facilitates interagency and interdisciplinary collaboration. An atmosphere of collaboration and shared goals helps promote a sense of hopefulness in families; this is in contrast to augmented hopelessness in families, often created by uncoordinated and even conflicting agency mandates and service plans. The complementary contributions of various team members function synergistically in identifying system and community resources to promote better outcomes. The team is able to determine who can be most effective to work toward each of the goals and assigns appropriate responsibility and accountability. Use of a strengths-based orientation and discussion of needs rather than problems is less stigmatizing and promotes more active engagement of families and youth in service-planning activities. Individualization of the care plan is emphasized by the fact that if a plan is not successful in achieving its goals, the expectation is that the plan was flawed and needs revision, not that the family is "noncompliant" and should be ejected as having failed the process. Furthermore, rather than being driven by priorities and limited service menus of the categorical agencies (education, child welfare, juvenile justice, and other agencies), the child and family team has access to a broad array of home- and community-based supports, such as home-based therapy, respite and mentoring services, and the like.

Interventions designed to reinforce strengths of the child or youth and family may include nontraditional therapies, such as specific skills training or mentored work experiences that remediate or offset areas of challenge. For example, a youth at risk for substance abuse might receive funding for prosocial activities, such as a health club membership or computer training. These interventions generally are not included in traditional categorical mental health funding and may require flexible funds that are not assigned to specific service types. Thus, the wraparound planning process must have access to flexible, noncategorical funding. Such funds should be available for addressing individual needs other than formal treatment needs (eg, assistance with housing). Within limits, the child and family team has authority to approve expenditures of flexible funds. The care coordinator has responsibility to remind the team of explicit guidelines regarding acceptable uses of flexible funding (eg, flexible funds are spent after other mechanisms are explored, with a clear relationship to improving the mental health of the child, and with a plan for long-term sustainability).

Wraparound is fundamentally not a clinical treatment but rather a team-based planning process, although it always needs to include clinical support, and the wraparound process itself is often psychotherapeutic in promoting increased self-esteem and adaptive functioning in the child and family. It has been noted that services are more likely to be effective if the wraparound process is informed by comprehensive clinical assessment addressing diagnostic and treatment issues, and if the specific interventions are evidence-based[27,28,29] and, above all, culturally relevant and able to promote sustained engagement of the family with the involved community-based supports.

A comprehensive description of the formal wraparound process has been recently summarized.[25] Four phases are described, including engagement and team preparation, with discovery of the strengths and needs of the child or youth and family; initial plan development by the team; plan implementation; and transition to address needs in additional domains (eg, school, behavior, housing, and so forth).

An important role in wraparound is that of the "parent partner," also called "family partner" or "family navigator." Parent partners provide critical peer support to parents and caregivers of youth receiving services. Parent partners are individuals whose own children have been through the service system and are able to share their own stories and knowledge of how to navigate the system. They provide culturally sensitive, nonjudgmental support to the family to help increase family involvement and serve as liaisons with professionals to decrease unintentional bias toward parents. Federal Medicaid has approved waivers in several State Medicaid plans to support payment of family partners as a medically necessary support.

A significant number of youth with SED served in systems of care are either in foster care or other out-of-home placements,[11] and consequently their most important relationships with family members may have been interrupted or even severed. Wraparound programs are increasingly striving to expand a youth's network of supportive relationships by using family searching methods that have become frequent in child-welfare systems. Rather than assuming that children have no family, wraparound teams work to locate extended family members who have lost contact with the youth or were unaware that he or she was in foster care. They are invited to become involved in case planning with the youth, and explore the possibility of creating more meaningful relationships that can endure, especially as formal services decrease. Expansion of the youth and family's network of supportive relationships is believed to be one of the most positive aspects of wraparound (Galloway A, personal communication, 2008). Another important value of wraparound is to provide positive support structures for the child or youth to help them find a place where they fit in and can be part of a community.[30]

Another important aspect of wraparound is the use of "natural" or "informal" community-based supports. These can be as varied as the communities in which the youth and family live. They include extended family, friends, the faith-based community, boys and girls clubs, teachers, neighbors, and other resources. A goal of wraparound is to move toward replacing formal supports as the means of addressing the needs of the child and family with informal supports as much as possible. Informal supports interface with professional services, and all services and supports are combined into a single care plan with clearly defined goals. The team is progressively constituted by individuals providing informal support. Participation of a professional on a child and family team does not require attendance at a team meeting. Professionals can be team members and participate in the team process via meetings and other communications held with the youth and family and care coordinator outside of the regular team meetings.

WRAPAROUND CASE ILLUSTRATIONS
Case #1

Juan is a 13-year-old Hispanic boy who lives with his mother, younger half brother, and stepfather. Juan has a diagnosis of attention deficit hyperactivity disorder (ADHD), combined type, severe, and oppositional defiant disorder. He was referred by his school for the wraparound service-planning program because of significant discipline problems at school, including some instances of aggression toward other students and teachers. Juan's mother and stepfather speak little English. His mother had previous involvement with child welfare, when Juan was younger, because of domestic violence in the home, and Juan was briefly placed in foster care until his birth father left the home. Juan's parents are suspicious of professionals and fear reinvolvement of child welfare. Furthermore, they have not been willing to consider a trial of medication for his ADHD as recommended by his pediatrician, primarily because Juan's stepfather does not believe in medicine for behavior problems. Other efforts to engage the family in treatment were also unsuccessful. When he enrolled in wraparound, Juan had been suspended from school twice.

Juan's mother reluctantly agreed to consider enrollment in Coordinated Family Focused Care, a wraparound child and family team-planning process that involves work with a parent partner and a care coordinator to create a child and family team, in partnership with the family, to help Juan function better at school. Juan's mother established some trust with the parent partner assigned to work with her because the parent partner had a similar cultural background, spoke Spanish as her first language, and had her own history of caring for a child with serious mental health issues.

In the course of the initial strengths and culture discovery, Juan noted that he liked to draw and said he was interested in becoming an artist when he grows up. He did especially well in art last year, in the 7th grade, when he got an A and had a very positive relationship with his art teacher. Early in the team planning process, furthering Juan's interest in art was identified as a primary goal. Flexible funding through the program was made available to pay for drawing lessons at the local art museum. However, there was concern that without a mentor to support his effort in the art classes, there was a high likelihood that oppositional and defiant behavior could result in Juan being asked to leave the class. His art teacher from the previous year was invited to participate on the child and family team. She came to a team meeting and agreed to accompany Juan to his art lessons for a nominal stipend, again paid for with flexible funding assigned to the program.

Juan had a dramatic response to taking the art lessons. A drawing he did received an award and was displayed in the art museum, which was a source of much pride for Juan, his mother, and his stepfather. Nevertheless, his difficulties in school continued. In the context of success with the art class and the emerging trusting relationship that Juan's parents had with the parent partner and care coordinator, they were willing to have a consultation with the child psychiatrist providing support to the program, especially as the parent partner offered to attend with the parents and provide support with translation. After reconfirming the diagnosis of ADHD and listening to the concerns about medicines voiced by the parents, the child psychiatrist provided information about the evidence supporting the benefit of medication. With additional support from the child and family team, including the pastor of their church, Juan's parents agreed to a trial of Concerta. There was an immediate benefit in both Juan's grades and behavior. He was thrilled, as were his parents.

Case # 2

Celia is a 17-year-old young woman who entered a wraparound project when she was 15 years old. As a child, she was removed from her parents' care because of neglect and subsequently was placed in a series of foster homes, without finding a successful long-term placement. She started having behavioral problems in early adolescence. Because of her mood difficulties, self-harming behaviors, inability to function in school, substance abuse, runaway episodes, and periodic aggression, she entered residential treatment when she was 12 years old. She spent most of the next 3 years in different residential programs, with periodic unsuccessful attempts to return to the community. The wraparound team met her when she was in residential treatment. The initial focus of their efforts was to find a highly experienced foster family who was a good match for Celia, guided by Celia's perception of what would work for her. The family they found was able to provide structure but were clear that they were not going to overwhelm her with rigid rules, which was what Celia had hoped for. They were motivated to form a relationship with her and to be emotionally available, but they understood that because of Celia's early attachment difficulties, they should not pressure her to get too close too quickly.

To help this foster placement succeed, Celia and the foster family were provided with an array of formal and informal supports, including crisis respite services, individual therapy, home-based family therapy, and mentoring. Efforts were made immediately to contact Celia's siblings and locate members of her extended family to expand her network of support. Because Celia's foster parents understood her needs and felt supported by the wraparound team, when her family members re-entered Celia's life the foster family did not experience it as a threat and were able to be supportive. During Celia's stay with the foster family, the wraparound team helped her develop her interest in art by advocating for her to take more art courses at her high school. She also developed her interest in music and began to perform at statewide conferences and meetings. Celia and her foster family connected so well that when they moved to an adjacent state, the child welfare agency, functioning as an integral part of the wraparound team, was willing to continue to support the placement. The team was able to stay together through a number of Celia's mental health setbacks, and Celia felt that she had a personal connection with every member of the team. Celia has now graduated from the wraparound program. She continues her interest in music and has ongoing contact with her siblings and some extended family members.

THE EVIDENCE BASE ON WRAPAROUND

One limitation of the research on wraparound relates to the fact that until recently it was not well-defined operationally and its applications varied across studies. Only recently has consensus been reached about the essential elements of the wraparound as an intervention.[22,25,31] Studies on wraparound have incorporated measures, such as the Wraparound Fidelity Index (WFI),[24] to ensure fidelity to the model as defined by the National Wraparound Initiative.[31] A recent study showed that higher fidelity, as measured by the WFI, was associated with better outcomes in multiple domains.[32]

The evidence base concerning wraparound generally characterizes the approach as promising.[11,29] Positive results from three randomized, controlled trials and a number of quasi-experimental studies in different communities with diverse populations of at-risk children and families have been described. These studies have generally reported positive outcomes in terms of reduction of externalizing behavioral problems, increased level of function, reduction of out-of-home placement, improved family management skills and function, and increased consumer and family satisfaction.[33,34] However, a randomized, controlled study found no difference in clinical outcomes for wraparound versus usual treatment.[35] Another study comparing wraparound to Multi-systemic Therapy (MST; see description below) found that youth who received only MST demonstrated more improvement in clinical symptoms than those who received only wraparound over the 18-month follow-up assessment.[29] It was noted by the investigators that because wraparound plans are individualized, the wraparound group may have had a mixture of effective and ineffective treatments, while the MST intervention is more standardized.

Interestingly, although wraparound is considered a promising but not yet strongly supported intervention, it has gained widespread acceptance as a planning approach, as evidenced by CMHS's requirement that it be used in system-of-care grant projects. Its popularity is likely because of its family-driven and strengths-based philosophical orientation. With such widespread use, however, it becomes difficult to obtain approval for randomized, controlled trials. This issue parallels the widespread adoption of the system-of-care model on the strength of its philosophy and values, which has required use of quasi-experimental designs.[36,37]

COMPARISON OF WRAPAROUND TO OTHER INTENSIVE COMMUNITY-BASED INTERVENTIONS

Several other intensive community-based interventions used in systems of care have been empirically evaluated, including MST, treatment foster care, and case management.[11,12,29] It is useful to examine how these models differ from wraparound (**Table 1**).

MST is an intensive home- and community-based family treatment model for children and adolescents at risk of out-of-home placement because of serious emotional and behavioral problems.[38] Originally developed for juvenile offenders, MST has been

Table 1
Overview of some intensive community-based interventions

Intervention	Essential Features	Who Provides Services	Where Services Provided
Multisystemic therapy	• Ecological case formulation, • 24/7 crisis availability, • high fidelity	Clinical MST team (mental health clinicians/ psychiatrist)	Primarily home-based or community-based
Wraparound planning process	• Family-driven team with facilitator; • strengths-based/ use of natural supports	• Any provider selected by team; • use of parent partners and natural supports	Community, home, or clinic
Intensive case management	• Intensive individualized services with assigned case manager	Varies	Usually home or community
Treatment foster care (Oregon MTFC model)	• Highly staffed; • use of intensive behavior modification; • family trained from outset	Foster family and behavioral consultants	Foster home and community consultation

applied to youth in the child welfare system, youth at risk for psychiatric hospitalization, and violent sex offenders. MST is an intensive intervention lasting 3 to 5 months in which all services are provided by the MST team. Interventions are based on systematic assessment of all aspects of the child and family using a social ecological perspective. MST has been carefully implemented to ensure adherence to the model. There have been nine randomized trials of MST demonstrating its efficacy.[39]

The evidence base for treatment foster care as a home-based alternative to residential treatment for youths with mental health needs or antisocial behavior derives primarily from research on the Oregon Social Learning Center model, called Multidimensional Treatment Foster Care (MTFC).[40] The Oregon model includes close supervision of foster parents by experienced therapists who train them in techniques of careful monitoring of behavior and consistent application of positive reinforcement and consequences. Two randomized, controlled trials demonstrated superiority of MTFC to treatment-as-usual for juvenile justice-involved youth, and a further study favored MTFC to treatment at a state psychiatric hospital.[11,41] MTFC has also been applied successfully to troubled youth in the child welfare system and to address the needs of preschoolers with aggressive and oppositional behavior.

Case management is a common strategy used in systems of care to coordinate care and ensure access to an array of services that will meet the child and family's needs. It includes various functions to meet these needs, including assessment, service planning and implementation, service coordination and monitoring, and advocacy.[42] Case-management approaches generally incorporate a specialist case manager or care coordinator who either functions as a broker of services or has a more intensive role, providing some direct support to the child and family, such as in the Children and

Youth intensive Case Management model.[43] There have been at least four random-ized, controlled trials of case management which have generally shown positive find-ings in relation to comparison groups.[11] However, the findings are somewhat difficult to assess as a group because of the variations in intensity of case management models tested (**Table 2**).

APPLICATIONS OF WRAPAROUND

Wraparound was developed in the late 1980s and expanded in the 1990s, and subse-quently has been used as a viable alternative to residential treatment. The Kaleido-scope Project in Chicago, Wraparound Milwaukie, and the states of Alaska and Vermont initiated some of the earliest and most successful wraparound programs in the country. Current SAMHSA system-of-care grants require high-fidelity wraparound. These grant communities now include tribal communities, a new wave of early childhood grants for children ages 0 to 8 (who hadn't been included in previous sys-tem-of-care programs), and state transformation grants. There is now a substantial literature on wraparound and the National Wraparound Initiative,[31] providing informa-tion and technical support. One of the most successful wraparound programs is Wraparound Milwaukie,[34] which has been used as a model for other states in devel-oping similar initiatives. Wraparound Milwaukie was implemented with a SAMHSA grant in Milwaukee County, Wisconsin in 1995 to serve high-risk youth in the Child Welfare and Juvenile Justice Systems who were at immediate risk of placement in res-idential, hospital, or correctional settings. The program uses a wide array of commu-nity-based interventions as alternatives to out-of-home placement. Wraparound Milwaukie was able to sustain its program after the grant period by developing a unique managed care entity in which four public agencies pool funding to create maximum flexibility and sufficient funding to meet the comprehensive needs of an average of 560 culturally diverse youth and families per year.[34]

A number of states, including Vermont, Oklahoma, Oregon, Mississippi, Massachu-setts, and Arizona, among others, have implemented wraparound on a statewide basis or are in the process of doing so. As noted above, litigation has played a role in imple-mentation of wraparound, such as occurred in Arizona in the J.K. consent decree in 2001 and in the recent Rosie D. settlement in Massachusetts.[44] There are unique challenges in statewide applications of wraparound, including development of state-level administrative mechanisms for blended funding, large-scale training of the work-force in wraparound methodology, and decision-making about allocation of resources to wraparound versus other community-based models.

Another issue that arises in applications of wraparound to larger populations is selection of an appropriate target population. In Oregon's statewide Wraparound

Table 2
Levels of evidence supporting intensive community-based interventions

Community-Based Intervention	Level of Evidence
Multisystemic therapy	5
Wraparound process	3
Intensive case management	4
Multidimensional treatment foster care	4

Definitions of levels of evidence:[59] 1, not evaluated; 2, evaluated but unclear (no or possibly negative effects); 3, promising (some evidence); 4, well established; 5, better or best.

Initiative,[45] a decision was made to include children who are at risk for serious mental health issues, as well as those already identifiable as having SED, to provide the benefits of wraparound as an early intervention strategy. In this application, modifications to wraparound, such as shorter-term applications and smaller teams may be appropriate. There has been little systematic examination of what might be considered "partial applications" of wraparound. However, there could be a role for applying the principles and some components of wraparound to different populations and in different contexts. This might include, for example, team-based processes in schools[46] or child welfare family decision-making meetings.[47] Interventions partially adhering to the wraparound model include incorporation of system-of-care values and principles into traditional psychotherapy and pharmacotherapy.[27]

POTENTIAL LIMITATIONS OF WRAPAROUND

It has been suggested that wraparound, a planning process which has a good record of engaging family and community support, would benefit from being combined with the strengths of specific evidence-based approaches.[48] It is thus likely that difficulties accessing specific clinical interventions needed by the youth and family will limit the effectiveness of wraparound.[29] The national shortage of mental health therapists, and especially child and adolescent psychiatrists, creates a problem in accessing these services, especially in rural areas and for those living in poverty.[49] Child and adolescent psychiatrists, who are needed to address complex diagnostic, psycho-pharmacologic, and other treatment needs of youth with SED, have limited opportunities to participate directly in wraparound teams, even in urban areas (Hedrick L, personal communication, 2008). There may also be gaps in access to evidence-based practices that should be included in the wraparound plan.

It has been noted that wraparound requires significant training and other supports.[50] A lack of systematic use of wraparound manuals by wraparound care coordinators, found in a recent study,[51] could limit the effectiveness of wraparound. Even beyond training in wraparound methodology, care coordinators need to have knowledge of evidence-based clinical interventions, and there is some evidence that wraparound providers are less familiar with some evidence-based practices than nonwraparound providers.[51] Administrative issues also impinge on the effectiveness of wraparound. Limitations to interagency collaboration may extend from local, state, or federal administrative barriers to key aspects of wraparound, including blending of funds, information sharing, and development of interagency service plans. Competing agency mandates may also create barriers to effective collaboration and service integration. Lack of organizational and system supports, such as manageable caseloads, availability of flexible funds, and standards for team composition, may interfere with fidelity.[52]

Another access issue concerns the limited availability of foster parents who have the experience, skills, and motivation to parent youth with complex mental health needs and histories of disrupted relationships. As shown in Case #2 above, young people who have had many failed relationships may require a unique set of attributes on the part of the foster parents, including tolerance for behavioral and emotional instability. Needless to say, it is difficult to locate uniquely well-matched foster parents for each youth. Availability of respite and other supports to these foster homes is also needed to allow youth to remain in the community and may require significant financial investment. Expanding their network of supportive relationships can allow youth to sustain treatment gains over time, but this process can be resource intensive as well.

FUTURE DIRECTIONS FOR RESEARCH AND IMPLEMENTATION

Given the significant national investment that has been made in wraparound, further research on high-fidelity wraparound is clearly needed. Future research should focus on identifying the most important ingredients for positive outcomes, and emphasis should be placed on the specificity of clinical interventions, particularly incorporation of evidence-based practices.[29,48]

Wraparound methodology will need to be refined for new and diverse populations, such as tribal communities, young children, and children who are showing early signs of developing more serious emotional or behavioral difficulties. Another challenge in application of wraparound is the frequent difficulty of engaging youth and families who may be quite isolated and mistrustful of "the system" to participate in services in the system-of-care. Callejas and colleagues[53] have described access to services as the "front porch" of a continuum of culturally competent mental health services; the front porch is built through outreach activities in the community, reciprocal linkages with community services, and creation of a welcoming reception area in an agency. A related issue is the need to create mechanisms to provide services to parents of SED youth who may need mental health and addictions services. Given the substantial literature on effects of parental depression and other mental disorders on children, this should be a central focus of systems of care.[54,55]

As noted above, future expansion of wraparound by states will need to address barriers to blended funding and integrated service planning and delivery, cross-training of an interdisciplinary workforce, and defining which specific subgroups should receive high-fidelity wraparound versus partial applications. Finally, as the national agenda moves toward comprehensive care that integrates mental and physical health care,[17,56] wraparound interventions within systems of care will have to do a better job of interfacing with primary care providers. The Academy of Pediatrics "medical home" model is very compatible with wraparound's coordinated, comprehensive, family-driven approach and closely overlaps with system-of-care values and principles.[57]

SUMMARY

The wraparound approach has become a national standard for service planning for children and youth with complex mental health needs and their families. Its philosophy and methods are consistent with national trends toward family-driven care and more positive, less-pathologizing approaches to mental health services. Aspects of wraparound that account for its appeal and positive outcomes likely operate at multiple levels. At the system level, wraparound requires administrative modifications that allow different agencies to work closely together, develop single, coordinated service plans, and create mechanisms for combining funds and creating opportunities for flexible funding in the interest of the youth and families served. At the level of the child and family, the values of wraparound truly put the child or youth and parents at the center of the process and allow them to chart their own course. By virtue of its strengths-based approach, the youth's self-esteem and sense of self-agency are reinforced by professionals, family members, and the network of people that wraparound builds around the child. This network of supports can remain with the child even after the team process is no longer part of a wraparound program. Just as it has been demonstrated that child-therapist relationship variables are predictive of youth mental health-treatment outcomes,[58] it makes sense that the relationship-building aspect of wraparound is helpful in promoting positive outcomes for children and families. Provision of an atmosphere of acceptance and encouragement in which the youth and parents feel a growing sense of personal agency and enhancement of their self-esteem and competence is a critical ingredient of any successful psychotherapy.

In terms of its evidence base, wraparound is still at the level of a promising intervention. The resources required for high-fidelity implementation of wraparound are considerable. To better understand its value, research examining specific components of wraparound, both formal and informal, is needed to determine which are most strongly associated with positive outcomes.

WEB REFERENCES ON WRAPAROUND

Focal point issue on quality and fidelity in wraparound. Available at: www.rtc.pdx.edu/pgFocalPoint.shtml.
Promising Practices (system of care) monographs on wraparound. (2001, vol. 1; 1998, vol. 4): Available at: www.mentalhealth.samhsa.gov/cmhs/ChildrensCampaign/practices.
National Wraparound Initiative. Available at: www.rtc.pdx.edu/nwi.
Wraparound Fidelity Index. Available at: www.uvm.edu/~rapvt.
Walker and Koroloff, Schutte monograph on necessary supports for ISP/wraparound. Available at: www.rtc.pdx.edu.

REFERENCES

1. Friedman RM, Katz-Leavy JW, Manderscheid RW, et al. Prevalence of serious emotional disturbance: an update. In: Manderscheid RW, Henderson MJ, editors. Mental health, United States, 1998. Rockville (MD): U.S. Department of Health and Human Services; 1999. p. 110–2.
2. Joint Commission on the Mental Health of Children. Crisis in child mental health: challenge for the 1970s. New York: Harper and Row; 1969.
3. Knitzer J. Unclaimed children: the failure of public responsibility to children and adolescents in need of mental health services. Washington, DC: The Children's Defense Fund; 1982.
4. Stroul B, Friedman R. A system of care for children and youth with severe emotional disturbances (rev ed) 1986. Washington, DC: Georgetown University Child Development Center, National Technical Assistance Center for Children's Mental Health; 1986.
5. Center for Mental Health Services Comprehensive Community. Mental Health Services for Children and Their Families Program. Available at: http://mentalhealth. samhsa.gov/cmhs/childrenscampaign/ccmhs.asp. Accessed September 7, 2008.
6. Center for Mental Health Services. Annual report to Congress on the evaluation of the Comprehensive Community Mental Health Services for Children and their Families Program. Atlanta (GA): ORC Macro; 2001. Available at: http://mentalhealth.samhsa.gov/cmhs/ChildrensCampaign/practices.asp.http:// mentalhealth.samhsa.gov/publications/allpubs/CB-E201/default.asp. Accessed September 6, 2008.
7. American Psychiatric Association. Diagnostic and statistical manual of mental disorders. text revision. 4th edition. Washington, DC: American Psychiatric Association; 2000.
8. SAMHSA Mental health information center under systems of care. Available at: http://mentalhealth.samhsa.gov/publications/allpubs/CA-0014/default.asp. Accessed September 7, 2008.
9. US Department of Health and Human Services. Mental health: a report of the surgeon general. Rockville (MD): U.S. Department of Health and Human Services,

Substance Abuse and Mental Health Services Administration, Center for Mental Health Services, National Institutes of Health, National Institute of Mental Health; 1999.

10. Federation of Families for Children's Mental Health. The vision and mission of the Federation of Families for Children's Mental Health. Claiming children. 2001 Summer. Available at: http://www.ffcmh.org/Claiming%20Children%20Summer% 2001.pdf. Accessed September 7, 2008.

11. Farmer MZ, Mustillo S, Burns BJ, et al. Use and predictors of out-of-home placements within systems of care. J Emot Behav Disord 2008;16(1):5–14.

12. Burns BJ, Hoagwood K. Community treatment for youth: evidence-based interventions for severe emotional and behavioral disorders. New York: Oxford University Press; 2002.

13. Pumariega AJ. Residential treatment for children and youth: time for reconsideration and reform. Am J Orthop 2007;77(3):343–5.

14. Friesen BJ, Koroloff NM. Family perspectives on systems of care. In: Stroul BA, editor. Children's mental health: creating systems of care in a changing society. Baltimore (MD): Paul H. Brookes; 1990. p. 41–67.

15. Osher T, deFur E, Nava C, et al. New roles for families in systems of care. In: Systems of care: promising practices in children's mental health. 1998 series, vol I. Washington, DC: Center for Effective Collaboration and Practice, American Institutes for Research; 1999.

16. Federation of Families for Children's Mental Health. Definition of "family-driven." Available at: http://www.ffcmh.org/systems_whatis.htm. Accessed September 10, 2008.

17. New Freedom Commission on Mental Health. Achieving the promise: transforming mental health care in America. Final Report. Rockville (MD): DHHS; 2003. Pub. No. SMA-03-3832.

18. Huffine C, Anderson D. Family advocacy development in systems of care. In: Pumariega A, Winters NC, editors. The handbook of child and adolescent systems of care: the new community psychiatry. San Francisco (CA): John Wiley & Sons; 2003. p. 35–65.

19. Samhsa. Definition of "youth-guided care." Available at: http://www.systemsofcare. samhsa.gov/ResourceGuide/systems.html. Accessed September 7, 2008.

20. Youth M.O.V.E. Available at: http://www.youthmove.us. Accessed September 7, 2008.

21. Behar L. Changing patterns of state responsibility: a case study of North Carolina. J Clin Child Psychol 1985;14(3):188–95.

22. Burns BJ, Goldman SK. Promising practices in wraparound for children with serious emotional disturbance and their families. Systems of care: promising practices in children's mental health. Washington, DC; Center for Effective Collaboration and Practice, American Institute for Research 1998 series; vol 4:77–100. Available at: http://mentalhealth.samhsa.gov/cmhs/ChildrensCampaign/practices.asp. Accessed September 27, 2008.

23. VanDenBerg JE, Grealish ME. Individualized services and supports through the wraparound process: philosophy and procedures. J Child Fam Stud 1996;5:7–21.

24. Bruns EJ, Burchard JD, Suter JC, et al. Assessing fidelity to a community-based treatment for youth: the wraparound fidelity index. J Emot Behav Disord 2004;12: 79–89.

25. Walker JS, Bruns EJ. Building on practice-based evidence: using expert perspectives to define the wraparound process. Psychiatr Serv 2006;57(11): 1579–85.

26. Nelson G, Ochocka J, Griffin K, et al. "Nothing about me, without me:" participatory action research with self-help/mutual aid organizations for psychiatric consumer/survivors. Am J Community Psychol 1998;26(6):881–912.

27. AACAP. Practice parameter for child and adolescent mental health care in community systems of care. J Am Acad Child Adolesc Psychiatry 2007;46(2):284–99.

28. Solnit AJ, Adnopoz J, Saxe L, et al. Evaluating systems of care for children: utility of the clinical case conference. Am J Orthop 1997;67:554–67.

29. Stambaugh LF, Mustillo SA, Burns BJ, et al. Outcomes from wraparound and multisystemic therapy in a center for mental health services system-of-care demonstration site. J Emot Behav Disord 2007;15:148–55.

30. Oregon Wraparound. Video: "I fit in: wraparound Oregon works for kids and families". Available at: www.youtube.com/watch?v=MPzTRZqIIEw. Accessed September 18, 2008.

31. National Wraparound Initiative. Available at: www.rtc.pdx.edu/nwi. Accessed September 15, 2008.

32. Bruns EJ, Suter JC, Force MM, et al. Adherence to wraparound principles and association with outcomes. J Child Fam Stud 2005;14:521–34.

33. Burchard JD, Bruns EJ, Burchard SN. The wraparound approach. In: Burns BJ, Hoagwood K, editors. Community treatment for youth: evidence-based interventions for severe emotional and behavioral disorders. New York: Oxford University Press; 2002. p. 69–90.

34. Kamradt B, Gilbertson SA, Lynn N. Wraparound Milwaukie. In: Epstein MH, Kutash K, Duchnowski A, editors. Outcomes for children and youth with emotional and behavioral disorders and their families: programs and evaluation best practices. 2nd edition. Austin (TX): PRO-ED, Inc; 2005. p. 307–28.

35. Bickman L, Smith CM, Lambert E, et al. Evaluation of a congressionally mandated wraparound demonstration. J Child Fam Stud 2003;12:135–56.

36. Duchnowski AJ, Kutash K, Friedman RM. Community-based interventions in a system of care and outcomes framework. In: Burns BJ, Hoagwood K, editors. Community treatment for youth: evidence-based interventions for severe emotional and behavioral disorders. New York: Oxford University Press; 2002. p. 16–38.

37. Reich S, Bickman L. Research designs for children's mental health services research. In: Epstein MH, Kutash K, Duchnowski AJ, editors. Outcomes for children and youth with emotional and behavioral disorders and their families: programs and evaluation best practices. 2nd edition. Austin (TX): Pro-ed; 2005. p. 71–100.

38. Henggeler SW, Shoenwald SK, Borduis CM, et al. Multisystemic treatment of antisocial behavior in children and adolescents. New York: Guilford; 1998.

39. Curtis NM, Ronan KR, Borduin CM. Multisystemic treatment: a meta-analysis of outcome studies. J Fam Psychol 2004;18(3):411–9.

40. Chamberlain P. Family connections: treatment foster care for adolescents. Eugene (OR): Northwest Media; 1994.

41. Shepard SA, Chamberlain P. The Oregon multidimensional treatment foster care model. In: Epstein MH, Kutash K, Duchnowski AJ, editors. Outcomes for children and youth with emotional and behavioral disorders and their families: programs and evaluation best practices. 2nd edition. Austin (TX): Pro-ed; 2005. p. 551–72.

42. Stroul B. Case management in a system of care. In: Friesen B, Poertner J, editors. From case management to service coordination for children with emotional, behavioral, or mental disorders: building on family strengths. Baltimore (MD): Paul H. Brooks; 1995. p. 3–25.

43. Evans ME, Armstrong MI, Kuppinger AD. Family-centered intensive case management: a step toward understanding individualized care. J Child Fam Stud 1996;5:55–65.
44. Judge David L. Bazelon center for mental health law. Available at: http://www.bazelon.org/. Accessed September 27, 2008.
45. Oregon Statewide Wraparound Initiative. Available at: www.wraparoundoregon.org/statewide. Accessed October 10, 2008.
46. Quinn KP, Lee V. The wraparound approach for students with emotional and behavioral disorders: opportunities for school psychologists. Psychology 2007;44(1):101–11.
47. Ryburn M. A new model for family decision making in child care and protection [Journal; Peer Reviewed Journal]. Early Child Dev Care 1993;86:1–10.
48. Weisz JR, Sandler IN, Durlak JA, et al. A proposal to unite two different worlds of children's mental health. Am Psychol 2006;61(6):644–5.
49. Thomas CR, Holzer CE 3rd. The continuing shortage of child and adolescent psychiatrists. J Am Acad Child Adolesc Psychiatry 2006;45(9):1023–31.
50. Walker JS, Bruns E. Quality and fidelity in wraparound. Focal point, research and training center on family support and children's mental health. Focal Point 2003; Fall: 3–28.
51. Bruns EJ, Walrath, Sheehan AK. Who administers wraparound: an examination of the training, beliefs, and implementation supports for wraparound providers. J Emot Behav Disord 2007;15(3):156–68.
52. Bruns EJ, Suter JC, Leverentz-Brady MA. Relations between program and system variables and fidelity to the wraparound process for children and families. Psychiatr Serv 2006;57(11):1586–93.
53. Callejas LM, Nesman T, Mowery D, et al. Creating a front porch: strategies for improving access to mental health services. In: Making children's mental health services successful series, FMHI publication no. 340–3. Tampa (FL): University of South Florida Louis de la Parte Florida Mental Health Institute, Research and Training Center for Children's Mental Health, 2008.
54. Beardslee WR, Gladstone TR, Wright EJ, et al. A family-based approach to prevention of depressive symptoms in children at risk: evidence of parental and child change. Pediatrics 2003;112(2):e119–31.
55. Nicholson J, Hinden BR, Biebel K, et al. A qualitative study of programs for parents with serious mental illness and their children: building practice-based evidence. J Behav Health Serv Res 2007;34(4):395–413.
56. Institute of Medicine. Improving the quality of health care for mental and substance-use conditions. Quality Chasm Series. Washington, DC; National Academies Press 2005. Available at: http://www.iom.edu/?id=30858. Accessed October 15, 2008.
57. American Academy of Pediatrics. Policy statement: the medical home. Pediatrics 2002;110(1):184–6.
58. Shirk SR, Karver M. Prediction of treatment outcome from relationship variables in child and adolescent therapy: a meta-analytic review. J Consult Clin Psychol 2003;71:452–64.
59. Kazdin AE. Evidence-based treatments: challenges and priorities for practice and research. Child Adolesc Psychiatr Clin N Am 2004;13(4):923–40.

Disparities in Treating Culturally Diverse Children and Adolescents

David S. Rue, MD[a,b,]*, Yuhuan Xie, MD[c]

KEYWORDS

- Minority • Children • Mental health • Disparities
- Under-utilization • Cultural competence

In 2001, the United States Surgeon General's Report on Mental Health decried the state of under-utilization of mental health services by racial and ethnic minorities of all ages.[1] The Surgeon General challenged the field to find ways to reduce disparities in access to the psychiatric treatment of the rapidly increasing minority populations in the United States. Since then, many clinicians, professional organizations, and governmental agencies at the local, state, and federal levels have responded to the Surgeon General's call to action, with increased efforts to define the nature and extent of disparities, to understand fully the causes of under-utilization, and to advance clinical research for culturally competent psychiatric treatments. This article considers disparities in the psychiatric care of racial and ethnic children and adolescents, with respect to their under-utilization of services and under-treatment, especially with psychotropic medications. Culturally adapted psychotherapeutic approaches are discussed, as well as the notion of a culturally competent clinician who strives to apply his or her clinical skills while constantly making adjustments to the beliefs, habits, and circumstances of culturally diverse children and their parents, one patient at a time.

EVOLVING DIVERSITY IN THE UNITED STATES: SOME BACKGROUND

The United States is the destination country for immigrants from all over the world. Welcoming new immigrants has long been an American cultural heritage. By and

[a] Department of Psychiatry and Behavioral Sciences, University of California Davis School of Medicine, 2230 Stockton Boulevard, Sacramento, CA 95831, USA
[b] Child and Adolescent Services, Sutter Center for Psychiatry, Sutter Medical Center, 7200 Folsom Boulevard, Sacramento, CA 95826, USA
[c] Division of Child and Adolescent Psychiatry, Department of Psychiatry and Behavioral Sciences, University of California Davis School of Medicine, 2230 Stockton Boulevard, Sacramento, CA 95831, USA
* Corresponding author. 2701 Del Paso Road, Suite 130–175, Sacramento, CA 95835.
E-mail address: rued@sutterhealth.org (D.S. Rue).

Psychiatr Clin N Am 32 (2009) 153–163
doi:10.1016/j.psc.2008.11.001
0193-953X/08/$ – see front matter © 2009 Elsevier Inc. All rights reserved.

psych.theclinics.com

large, most European immigrants were well received and readily assimilated into the mainstream American social and cultural fabric.[2] In contrast, non-European immigrants were not always welcomed. In fact, non-European immigration was legally curtailed or actively controlled. The Chinese Exclusion Act of 1882 is one example; this federal law legalized the governmental practice of discrimination against Chinese immigrants entering the United States. Later in 1924, the "quota" system (based on country of origin) was established, allowing only a very limited number of nonwhite immigrants into the United States, while white immigrants were not affected by the system. This race-based practice continued until 1965, when the quota system was replaced with the Immigration and Nationality Act. The new law has since facilitated the increase in the number of non-European immigrants to the United States.

The racial and ethnic landscape of the United States is clearly changing: it is not black and white anymore. Over the past three or four decades, the growth of ethnic and racial minorities is most notable among Hispanic and Asian immigrants, with their children being the most rapidly expanding segment of the American population. In 2000, racial and ethnic minority children and youths under age 20 were near a majority in about one-fifth of American counties. In 2007, they were a majority in one in four counties. Nationwide, they now represent 43% of the under-20 age group in the United States.[3]

The recent changes in the United States population make-up have resulted in a racially and culturally diverse society. The cultural diversity in the United States permeates music, sports, food, entertainment, education, and the work place. This diversity is reflected in the variety of the faces of children and their parents, who live not only in major urban centers but also in suburban and rural areas across the country.[4] Contemporary children and adolescents in the United States are likely to have friends and classmates whose cultures and primary languages spoken at home are different from their own, and they seem more at ease in different cultural milieus than their parents might have been at the same age.[5] Before proceeding to discuss disparities in care, it is necessary to first provide working definitions for the terms "race," "ethnicity," and "culture."

RACE, ETHNICITY, AND CULTURE

Race, ethnicity, and culture are social constructs. Race refers to a population considered distinct from others for certain outward, physical characteristics. Ethnicity is a term representing "social groups with a shared history, sense of identity, geography, and cultural roots."[6] Culture is defined as a group of people's "shared patterns of belief, feeling, and knowledge that ultimately guide everyone's conduct and definition of reality."[7] There are no established biological criteria for dividing races into distinct groups. Racial categories sometimes serve as proxy for socioeconomic risk factors, or as a substitute for culture.[8] Racial and ethnic minorities in the United States include "blacks, American Indians, Hispanics, Asians, Pacific Islanders, and people of mixed races."[3]

DISPARITIES IN PSYCHIATRIC CARE
Under-Utilization of Services

The outstanding issue in minority mental health is that racial and ethnic minorities— children and adults alike—do not use mental health services as often as Caucasians do. In 2001, the Office of the United States Surgeon General released its *Report on Mental Health* and its supplement, "Mental Health: culture, race, and ethnicity." The *Report* states that the under-utilization of mental health services by racial and ethnic minorities is "a major public health threat."[1] It continues, "Minorities have less access to, and availability of, mental health services; minorities are less likely to receive needed mental health services; minorities in treatment often receive a poorer quality of mental health care." In 2003, the President's New Freedom Commission on Mental Health concluded that minorities suffer from a "higher burden of disability" because of difficulty with access to mental health care.[9] In short, culturally diverse children and adolescents, like their parents, have more difficulty in the United States accessing mental health services than Caucasians, and they often go untreated.

Elster and colleagues[10] reviewed the literature, published from 1991 to 2003, to identify the extent of racial and ethnic disparities among adolescents who were treated in ambulatory adolescent health care settings, including mental health care. Eleven of 61 studies on mental health met the inclusion criteria, and 4 of 11 articles were considered scientifically rigorous. The authors of these four articles concluded that African American adolescents received fewer mental health care services than non-Hispanic white youths did. However, the data suggested that there were no significant disparities between Hispanic adolescents and non-Hispanic white youths.

Another study involved 1,256 high-risk youths aged 6 to 18 who were receiving services in a publicly funded system of care, including child welfare, juvenile justice, special education, alcohol and drug abuse, and mental health services. The study investigated the disparities in mental health service use, with other sociodemographic or clinical variables being held constant, such as family income, functional impairment, and caregiver strains. The investigators found significant racial and ethnic group differences in the likelihood of any mental health service provided. In this study, 79% of non-Hispanic white youths received mental health services, compared with 59% of Asian/Pacific Islander Americans, 64% of African Americans, and 70% of Latino Americans. But after controlling for the effects of socio-demographic factors, African American and Asian and Pacific Islander American youths were approximately one-half as likely as non-Hispanic white youths to receive any mental health services, including formal outpatient mental health services. However, race and ethnicity were not factors in the use rate of 24-hour care services, such as in-patient psychiatric unit service, residential treatment center, or group home services.[11]

Disparities in Psychotropic Medication Treatment

With the ever-increasing influence and intrusion of pharmaceutical companies through aggressive marketing, the prescription rates for children and adolescents with psychiatric disorders in many countries have risen sharply over the past decade.[12] While the use of psychotropic medication for children and adolescents with psychiatric disorders is variable from one country to the next around the world, it is astounding that the United States is accountable for over 80% of the world's use of stimulant medications. Antidepressants and antipsychotics are prescribed for use in children and adolescents many times greater in the United States than in other countries. Variability in psychiatric drug use is said to reflect differences in social and cultural context, in which childhood psychiatric disturbances are perceived, interpreted, and managed in different ethnic groups.[13]

While the United States leads the world in prescribing psychoactive agents for minors, it is ironic to note that racial and ethnic children are under-treated with medications at outpatient settings. One study examined rates of psychotropic medication use by high-risk youths in public sector services in southern California. In the study, race and ethnicity predicted psychotropic medication use by these youths, with all other factors (age, gender, household income, insurance, diagnosis) being held constant. The conclusion of the study was that African American and Latino youths and "others" (mostly Asian and Pacific Islander children) were less likely to use psychotropic medications than Caucasian youths.[14] The investigators suggested that the interplay of a variety of barriers to care, and not any single factor—such as parent's cultural be-liefs—are responsible for mental health disparities. Racial and ethnic minority youths are treated with psychotropic medications at rate much lower than that of whites.

Disparities in Treatment of ADHD

In the United States, ADHD is one of the most common and most researched child-hood mental disorders, with an incidence rate of about 3% to 7% in school-aged chil-dren.[15] Several studies summarized below confirm that African American, Latino, and Asian/Pacific Islander American children and adolescents are less likely to receive psychotropic medications for ADHD than their non-Hispanic white counterparts.

Zito and colleagues[16] reported that compared with non-Hispanic white children, African American children with Medicaid insurance had a distinctly lower rate of treat-ment with psychotropic medication (39% versus 52%). Racial and ethnic children at risk for ADHD were nearly twice as unlikely to have their service needs met, including the administration of appropriate medication treatment.[17] Safer and Malever[18] re-ported that African American and Latino students in a statewide survey of Maryland public school students received methylphenidate at approximately half the rate of their white counterparts. In North Carolina, Rowland and colleagues[19] found that, com-pared with non-Hispanic white children, the caregivers of African American (70%) and Hispanic children (30%) were less likely to report use of ADHD medication, even after adjusting for gender, grade, and past diagnosis of ADHD.

Pediatric Ethnopsychopharmacology

There is a small body of literature on cross-cultural, inter-ethnic child and adolescent psychopharmacology, such as pharmacokinetics, pharmacodynamics, efficacy, and side-effects. These articles are reviewed to examine if there is a difference in pharma-cologic response that may be associated with disparities in use of medications among different ethnic groups.

The Multimodal Treatment Study of Children with Attention-Deficit/Hyperactivity Disorder is a landmark study involving 579 children of different racial and ethnic back-grounds, aged 7 to 9 years, receiving 14 months of medication management, behav-ioral treatment, combination, or community care. The study raised a hypothesis at the outset that African American children would have a lower response rate to methylphe-nidate in initial titration. Arnold and colleagues[20] analyzed the data and found that "the methylphenidate response rate for African American children was almost identical (76% versus 78%) to that of Caucasian children." Thus, the hypothesis of lower response rate among African American children was not supported in this study. In addition, the titration response profile for Latino children was also similar to those of other groups. Based on the results of this multi-site, federally funded research, the in-vestigators recommended that children of all ethnicities with ADHD be treated with carefully monitored medication trials.

The Research Units on Pediatric Psychopharmacology Anxiety Study[21] examined whether the ethnicity of a child, along with many other demographic and clinical factors (age, gender, type of anxiety disorder, severity of illness, comorbidity, intellectual level, family income, or parental education), may affect the outcome of the pharmacological treatment effect in children and adolescents with anxiety disorders. The study found that fluvoxamine was highly efficacious in improving children and adolescents with anx-iety disorders, independent of the ethnic or cultural variables of the study subjects.

Tamayo and colleagues[22] studied the pharmacological response to atomoxetine in Latino versus Caucasian pediatric outpatients in two multicenter, open-label trials during the first 10 to 11 weeks of treatment. They found that Latino and Caucasian children with ADHD demonstrated a similar pattern of efficacy and tolerability with atomoxetine. Treatment-emergent adverse-event profiles revealed a divergence of complaints. Non-Hispanic whites frequently reported abdominal and throat pain, while Latinos complained of decreased appetite and dizziness. However, Latino subjects reported fewer adverse events than Caucasians. It is important to note that mean doses of atomoxetine were comparable between the two groups. The authors believe that the study data challenges the notion that Latino patients, compared with Caucasians, require lower doses of psychotropic medications.

The three inter-ethnic studies reviewed here indicate that there are no demonstrable differences in the pharmacological response of methylphenidate and atomoxetine among different racial and ethnic groups. There appears to be no association between under-treatment of minority youth with medications and ethnopharmacology of these drugs.

Under-utilization of mental health services by minorities is both concerning and confounding. It is disconcerting that a large segment of the United States populations goes untreated for their mental and emotional suffering, despite the increased attention that is being paid to disparities. It is important to point out the statistical data on disparities. The data challenge us to first understand the root causes of uneven care and then, to correct the disparities. However, it has turned out to be a daunting task to fully understand what contributes to the under-utilization in the United States. Cultural factors are considered as one of the many contributors.

CULTURAL FACTORS IN UNDER-UTILIZATION

The under-utilization of mental health care by ethnic minorities stems from the interplay of a myriad of sociocultural issues not only in initiating the treatment, but also in staying in treatment, once started. Because mental health care takes place in a cultural context involving both the giver and the receiver of care, much research has been done to explore and understand what cultural factors in the dyadic relationship might serve as the root causes of the under-utilization phenomenon. Snowden and colleagues[23] identified multiple cultural factors to possibly explain the disparities in mental health care: "trust and treatment receptiveness, stigma, culturally distinctive beliefs about mental illness and mental health, culturally sanctioned way of expressing mental heath-related suffering and coping styles, and client preferences for alternative interventions and treatment-seeking pathways, as well as unresponsive programs and providers." These cultural factors and possibly others are important to fully understand, both individually and in totality. This section focuses on one of these cultural factors and discusses how cultural beliefs and attitudes affect parents in seeking help for their children.

Cultural Beliefs About Causes and Treatments

Culture influences how people interpret their illness.[24] For example, the Vietnamese parents in an Australian community sample believe that "biological/chemical imbalance, trauma, and spiritual imbalance might cause child mental illness."[25] The following vignette illustrates how one Vietnamese mother interpreted her only son's mental illness.

A 16 year-old Vietnamese-born male, residing in northern California, became mute and immobile during a family banquet at a restaurant, and then suddenly began shouting obscenities at no one in particular. As his startled mother attempted to calm him down, he got up from his seat and started to run to the door. His relatives held him down on the floor while police help was sought. He fought with the police, but was eventually taken to the Emergency Department of a local hospital. Upon arrival, he received 10-mg Haldol and 2-mg Ativan intramuscularly and was transferred to an adolescent psychiatric facility about 100 miles away on an emergency hold. His mother, who did not speak intelligible English, was petrified. She later said that she thought her son had died. When she separately arrived at the hospital a day later, the patient was recovering from the sedating effect of the psychotropic medications he had received and was becoming agitated again. He began running down the hallways of the hospital unit, screaming in Vietnamese, which is his primary language. His mother stated that her son was "invaded by an evil spirit." She insisted that what he needed was the intervention by a Vietnamese spirit healer, a ba dong, and she refused to agree to the use of medications. However, thanks to persuasive counsel by her relatives, she reluctantly conceded to the administration of the medications in the hospital. He was first treated with an atypical antipsychotic medication, which was then replaced with another atypical neuroleptic a week later, without much improvement. When a minor tranquilizer was added to the regimen, he seemed to improve and his mind was almost lucid, but only for a half of a day. He became mute again in a day. He would eat only the Vietnamese food his mother brought in. He otherwise was engaged in his private thoughts, talking and making odd noises, while remaining in bed. After a few weeks of maintaining this status quo, his mother became anxious and started raising concerns about the toxic effects of the psychotropic medications "on his mind," referring to the sedative side effect of the medications. She then reversed her earlier consent to the administration of psychoactive agents. She requested that a spiritual healer be consulted. After two special visits by the most highly respected ba dong in the region failed to quicken his recovery, the mother was very disappointed and confused. She began talking about taking him back to Vietnam. "America is too hard," she said. She once again consented to the physician's request to restart the previous medications. The patient gradually became stabilized during the ensuing 2 weeks. He and his mother were "homesick." He was discharged to the care of a Vietnamese-speaking psychiatrist in the community mental health center in their hometown.

Yeh and colleagues[26] reported racial and ethnic patterns in parental beliefs about the etiologies of child problems in southern California. They used a questionnaire with 11 etiological categories. The investigators found that racial and ethnic parents were less likely than white parents to endorse biopsychosocial categories of etiology, such as physical causes, personality, relational issues, familial issues, and trauma. In the case of Asian/Pacific Islander and Latino parents, they were in favor of sociological causes, such as friends, American culture, prejudice, and economic problems. Both African American and Asian/Pacific Islander parents believed that prejudice caused child mental and emotional problems. Asian and Pacific Islander parents particularly emphasized that American culture was a major contributor to child problems, as was the case with the mother of the Vietnamese-born patient in the vignette. This study suggests that the conventional, "one-size-fits-all," biopsychosocial explanatory model may not serve well for most racial and ethnic children and their families. It leads one to consider that with their belief in a sociological explanatory model, Latino and Asian/Pacific Islander American parents initially may be inclined to accept a sociologically oriented approach, such as explorations of prejudice, discrimination, trauma, economic stresses, school pressures, or peer conflicts.

In another study, the investigators concluded that Asian/Pacific Islander and African American parents were less likely than non-Hispanic white parents to agree with teachers that their children's behavior was an outward manifestation of an underlying disorder.[27] Many racial and ethnic parents may not share the mainstream culture's scientific explanations for mental or behavior disorders, and may be reluctant to engage in a discussion of a child's behavior problems in scientific terms.

Bussing and colleagues[28] reported that both Caucasian and African American parents offered similar causal explanations for child problems, although Caucasian parents were more likely than African American parents to use medical terminology to describe their child with disruptive behavior problems, such as ADHD. Labeling a child with medical terms does not sit well with many ethnic parents because to them medical terms are impersonal and tend to foreclose any alternative explanations. For example, when one speaks of "hyperactivity," an ethnic parent may well think of "too much energy" or of "being rambunctious."

It is not unusual that parents from the same culture don't necessarily agree on which symptom is most concerning to them, among the many symptoms of a disorder, such as autistic disorder. It is not surprising then that parents of different cultural backgrounds are concerned with different aspects of same disorder. For example, South Asian Indian parents tend to initially notice the social difficulties of their children with autistic disorder, followed by noticing delays in speech ability.[29] So they would tend to first seek behavioral or socialization therapy. In contrast, mainstream American parents are concerned more with general developmental delay or regression in language skills than social or communicative deficits.[30] Consequently, United States parents might first seek language therapy. These differences most likely reflect cultural values held in the respective culture. For Asian Indians, their culture emphasizes proper social behaviors, while for American parents, individual competence in their child is higher on the scale of desirable qualities than is sociability.

CULTURALLY COMPETENT PSYCHOTHERAPY RESEARCH

In their recent review article, "The Case for Cultural Competency in Psychotherapeutic Interventions," Sue and colleagues[31] state that "culturally adapted interventions provide benefit to intervention outcomes. This added value is more apparent in the research on adults than on children or youths…" In the following sections, three culturally adapted treatment approaches for minority children and their families are reviewed. These studies or their variations may be applicable to other treatment settings for racial and ethnic children and adolescents.

Storytelling Therapy

The culturally adapted storytelling technique, called "cuento therapy," was first introduced by Constantino and colleagues.[32] The therapy was provided for Puerto Rican children to promote self-esteem, emotional well-being, and adaptive behaviors. The adults would read *cuentos* (Puerto Rican folktales) or biographies of heroic individuals during their sessions with children at risk for emotional or behavioral problems. Children were randomly assigned to either a *cuento* intervention group or other groups (art/play therapy group or no-intervention control group). Favorable emotional and behavioral outcomes were noted in the children in the culturally adapted *cuento* intervention group, compared with other groups.

Family Therapy

Santisteban and colleagues[33] and Szapocznik and colleagues[34] created Brief Structural Family Therapy (BSFT) in the course of working with Hispanic families, but later it was adapted to other urban minority group families, such as African Americans and Puerto Ricans. The model is flexible and is focused on problem solving. Specific issues unique to certain families, such as prejudice and immigration, are discussed together as a family. The model's structural family approach resonates well with the ethnic culture's preference for well-defined hierarchies within the family. BSFT was found to be effective in improving youth conduct, family functioning, and treatment adherence, compared with no-intervention controls.

Cognitive Behavioral Therapy

The efficacy of culturally adapted forms of cognitive behavioral therapy (CBT) in culturally diverse populations[35] has been examined. However, most studies were conducted on adult patients, with an exception of Rossello and colleagues.[36] They found that culturally adapted forms of CBT and interpersonal psychotherapy (IPT) for Puerto Rican youths with depression were effective, compared with a wait-list control group, in terms of decreases in depressive symptoms. They discussed how CBT and IPT appeal to the cultural mind-set of Latino adolescents, by listing five structural and treatment characteristics of CBT: a didactic orientation, a classroom arrangement, an active intervention by the therapist, focus on the present and on problem-solving, and concrete techniques to be used in facing problems. On the other hand, IPT involves focusing primarily on the present and pressing interpersonal conflicts that are pertinent to Latino values of *familismo* (family) and *personalismo* (personal considerations). It appears the culturally adapted content and approaches of CBT and IPT seem quite consistent with Latino values. Positive outcomes are possible with other racial and ethnic children and youths, who share with Latinos similar cultural appreciations of *familismo* and *personalismo*.

THE CULTURALLY COMPETENT CLINICIAN

Sue and colleagues[31] offer an operational definition of cultural competence in clinicians as follows: "Competence is usually defined as an ability to perform a task or the quality of being adequately prepared or qualified. If therapists or counselors are generally competent to conduct psychotherapy, they should be able to demonstrate their skills with a range of culturally diverse clients." Cross and colleagues[37] delineated the functional qualities of a culturally competent clinician more specifically as: being aware of his or her own culture and its biases, being aware and accepting of cultural diffferences, understanding the dynamics in working across cultures, obtaining new cultural knowledge, and acquiring and adapting clinical practice skills to adjust to the patient's cultural context. A clinician acquires these qualities added to his or her general clinical competence through reflective living experiences and through intentional learning of different cultures. His or her daily encounters with multicultural patients are occasions for learning about the persons and their cultures. One becomes comfortable and competent with patients from different cultures over time, as one's world view enlarges and becomes more inclusive of humanity.

The learning curve on cultural competence is not always linear, but it does resemble the epigenetic progression of Eriksonian psychosocial developmental theory.[38] It starts with one's conscious awareness of his or her own culture and its biases. Cultural humility is the beginning of one's journey to cultural competence in life as well as in clinical practice. The clinician ultimately finds culturally sensitive and relevant ways to treat patients effectively, regardless of culture and ethnicity.

A recently published study of adult patients with diabetes illustrates how a physician's cultural blindness was a determining factor in the poor outcomes for black patients more frequently than for white patients. Sequist and colleagues[39] recruited 90 primary care physicians, treating 6,814 patients with diabetes, in a large health care system in eastern Massachusetts. To be included in the study, each physician treated a minimum of five white patients and five black patients. In the study, they identified three potential contributors to black-white outcome differences in achieving ideal diabetes control: within-physician effects, between-physican effects, and patient effects. Patient effects included such demographic data as patient age, sex, income, insurance, body mass index, glomerular filtration rate, and presence of cardiovascular disease. They found that within-physician effects contributed to overall racial disparities in outcomes more decidedly than patient factors and between-physician effects combined. The investigators concluded that "the problem of racial disparities is not characterized by only a few physicians providing markedly unequal care, but that such differences in care are spread across the entire system, requiring the implementation of system-wide solutions." In other words, this research finding bears witness to the assertion that possibly unaware but certainly unwittingly, most physicians, including psychiatrists, impose both individual and institutional ethnocentrism, if not the overt racism of yesteryear, while treating minority patients in the trenches of American medicine in the twenty-first century. The authors agree with the study's recommendations that "system-wide interventions will be needed to improve care for minority patients across all physicians." Clinically competent physicians also need to become culturally competent by learning to adapt their clinical skills to the cultural context of their patients. Much can be learned from this study that applies to psychiatric practice, not just in the Eastern Seaboard states but all over the United States.

SUMMARY

"The Child is father of the Man," a poet once said. How a child is treated by society determines not only the child's future but the future of the society. In the United States, a large segment of its future "father of the Man" is deprived of psychiatric care, which they need. This article discusses how racially and ethnically diverse children in the United States are denied access to psychiatric services. Many of them often go under-treated or untreated, especially in out-patient psychiatric settings. Still, culturally competent care for these children is possible through the combined efforts of both individual clinicians and institutions, bringing down the barriers of ethnocentrism and creating mental health services that treat all children and their families fairly, respectfully, and appropriately.

REFERENCES

1. Mental Health. Culture, Race, and Ethnicity—a supplement to mental health: a report of the Surgeon General. Rockville (MD): US Department of Health and Human Services; 2001.
2. Pumariega AJ, Rothe E. Cultural considerations in child and adolescent psychiatric emergencies and crises. Child Adolesc Psychiatr Clin N Am 2003;12(4): 723–44, vii.
3. Pollard K, Mather M. 10% of U.S. counties now 'majority-minority.' Washington (DC): Population Reference Bureau; August 2008.
4. Canino IA, Inclan JE. Culture and family therapy. Child Adolesc Psychiatr Clin N Am 2001;10(3):601–12.
5. Canino IA, Spurlock J. Culturally diverse children and adolescents: assessment, diagnosis, and treatment. 2nd edition. New York: The Guilford Press; 2000.
6. Chaudhry I, Neelam K, Duddu V, et al. Ethnicity and psychopharmacology. J Psychopharmacol 2008;22(6):673–80.
7. Griffith EEH, Gonsales CA. Essentials of cultural psychiatry. In: Hales RE, Yudofsky SC, Talbot JA, editors. American Psychiatric Press Textbook of Psychiatry. 2nd edition. Washington, DC: American Psychiatric Press; 1994. p. 1379–404.

8. Lillie-Blanton M, Laveist T. Race/ethnicity, the social environment, and health. Soc Sci Med 1996;43(1):83–91.

9. Hogan MF. The President's new freedom commission: recommendations to transform mental health care in America. Psychiatr Serv 2003;54(11):1467–74.

10. Elster A, Jarosik J, VanGeest J, et al. Racial and ethnic disparities in health care for adolescents: a systematic review of the literature. Arch Pediatr Adolesc Med 2003;157(9):867–74.

11. Garland AF, Lau AS, Yeh M, et al. Racial and ethnic differences in utilization of mental health services among high-risk youths. Am J Psychiatry 2005;162(7): 1336–43.

12. Vitiello B. An international perspective on pediatric psychopharmacology. Int Rev Psychiatry 2008;20(2):121–6.

13. Sussman LK, Robins LN, Earls F. Treatment-seeking for depression by black and white Americans. Soc Sci Med 1987;24(3):187–96.

14. Leslie LK, Weckerly J, Landsverk J, et al. Racial/ethnic differences in the use of psychotropic medication in high-risk children and adolescents. J Am Acad Child Adolesc Psychiatry 2003;42(12):1433–42.

15. American Psychiatric Association. Diagnostic and Statistical Manual of Mental Disorders DSM-IV-TR. Arlington (VA): American Psychiatric Association; 2000.

16. Zito JM, Safer DJ, dosReis S, et al. Racial disparity in psychotropic medications prescribed for youths with Medicaid insurance in Maryland. J Am Acad Child Adolesc Psychiatry 1998;37(2):179–84.

17. Pumariega AJ, Glover S, Holzer CE 3rd, et al. Administrative update: utilization of services. II. Utilization of mental health services in a tri-ethnic sample of adolescents. Community Ment Health J 1998;34(2):145–56.

18. Safer DJ, Malever M. Stimulant treatment in Maryland public schools. Pediatrics 2000;106(3):533–9.

19. Rowland AS, Umbach DM, Stallone L, et al. Prevalence of medication treatment for attention deficit-hyperactivity disorder among elementary school children in Johnston County, North Carolina. Am J Public Health 2002;92(2):231–4.

20. Arnold LE, Elliot M, Sachs L, et al. Effects of ethnicity on treatment attendance, stimulant response/dose, and 14-month outcome in ADHD. J Consult Clin Psychol 2003;71(4):713–27.

21. Walkup J, Labellarte M, Riddle MA, et al. Treatment of pediatric anxiety disorders: an open-label extension of the research units on pediatric psychopharmacology anxiety study. J Child Adolesc Psychopharmacol Fall 2002;12(3):175–88.

22. Tamayo JM, Pumariega A, Rothe EM, et al. Latino versus Caucasian response to atomoxetine in attention-deficit/hyperactivity disorder. J Child Adolesc Psychopharmacol 2008;18(1):44–53.

23. Snowden LR, Yamada AM. Cultural differences in access to care. Annu Rev Clin Psychol 2005;1:143–66.

24. Kleinman A. Rethinking Psychiatry: from cultural category to personal experience. New York: Macmillan/The Freepress; 1988.

25. McKelvey RS, Baldassar LV, Sang DL, et al. Vietnamese parental perceptions of child and adolescent mental illness. J Am Acad Child Adolesc Psychiatry 1999; 38(10):1302–9.

26. Yeh M, Hough RL, McCabe K, et al. Parental beliefs about the causes of child problems: exploring racial/ethnic patterns. J Am Acad Child Adolesc Psychiatry 2004;43(5):605–12.

27. Yu SM, Nyman RM, Kogan MD, et al. Parent's language of interview and access to care for children with special health care needs. Ambul Pediatr 2004;4(2): 181–7.

28. Bussing R, Schoenberg NE, Perwien AR. Knowledge and information about ADHD: evidence of cultural differences among African-American and white parents. Soc Sci Med 1998;46(7):919–28.

29. Daley TC. From symptom recognition to diagnosis: children with autism in urban India. Soc Sci Med 2004;58(7):1323–35.

30. Coonrod DV, Bay RC, Balcazar H. Ethnicity, acculturation and obstetric outcomes. Different risk factor profiles in low- and high-acculturation Hispanics and in white non-Hispanics. J Reprod Med 2004;49(1):17–22.

31. Sue S, Zane N, Nagayama Hall GC, et al. The case for cultural competency in psychotherapeutic interventions. Annu Rev Psychol 2009;60:10.1–10.24.

32. Constantino G, Malgady RG, Rogler LH. Cuento therapy: a culturally sensitive modality for Puerto Rican children. J Consult Clin Psychol 1986;54(5):639–45.

33. Santisteban DA, Suarez-Morales L, Robbins MS, et al. Brief strategic family therapy: lessons learned in efficacy research and challenges to blending research and practice. Fam Process 2006;45(2):259–71.

34. Szapocznik J, Prado G, Burlew AK, et al. Drug abuse in African American and Hispanic adolescents: culture, development, and behavior. Annu Rev Clin Psychol 2007;3:77–105.

35. Jackson B, Lurie S. Adolescent depression: challenges and opportunities: a review and current recommendations for clinical practice. Adv Pediatr 2006;53: 111–63.

36. Rossello J, Bernal G, Rivera-Medina C. Individual and group CBT and IPT for Puerto Rican adolescents with depressive symptoms. Cultur Divers Ethnic Minor Psychol 2008;14(3):234–45.

37. Cross T, Bazron B, Dennis K, et al. Towards a culturally competent system of care: a monograph on effective services for minority children who are severely emotionally disturbed. CASSP Technical Assistance Center, Georgetown University Child Development Center, 3800 Reservoir Road, N.W, Washington, DC 20007; 1989.

38. Erikson EH. Childhood and society. 2nd edition. New York: W.W. Norton; 1963.

39. Sequist TD, Fitzmaurice GM, Marshall R, et al. Physician performance and racial disparities in diabetes mellitus care. Arch Intern Med 2008;168(11):1145–51.

The Psychiatrist as Consultant: Working Within Schools, the Courts, and Primary Care to Promote Children's Mental Health

Susan Milam-Miller, MD[a,b,c]

KEYWORDS

• Consultation • School • Juvenile justice • Primary care • Child

Although modern psychiatrists are trained in the medical model of direct patient care where doctor and patient meet in the hospital or clinic, today's child psychiatrists are also being asked to step out of this model to serve as consultants in the community.[1] In schools, in the courts, and in primary care clinics, child psychiatrists work outside of the traditional framework of direct patient care, following a tradition that traces its roots to the early child guidance movement. This movement began with attempts to understand and change disruptive behavior of children in the community and laid an early foundation for the present-day specialty of Child and Adolescent Psychiatry. The first child guidance clinic in the United States, the Juvenile Psychopathic Institute, founded in Chicago in 1909, was the result of one physician's efforts to assist the juvenile court in designing treatment for children displaying delinquent behavior. Decades later, beginning in the mid-twentieth century, several child psychiatrists, including Caplan and Berlin, made important contributions to the practice of mental health consultation in schools and other agencies by delineating practical steps in the consultative process.[2] Psychiatrists have historically worked alongside other physicians caring for children in the hospital setting, and as an increasing number of children present in the pediatrician or family doctor's office with problems requiring mental health treatment, consultation by psychiatrists in or to outpatient primary care settings has become more common.[3] Motivated by ongoing need in the community,

[a] University of California Davis School of Medicine, Davis, CA, USA
[b] Sonoma County Mental Health, 3333 Chanate Road, Santa Rosa, CA 95405, USA
[c] Private Practice, 725 Farmers Lane, Suite 16, Santa Rosa, CA 95405, USA
E-mail address: susan.milam@stanfordalumni.org

Psychiatr Clin N Am 32 (2009) 165–176
doi:10.1016/j.psc.2008.10.002
0193-953X/08/$ – see front matter © 2009 Elsevier Inc. All rights reserved.

psych.theclinics.com

psychiatrists continue to join with a diverse group of professionals to improve the mental health of children where the children are located.

Given the well-documented shortage of child and adolescent psychiatrists in the United States, it is conceivable that the general psychiatrist may receive requests for consultation related to the mental health needs of children. Many lessons learned in traditional adult consult/liaison psychiatry can be translated to the community setting to serve children's needs.[2] In responding to such a request, the general psychiatrist also finds several issues unique to community mental health consultation focused around children. In the best-case-scenarios, each child who is a focus of consultation comes with a family—a family that contains potential allies and forces that resist change. Children and adolescents are by definition undergoing rapid development and knowledge of normal development is essential in evaluation and treatment of childhood emotional and behavioral problems. Laws of consent for treatment of minors vary depending on the state and the consultation question at hand and the consultant must also be familiar with mandated reporting of child abuse and neglect. Finally, the network of intersecting agencies that touch the lives of children offers complexity at the systems level that can be fascinating and perplexing. Fortunately, agencies approach psychiatrists not for their expertise in a particular child-serving agency, but for their more general ability to work within systems to effectively offer their expertise in mental health issues.

In schools psychiatric consultants learn to apply the skills of the psychiatrist to help not "patients," but students, faculty, and administrators. In the juvenile justice system, the psychiatric consultant learns a new set of rules that apply to confidentiality, consent for treatment, and court-ordered evaluation versus parent-requested treatment. In the primary care clinic, the psychiatric consultant discovers how to translate diagnosis and treatment recommendations into language that is useful for the primary care provider and the patient. In all of these settings, once invited, the psychiatric consultant gains a privileged position. Both a part of and also separate from the system requesting consultation, the psychiatric consultant can bridge understanding between specialty mental health services and mainstream child-serving agencies to ultimately benefit children in these diverse systems.[4]

This article describes consultation to schools in some depth to introduce practice issues relevant in all psychiatric consultation around the needs of children that occurs outside of the hospital setting. In the school setting, and in other systems, an essential piece of the work of the psychiatric consultant lies in establishing and maintaining the unique role of consultant. The consultant draws on traditional psychiatric knowledge and skills, but adapts these according to the needs of the system requesting consultation. Discussion of case examples from consultation to schools, the juvenile justice system, and primary care provide further illustration of contemporary psychiatric consultation in the community.

THE CONSULTANT'S ROLE

In a consultative relationship, a professional in one system requests the aid of another professional to achieve some aim in which the expertise of the consultant is relevant. The consultant accepts such a request because he or she shares this belief—that he or she can indeed bring a new perspective to the problem at hand. Far from a simple one-way transfer of knowledge, however, a successful consultative relationship involves bidirectional teaching and learning. Although most accustomed to the hierarchical authority of the doctor within the medical system, the psychiatric consultant assumes a much more collaborative position as he or she learns about the problem and the relevant system from the consultee. Two experts, side by side, view a problem and the consultant offers recommendations that the consultee may or may not choose to follow. In consultative work, there are no physician orders, no issues of compliance, and no absolute authority claimed by the consultant.

The differences between the traditional role of psychiatrist and the roles occupied by psychiatrists as consultants outside the medical system can be stark, but the basic tools are the same. The consultant brings a specific knowledge base to the work: principles of child development, systems-based practice, diagnosis and treatment of mental disorders, and an appreciation of psychodynamic forces within the group, family, and individual. These areas of knowledge find application on the school campus as they are applied to the problems identified by the consultee. Principles of child development may be invoked when a middle school administrator asks for assistance in designing a health curriculum appropriate for her students in early adolescence. An orientation toward system-based practice becomes relevant when an inner-city high school requests input about how best to serve a 15-year-old boy who has been violent on campus and is currently on probation. Knowledge about the diagnosis and treatment of mental disorders is used when consulting around an 8-year-old girl who has symptoms of ADHD and is disruptive in the classroom. Psychodynamic principles come to bear in identifying resistance to change and then facilitating change in the consultees and the school as a whole.

THE CONSULTANT'S ENTRY INTO THE SYSTEM

In any consultative setting, the psychiatric consultant follows a basic pattern to establish and make use of the relationship with the consultee to the benefit of the system as a whole and individuals within the system. A cycle of joining, needs assessment, and intervention forms the foundation of consultative work.

The initial joining process followed by the consultant parallels that of the cultural anthropologist who investigates a society to reveal the agreed-on rules that govern and distinguish a specific group of people. As described by anthropologist Franz Boas, this type of investigation is based on the assumption that different groups and institutions maintain distinct cultures that must be understood to make sense of individuals' conduct within that culture.

> Courtesy, modesty, good manners, conformity to definite ethical standards are universal, but what constitutes courtesy, modesty, very good manners, and definite ethical standards is not universal. It is instructive to know that standards differ in the most unexpected ways.[5]

The consultant joins with the system to gain the trust of the consultee and to learn the standards, or the basic ins and outs of the system. This process is followed by a careful assessment of strengths and weaknesses of the consultee and system in managing the problems raised by the consultation question. Finally, a consultant brings his or her professional expertise informed by the first two steps to advise intervention at appropriate levels of the system.

As in anthropologic research, there is no such thing as pure observation. A psychiatric consultant cannot join with an institution requesting help without some perturbation of the system and the consultant must be aware of the potential impact of his or her simple presence and interest in the system. The following is an example of a school crisis that might prompt requests for help from general psychiatrists and other mental health professionals in the community.

Early in the school year at an inner-city high school, a student was shot and killed off campus. Remembering the general psychiatrist who had once done a presentation about teen mental health for the school counseling staff, the staff immediately contacted this psychiatrist to request support in addressing current and future mental health needs of students related to violence in their community. As school staff quickly mobilized and provided grief counseling to students without specific input from the consultant, the psychiatric consultant met with staff to discuss how students were using counseling services and how staff and administration had been affected by the student's death. As the campus environment returned to normal, school staff commented on the helpfulness of having the perspective of a professional outside of the school. Several related that simply having the opportunity to reflect on this event as staff had strengthened their efforts to help the students cope. In the following weeks, the school counselor and principal enlisted the consultant's help in reviewing crisis response procedures for the school.

In this example, the consultant had little time to become acquainted with the school system, but through a crisis involving the mental health of students and staff, the consultant was invited further into the system, into a position and role that allowed the consultant to provide support and leadership to the staff and, indirectly, to the students.

Before a psychiatric consultant begins the work of joining with an agency or another professional, a connected series of questions should be answered to help frame these efforts. As described by Petti, these include the following:

Why is the request being made now?
Who is the consultee?
What is the role of the requesting program in this process?
How will this consultation be viewed by program administrators?
What are the expectations of the consultee?
What possible conflicts of interest exist?[6]

At times these questions can only be answered fully in retrospect, as a consultant proceeds to learn more about the system through actively working with the consultee. Proceeding too quickly after a request for help, however, may lead to misunderstandings and frustration on the part of the consultant and the consultee.

A consultant to schools typically has many opportunities to gather information about the school, just as a traditional consult-liaison psychiatrist gradually gets to know the medical team requesting psychiatric consultation and their particular hospital setting. For the school consultant, this happens primarily through careful observation while on campus. The process typically begins with formal meetings with administration or staff. Later, the consultant may be invited to observe classrooms and attend school events. Often, the most information can be gleaned by unobtrusively observing students in the hallway or at the lunch period. At all of these times, data are gathered about the structure, mission, and specific history and culture of the school, as well as characteristics of its administration, staff, and the students and families that are served by the school. The consultant uses all of this information to understand the context in which a problem exists.

DEFINING THE QUESTION

The psychiatric consultant's role is defined by the types of questions asked and the types of input requested by the consultee. The agreed-on focus of consultation may be case-based, consultee-based, or a combination of both. Case-based consultation is most closely related to traditional hospital consultation focusing on one patient, whereas consultee-based consultation parallels the liaison role of the hospital psychiatric consultant supporting the medical team. Case-based consultation, closest to the medical model, focuses on a problem related to one student, as in this example.

The preschool teacher asks for help in responding to a 4-year-old girl who has recently become aggressive toward other children in the class after the birth of a younger sibling. The consultant clarifies the behavior in question through classroom observation, carefully inquires about strategies already tried by the teacher, interviews the family, and reviews further information about the student with the parents' consent. No other specific developmental concerns are identified and a strategy involving rewards and consequences is recommended by the consultant.

Although a request like this is less likely to come to a general psychiatrist, the approach to this preschool-aged child demonstrates the importance of direct observation and obtaining collateral information from as many sources as possible.

In consultee-based consultation, the consultee invites more general input from the consultant to indirectly benefit students. Consultee-based consultation in the schools might focus on professional development for staff or an ongoing liaison with administrative or counseling staff of the school.[7]

A group of middle-school teachers identify high levels of test-taking anxiety in their students and approach a local psychiatrist known for his expertise in cognitive behavioral therapy for general tips in helping students cope with taking standardized tests. During a staff development presentation by the consultant on anxiety management strategies, staff members voice their own anxieties about the outcome of the standardized tests that serve as measurement of the school's success. Teachers report after the presentation that they feel more confident in their skills to help students to prepare for the examinations.

At times, a question that seems to be related to a specific child may reveal more general concerns at the school and the consultant may help the consultee to determine where to begin when multiple levels of intervention are possible.

A high school principal requests help in accessing counseling services for a student who seems depressed. As the problem is discussed with the consultant, the principal offers several other examples of students he believes would benefit from mental health services but whose needs exceed the school's current capacity. After suggesting possible referral agencies for the student originally discussed, plans for a new program evolve with the principal's leadership and continued input from the consultant. Through collaboration with the local university psychology training program, on-site psychotherapy services are provided.

This case describes a trend in school consultation whereby a consultant becomes an active collaborator with the school in implementing a program to address identified mental health needs of the students. Many school consultation programs across the United States now have psychiatrists not only advising administrators and teachers but also directly developing intervention programs with the school's invitation. Rappaport[8] describes several such programs. Psychiatrists participate in school-based clinics where they provide direct clinical care to students and serve as consultants to administrators, teachers, and other health care providers. Early intervention programs that match at-risk youth with positive adult role models have turned to psychiatric consultants for help in program planning. Psychiatrists have also provided consultation in novel outreach efforts that use the tools of telepsychiatry to expand the reach of the consultant to more schools.[8]

MEASURING OUTCOMES

In psychiatric consultation, as in all areas of medicine, physicians, consultees, and funding agencies are interested in the demonstration of positive outcomes.[9]

In the schools, an individual consultant may measure outcome through feedback from consultees, formal student health and academic measures, or program evaluation that measures success in multiple relevant domains. From a practical standpoint, outcomes research in psychiatric consultation give the consultant direct feedback about the extent of influence on the system and can help to determine which methods of consultation are most effective. Data about outcomes can also help the consultant to gain the support of administrators and potential sources of organizational and financial support.[10]

Schools have proved to be challenging systems in which to conduct consultation outcomes research. The availability of control groups has been limited as is the ability to account for the multiple intersecting variables found on each campus. Despite these challenges, positive outcomes have been registered for as many as 75% of all school consultation programs studied.[11] Debate exists as to the relative success of student-centered consultation as compared with consultee-centered consultation, and current models of school consultation frequently incorporate elements of both.[12]

For the independent consultant not affiliated with an academic center, the task of outcomes measurement in school consultation may be particularly daunting. Simple self-report data from administrators, teachers, and students can be obtained to direct the focus of consultation in its beginning stages.

At the start of the year, a consultant to the local high school collected data on teachers' knowledge and awareness about mental health concerns in their students. After a consultation program that provided specific in-service training for teachers, repeat measures were completed to evaluate changes in teachers' knowledge and attitudes demonstrating gains in this group. The next year, the consultant was able to collect data from a control group of teachers from within the same school and documented significant differences between the groups that were attributable to the trainings delivered by the consultant.

At the end of a round of outcomes evaluation, the psychiatric consultant moves forward, again assessing the needs and strengths of the school system and joining with multiple stakeholders in determining where the next steps will be taken to help improve children's mental health on campus.

PROFESSIONAL AND ETHICAL ISSUES IN CONSULTATION

As the psychiatric consultant works to maintain a defined role within the school setting, several potentially charged professional and ethical issues emerge. Physicians have strict codes of professional responsibility toward patients, but what is the consultant's role in the safety and welfare of students, family members, teachers, or administrators? How is confidentiality handled between different stakeholders on campus? Which actions by the consultant require parent consent? To whom is the psychiatrist ultimately responsible as a consultant and where might conflicts of interest arise? Are the duties performed as a consultant covered by professional liability insurance? To answer these questions, the consultant may be forced to examine his or her role again and again during the course of consultation.

At a small community's only day treatment school for emotionally disturbed adolescents a psychiatrist is contracted to provide medication management to students on site. The psychiatrist routinely attends staff meetings where mental health treatment staff and school staff discuss students' progress. This week, the program director raises a sensitive issue: it has just been discovered that a younger student, Vincent, who is scheduled to begin at the school next week, may have been involved in an incident of sexual abuse years ago with a current student at the school, Chris. This information was inadvertently learned when

Vincent's father attended a meeting with the school intake coordinator on the school campus and recognized Chris's mother who was there to pick up Chris for a dentist appointment. The two parents met 6 years ago during a conference at the boys' elementary school held to discuss suspicions that 7-year-old Vincent had been touched inappropriately by then 10-year-old Chris in the school bathroom. Chris has never revealed this history during sessions with his school therapist and Vincent similarly has not discussed the incident recently. The program director asks the psychiatrist for an opinion about the best way to handle this situation.

In the above example, to decide the best way to address the director's questions the consultant must consider issues of confidentiality (who has the right to know about this potential conflict?), inherent conflicts of interest for the consultant (how can the consultant simultaneously advise to the program director while also maintaining his responsibilities as the treating psychiatrist for Chris?), and concerns related to distributive justice (who has the right to receive treatment at the school?).

Although the role of the consultant may shift significantly during the course of consultation, standard guidelines do exist for psychiatrists working in the school setting and other consultative settings.[13–15] This expanded role for the psychiatrist can bring great rewards to the consultant and the system, despite the complexities of consultative work.

CURRENT TRENDS IN PSYCHIATRIC CONSULTATION TO SCHOOLS, COURTS, AND PRIMARY CARE

Consultation to community agencies traces a significant heritage from the beginnings of the child guidance movement.[16] As the needs and resources of communities have shifted over the past 50 years, so has the work of the psychiatric consultant. Despite the trend toward collaborative work with agencies rather than indirect consultative work, the basic roles of the psychiatric consultant remain constant. In the agencies they serve, psychiatrists function as teachers, as direct clinical evaluators and treaters for children, and as advocates and leaders, developing innovative solutions to promote children's mental health.

Consultant as Teacher

A psychiatrist beginning a consultative relationship with a large community health center begins seeing children referred for evaluation at a clinic site geographically separate from the main clinic where referring primary care clinicians work. While working with administration to determine when an office may be available in the main clinic, the consultant notes that most referrals center around questions of diagnosis and treatment of ADHD in school children and depression in adolescents. The consultant suggests offering monthly lunchtime children's mental health lectures at the main clinic, beginning first with these two commonly encountered diagnoses, and later broadening the topics covered by informally assessing the needs of the clinicians attending the lectures.

Over time, resources are found by the administration to provide free lunch for each lecture and attendance increases to include not only primary care clinicians but also therapists, health educators, and community organizers affiliated with the clinic. Informal "curbside" consultations increase as clinicians feel more comfortable contacting the consultant by e-mail or phone.

This example illustrates how intertwined consultee-based skills development and case-based consultation may be. The monthly lecture series not only provided relevant content related to children's mental health but also became an opportunity for building liaison relationships with referring clinicians. The consultant was able to informally assess the clinicians' comfort with evaluating mental health complaints, and, as a result, recommendations given after future consultation evaluations could be tailored to the referring clinician. At the same time, each lunchtime meeting became an opportunity to indirectly address providers' resistance to acknowledging the unmet mental health needs in their pediatric patients. With the consultant providing information and actively gathering information from the clinicians, authority and anxiety were shared.

Consultant as Clinician Providing Direct Evaluation or Treatment of Children

A psychiatric consultant participates in an interdisciplinary team charged to evaluate juveniles exhibiting signs of emotional or mental disorder before placement by the courts. This service is provided in a small group home setting where juvenile wards spend 2 to 3 weeks attending school on site and meeting with mental health, probation, and social services professionals whose job it is to assess needs of the child and recommend the most appropriate treatment and setting for rehabilitation. A 15-year-old girl is admitted to the assessment center from juvenile hall. Her charges include vandalism, breaking and entering, and assault against another minor. During her evaluation, the psychiatric consultant determined that during the past month, the 15-year-old had a history of impulsive running away, reckless spending, and had been sexually active with many partners. Her parents described these behaviors as not at all characteristic of this teen and reported that the behaviors had an abrupt onset in the spring of her sophomore year of high school. Before that, she had been a focused student, well liked by her peers and her peers' parents, and involved in several community activities. When interviewed by the psychiatric consultant, the 15-year-old seemed depressed and on further questioning met full criteria for a major depressive episode. With her parents' description of the sudden change in behavior along with the youth's own reports of the time immediately before being taken into custody and a negative urine drug screen, it seemed likely that in addition to her current depression, she had previously met criteria for a manic episode. These findings were discussed with the interdisciplinary team and when further collateral information and psychological testing supported the psychiatrist's findings, the girl was ordered by the court to a residential treatment setting where she received comprehensive treatment, including a trial of a mood stabilizer.

In this example, the psychiatric consultant functions in a role that is similar to that in the traditional doctor–patient relationship, although in this case the psychiatrist will not be the treating physician for the child. In the juvenile justice setting, where adolescents have a 10-fold increased likelihood of psychotic illness and increased prevalence of major depression and ADHD, the psychiatrist may play a crucial role in detecting untreated mental illness.[17] Evaluation conducted while a youth is in custody or on probation may be complicated by concerns about confidentiality. The knowledge that information from the evaluation will be shared with probation may compromise an adolescent's ability to reveal enough personal information for accurate diagnosis or treatment recommendations. At the same time, the involvement of multiple evaluators and often extensive access to collateral information from social services and probation may empower the team to reach a diagnostic formulation that can help determine appropriate placement recommendations. Working in this setting, it is essential for the psychiatric consultant to be familiar with the general orientation and goals of not only the juvenile justice system but also all other child-serving agencies represented around the table.[14]

Consultant as Systems Expert and Collaborator in Program Development

A child psychiatry division of a major medical center provided consultation to a local inner-city high school over the course of 5 years. During this time, the consultants evaluated many students who were then referred for ongoing mental health treatment at the local children's clinic. After an informal survey of students referred to these services, it was determined that a full 50% never made it for their first intake appointment. The school principal convened a meeting of teachers and parents and invited the psychiatric consultant to attend. During the meeting, the psychiatric consultant presented the idea of establishing a mental health clinic on campus. After a year of planning, grant-writing, and collaboration with the local children's mental health clinic, a school-based satellite mental health clinic was founded. The psychiatric consultant continued to provide psychiatric evaluation of students, but now instead of being referred out for treatment, the students could be followed by the consultant and newly-hired therapists on campus. Outcomes research at the end of the first year of the school-based mental health clinic indicated that the new program was associated with decreases in three meaningful measures: absences, course failures, and disciplinary referrals.[1]

In the above case, the psychiatric consultant moved from case-based consultation into providing consultation to the system and did so by engaging directly in program planning by invitation of the school administration. A need for services that students and families would find acceptable and convenient was filled successfully because school personnel, families, the psychiatric consultant, and the local community mental health agency collaborated. In helping to initiate novel programs to address children's mental health needs, psychiatrists act as consultants to the system, clinical team leaders, supervisors for allied professionals on the treatment team, and clinicians providing direct service. Management of overlapping but distinct roles presents a central challenge and an opportunity in psychiatric consultation.

TRAINING FOR PSYCHIATRIC CONSULTANTS

During general psychiatry residency, rotations in consultation/liaison psychiatry take place predominantly in the inpatient general hospital setting. With few exceptions, general psychiatry trainees have little opportunity for exploration of the role of the psychiatrist in consulting to public agencies, the courts, or primary care.[18] General psychiatrists with interest in working as consultants to child-serving agencies and primary care must seek training and experience outside of their formal residencies. Completion of a 2-year child and adolescent psychiatry residency offers broad experience in consultation through formal didactics and clinical rotations.[19] Forensic fellowship provides another path for in-depth training in consultation to adult, juvenile, and family courts. Community psychiatry fellowships also exist and train fellows to apply system-based care principles in interagency work.[20] Most general psychiatrists with an interest in consultation to schools, juvenile court, or primary care gain their experience on the job. To support psychiatric consultants, the American Psychiatric Association, the American Academy of Child and Adolescent Psychiatry, the American Academy of Psychiatry and the Law, and the American Association of Community Psychiatrists offer continuing medical education in consultation at their regional and national annual meetings and through their journals. Several references included in this article offer a general overview and specific techniques for the psychiatrist building a practice as a consultant.

SUMMARY

Never doubt that a small group of thoughtful, committed people can change the world.

—Margaret Mead[21]

As consultants, psychiatrists form relationships with and work alongside other professionals serving children with one main goal in mind: to promote children's mental health. As physicians, these consultants could arguably accomplish the same goal by staying comfortably within their hospitals, offices, and clinics to evaluate and treat the steady stream of children presenting for psychiatric care. Instead, psychiatric consultants enter the foreign territories of the schools, juvenile courts, and primary care clinics to offer their specialized skills, help build the skills of their consultees, and provide vision and leadership for creating systems that truly serve children where the children are. By joining with "small groups of thoughtful, committed people," the psychiatrist may extend his or her impact beyond that of the traditional physician providing patient care.

It is clear that separate agencies with bureaucratic walls built up between them cannot effectively serve the needs of children and families whose lives are affected by mental illness, chronic psychosocial stressors, and other social ills. The psychiatrist as consultant stands as a potential bridge between agencies, keeping open a dialog that is crucial to promoting children's emotional well-being and advocating for early identification and intervention for childhood mental illness.

ACKNOWLEDGMENTS

The author thanks Robert Horst, MD for his assistance in the preparation of this manuscript.

FURTHER READINGS

Berkovitz IH, Sinclair E. Training programs in school consultation. Child Adolesc Psychiatr Clin N Am 2001;10(1):83–92.

Bostic JQ, Rauch PK. The 3 Rs of school consultation. J Am Acad Child Adolesc Psychiatry 1999;38(3):339–41.

Daws D. Standing next to the weighing scales. J Child Psychother 1999;11(2):77–85.

Rappaport N. Psychiatric consultation to school-based health centers: lessons learned in an emerging field. J Am Acad Child Adolesc Psychiatry 2001; 40(12):1473–5.

School Mental Health Project, Department of Psychology, UCLA. The current status of mental health in schools: a policy and practice analysis. Los Angeles (CA): Center for Mental Health in Schools; 2006.

American Academy of Child and Adolescent Psychiatry. Available at: http://www.aacap.org/. This site is the source for the consultation practice parameters referenced above and the family children's mental health information sheets "Facts for Families."

Massachusetts General Hospital, School Psychiatry. Available at: http://www.massgeneral.org/schoolpsychiatry/. This link provides tools for clinicians, families, and educators to support students who have complex mental health needs.

University of California, Los Angeles School Mental Health Project. Available at: http://smhp.psych.ucla.edu/. A site that provides a web search portal for topics related to school consultation and policy analysis regarding school mental health needs and interventions.

REFERENCES

1. Pearson G, Jennings J, Norcross J. A program of comprehensive school-based mental health services in a large urban public school district: the Dallas model. Adolesc Psychiatry 1998;23:207–31.
2. Berlin I. The field of child and adolescent psychiatry: an overview. In: Wiener JM, Dulcan MK, editors. The American psychiatric publishing textbook of child and adolescent psychiatry. Arlington (VA): American Psychiatric Publishing; 2004. p. 6–7.
3. Connor DF, Mclaughlin TJ, Jeffers-Terry M, et al. Targeted child psychiatric services: a new model of pediatric primary clinician–child psychiatry collaborative care. Clin Pediatr (Phila) 2006;45(5):423–34.
4. Fritz GK. Introduction. In: Fritz GK, Mattison RE, Nurcombe, editors. Child and adolescent mental health consultation in hospitals, schools, and courts. Washington, DC: American Psychiatric Press, Inc.; 1993. p. ix–xv.
5. Boaz F. Foreword. In: Mead M, editor. Coming of age in Samoa. New York: HarperCollins Publishers; 2001. p. xxi–xxii.
6. Petti TA. Working within communities. In: Petti TA, Salguero C, editors. Community child and adolescent psychiatry: a manual of clinical practice and consultation. Washington, DC: American Psychiatric Publishing, Inc.; 2006. p. 3–16.
7. Caplan G, Caplan RB. Consultee-centered case consultation in mental health consultation and collaboration. Langrove (IL): Waveland Press; 1993.
8. Rappaport N. Emerging models. Child Adolesc Psychiatr Clin N Am 2001;10(1): 13–24.
9. Sheridan SM, Welch M, Orme SF. Is consultation effective? A review of research. Remedial and Special Education 1996;17:341–54.
10. Berkovitz IH. Evaluations of outcome in mental health consultation in schools. Child Adolesc Psychiatr Clin N Am 2001;10(1):93–103.
11. Bostic JQ, Bagnell A. Psychiatric school consultation: an organizing framework and empowering techniques. J Am Acad Child Adolesc Psychiatry 2001; 40(12):1–12.
12. Practice parameter for psychiatric consultation to schools. Journal of the American Academy of Child & Adolescent Psychiatry 2005;44(10):1068–83.
13. Lee AR. Creating a mental health consultation package for community agencies. Hosp Community Psychiatry 1977;28:745–8.
14. Practice parameter for the assessment and treatment of youth in juvenile detention and correctional facilities. Journal of the American Academy of Child & Adolescent Psychiatry 2005;44(10):1085–98.
15. Practice parameter on child and adolescent mental health care in community systems of care. Journal of the American Academy of Child & Adolescent Psychiatry 2007;46(2):284–99.
16. Berlin IN. A retrospective view of school mental health consultation. J Am Acad Child Adolesc Psychiatry 2001;40(12):25–31.
17. Fazel S, Doll H, Langstrom N. Mental disorders among adolescents in juvenile detention and correctional facilities: a systematic review and metaregression analysis of 25 surveys. J Am Acad Child Adolesc Psychiatry 2008;47(9): 1010–9.
18. Brown MA, Astman JA. A novel partnership in psychiatric education. Acad Psychiatry 2007;31:375–9.
19. Diamond JM, Dogin J. Role of the child and adolescent psychiatrist. In: Petti TA, Salguero C, editors. Community child and adolescent psychiatry: a manual of

clinical practice and consultation. Washington, DC: American Psychiatric Publishing, Inc.; 2006. p. 57–71.

20. American Association of Community Psychiatrists. Guidelines for developing and evaluating public and community psychiatry training fellowships. AACP Newsletter 2008;22(2):4, 5,10.

21. Mead M. Specific source unknown. Available at: http://www.interculturalstudies.org/. Accessed August 15, 2008.

Clinical Implications of Current Findings in Neurodevelopment

Penelope Knapp, MD[a],*, Ann M. Mastergeorge, PhD[b]

KEYWORDS

- Neuroplasticity • Neurodevelopment • Biological factors
- Developmental trajectories • Early indicators

CURRENT FINDINGS IN NEURODEVELOPMENT
Biological Factors

Research in the last decade has increased our knowledge about biological factors underlying neurodevelopmental processes in childhood. Genetic research has gone beyond mapping the human genome to identifying epigenetic factors and explicating gene-environment interactions. Biological markers of vulnerability to specific disorders have been identified. The functions of and interactions between neuroanatomic regions have been illuminated by new imaging and other noninvasive techniques, such as EEG, event-related potentials (ERP), and functional magnetic resonance imaging (fMRI), that allow us to link earliest signs of disorders to neurological changes.

Genetic susceptibility and other factors that influence patterns of interaction between the child and his environment will influence the development of his neural circuitry. Recent descriptions of neural circuitry[1–4] present particular new information about the development of social and language capacities, and explain more about how brain organization and function are modified as a result of interaction with the environment.

Tools to study brain development have moved the field beyond detailing of behavioral phenomena (**Fig. 1**). Striking recent advances in the understanding of gene-environment interplay and its relation to psychopathology challenge received wisdom about how psychiatric disorders develop (**Fig. 2**). Effects of genes and environment can no longer be supposed to be separate, and, via epigenetic effects, environments moderate the expression of genes. Gene-environment correlations may, through

[a] Department of Psychiatry and Behavioral Sciences, University of California, Davis, Medical Investigation of Neurodevelopmental Disorders Institute, 2825 50th Street, Sacramento, CA 95817, USA
[b] Human Development and Family Studies, University of California, Davis, Medical Investigation of Neurodevelopmental Disorders Institute, Davis Medical Center, One Shields Avenue, 2323 Hart Hall, Davis, CA 95616, USA
* Corresponding author.
E-mail address: pkknapp@ucdavis.edu (P. Knapp).

Psychiatr Clin N Am 32 (2009) 177–197
doi:10.1016/j.psc.2008.11.006
0193-953X/08/$ – see front matter © 2009 Elsevier Inc. All rights reserved.

psych.theclinics.com

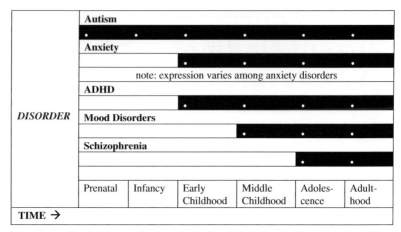

DISORDER	Autism					
	Autism					
	●	●	●	●	●	●
	Anxiety					
			●	●	●	●
	note: expression varies among anxiety disorders					
	ADHD					
			●	●	●	●
	Mood Disorders					
				●	●	●
	Schizophrenia					
					●	●
	Prenatal	Infancy	Early Childhood	Middle Childhood	Adoles-cence	Adult-hood

TIME →

Fig. 1. Typical symptom onset and expression of childhood psychiatric disorders.

effects of parent and child behaviors, influence environmental risk exposure and gene-environment interactions, as shown for disorders such as anxiety, depression, and conduct disorder, and are likely important in a range of multifactorial conditions. Our evolving understanding of complex gene-environment interplay may move the field farther from biological reductionism to understanding genetic contributions to risk and protective developmental trajectories.[5]

Neural underpinnings of human social behavior are investigated using electroencephalography and ERP methods to study neural correlates of infant processing of social information.[6] Such work can provide neurological data on the underpinnings of clinically observed developmental processes. This could better detail how maturational-modular cortical regions come "on line" in sequence, to allow development of perceptual,

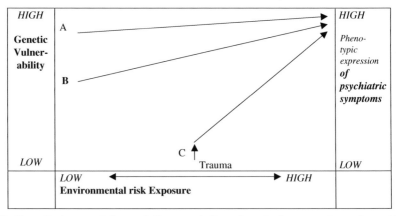

Fig. 2. Gene-Environmental correlations and the phenotypic expression of psychiatric symptoms. Curve A: Example of childhood autism: clinical picture present moderated only slightly by environmental factors. Curve B: Example of attention deficit hyperactivity disorder (ADHD): clinical picture can be influenced by environmental factors, such as structured classroom, behavioral approaches, and psychostimulant medications. Curve C: Example of posttraumatic stress disorder (PTSD): clinical picture results almost entirely from environmental factors.

cognitive, or motor abilities, such as how the maturation of the prefrontal cortex enables "theory of mind" computations. This could also provide specific information about how brain regions progress from broadly tuned to more finely tuned systems, or how some regions of the cortex gradually specialize for processing social stimuli.

Trajectories of anatomic brain development (ie, morphometric changes over time) can be understood with new imaging techniques. Noninvasive neuroimaging expands our understanding of how the cerebral cortex is organized over time. Shaw and colleagues[7] relate traditional cortical maps to new developmental data from sequential imaging to demonstrate differing levels of complexity in cerebral cortical growth. Longitudinal anatomic MRI studies of children with typical development, with ADHD, and with childhood onset schizophrenia begin to define trajectories of brain development. This enables visualizing a phenotypic bridge between genes and behavior in healthy children and in those with psychiatric illness.[8]

While some disorders, such as autism, have early and relatively invariant onset, most psychiatric disorders may evidence their onset over many years. This is because allostatic load, or the physiological costs of chronic exposure to neural or neuroendocrine stress, has relatively more influence. Consequently, heritability effects on behavior may increase across the lifespan.[9] Markers of biological vulnerabilities that moderate the effects of environment on behavior have been identified: for example, respiratory sinus arrhythmia, a measure of parasympathetic activity, predicts capability for emotion regulation that may protect children in high-risk environments from developing psychopathology.[10]

Markers of biological vulnerability[9] also improve prediction of psychopathology. For example, for children whose parents are schizophrenic, taxometric analyses of certain behavioral and endophenotypic markers, such as impaired attention, saccadic intrusions in smooth pursuit eye tracking, and spatial working memory deficits, may facilitate identifying premorbid schizophrenia at younger ages. Neurobiological markers of risk are beginning to be identified for bipolar disorder through neuroimaging. Dysregulated activity in the anterior network, affecting activity of hypothalamic nuclei, is hypothesized to bring about neurovegetative symptoms, such as altered appetite, energy, and sleep.[11] Specific genetic and neurobiological markers may identify particularly vulnerable individuals. Bryant[12] reviewed studies of heart rate as a marker for vulnerability to PTSD following trauma, and concluded that in combination with diagnostic status immediately after trauma—that is, whether or not the individual met criteria for acute stress disorder—heart rate predicted the emergence of PTSD.

New noninvasive techniques have expanded recent understanding of both how normal development and learning occur, and how psychopathology develops. Differences in emotional arousal to social stimuli have been shown to be associated with psychiatric symptoms.[13] Children with reduced emotional arousal had higher levels of conduct problems, and those with increased arousal had higher levels of anxiety symptoms at 1-year follow-up. Recent understanding of the more complex and specific role of the locus ceruleus-norepinehrine (LC-NE) system demonstrates that it influences not only arousal and engagement, but also disengagement from a task and movement toward alternative exploratory behaviors.[14]

Better understanding of neurobiological substrates informs us about how any child, not only the child with a psychiatric disorder, may learn and remember. In addition to the memory system that includes the hippocampus, the basal ganglia, in particular the dorsal striatum, plays a role in learning and memory.[15] Habitual or stereotyped learned behavioral routines could develop as a result of experience-dependent plasticity in basal ganglia-based circuits, and may influence cognitive activity as well as behavior.[16] Neuroanatomical correlates of temperament have been elucidated by demonstrating correlations between four core temperament dimensions, effortful control, negative affectivity, surgency and affiliativeness, temperamental characteristics and volumetric measures of anterior cingulated cortex (ACC), orbitofrontal cortex, amygdala, and hippocampus,[17] providing evidence for a neuroanatomical basis for individual temperament differences. Better understanding of the neurobiological mechanisms that may underlie the development of certain psychiatric disorders will move the field beyond clinical description to knowledge that is tactical for prevention and early intervention.

Neuroplasticity

Neuroplasticity is the term for alterations of time course of responses and of activation thresholds that occur through short-term synapse modulations and long-term neuro-anatomical growth and pruning. Neuroplastic processes allow experience-dependent adaptation, but neuroplastic changes to adapt to harmful experiences may lead to psychopathology. Recent research deepens our understanding of these processes. Molecular mechanisms for the influence of nurture upon nature, and ways that epigenetic effects on gene expression influence brain development are being explicated.[18]

For example, parental nurturance during infancy (eg, tactile stimulation of infant rodents) up-regulates glucocorticoid receptors in the hippocampus and frontal cortex, inhibiting input to hypothalamic neurons containing corticotropin-releasing hormone and increasing expression of a nerve growth factor-induced clone A, a critical transcription factor. Failure of such up-regulation, as in severe neglect, could bring about pervasive problems in self-regulation observed in maltreated children.[19]

Because the processes by which the child's brain continuously interacts with his social environment are dynamic, manifestations of emerging disorders change over time. This calls for conceptual changes to the categorical diagnostic descriptive scheme. Equifinality, the concept that diverse etiological factors may culminate in a single diagnosis (for example Conduct Disorder), is one example of such a change; multifinality, the concept that a single etiological factor may culminate in many diagnoses (for example sequelae of childhood abuse) is another.[20]

Comorbidity, defined as the co-occurrence of two or more psychological disorders, has been identified as one of the most pressing current issues in developmental psychology and psychiatry. The presence of comorbidity is considered to be a marker of risk.[21] The concept of comorbidity may describe, but not explain, the observation of the phenomenon that symptoms cross Diagnostic and Statistical Manual of Mental Disorders (DSM) diagnostic categories. More recent concepts of homotypic and heterotypic disorder patterns better explain this phenomenon.

Homotypic disorders co-occur within the externalizing spectrum, as when a child meets criteria for ADHD plus oppositional defiant disorder (ODD), or the internalizing spectrum, as when the child has both anxiety and depressive disorders. Though homotypic comorbidity among differently classified disorders is high,[22] very different treatment approaches have been promulgated for specific disorders. Yet it is now understood that a common dysfunction in the mesolimbic dopamine (DA) system, is a core neural substrate of risk for most if not all externalizing behaviors.[9,23] Positron emission tomography and fMRI studies have linked low DA levels with neural activity in the primary reward centers of the brain, and core clinical symptoms of externalizing psychophathology, such as sensation seeking, low motivation, irritability, and negative affectivity. Thus, central DA dysfunction is a probable endophenotype of genetic risk. Moreover, different internalizing or externalizing disorders may develop sequentially across the lifespan, as is the case for ADHD preceding Tourette syndrome or antisocial personality disorder, or the successive development of different anxiety disorders. This is termed "homotypic continuity." Central dopaminergic dysfunction may account for this.[24]

"Heterotypic disorder" is the term for the co-occurrence of an internalizing disorder, such as anxiety, with an externalizing disorder, such as ADHD. Common neural and genetic effects influence diverse classes of heterotypic disorders as well.[9] A common neural deficiency likely accounts for overlapping symptoms in these disorders.[23] Studying overlapping biological vulnerabilities for depression and conduct disorder (CD), we observe that both are characterized by irritability, negative affectivity, and anhedonia, and that each of these symptoms has been linked at the neural level with reduced activation in structures involved in approach motivation. Furthermore, blunted activation has been revealed by neuroimaging studies in mesolimbic and mesocortical regions during reward tasks in both CD and depression.[25–27]

Other biological traits moderate a deficiency in DA-mediated reward circuitry. Individuals with low behavioral inhibition present principally with CD, and those with high behavioral inhibition present principally with depression.[10] In individuals with blunted reward systems, high-trait anxiety modulated by the septohippocampal system, a different (primarily serotonergic) neural network potentiates depression, whereas low-trait anxiety potentiates delinquency.

Attachment: A Neurobiological Perspective

Another new approach in developmental psychopathology is work exploring a deeper understanding of the effect upon brain development of interpersonal interactions, particularly in infancy and early childhood. This builds on the concepts of attachment and attachment disorders. The attachment system is a goal-corrected motivational system that, optimally, buffers stress and that, when malfunctioning, fails to do so.[28] Not all interactions between parent and child will be integral to attachment motivations or affectivity. The attachment system has roots in a biological system that ultimately regulates behavior and is implicated in stress reactivity and self-regulation.[29,30]

Early positive and nurturing experience generally influences a developmental trajectory that allows the child to make positive adaptations to stress. This is mediated and moderated by biobehavioral interactions. For example, daily cortisol production has been shown to be influenced by positive parenting and sensitive discipline.[31] The success of a brief intervention focused on increasing parental sensitivity may be moderated by heritable factors: children's dopamine levels influence whether, if their mothers' behavior was insensitive, they developed externalizing behaviors, such as oppositionality and aggression, and their response to treatment.[32] The fact that there are children who respond differentially to both sensitive and insensitive parenting, depending on whether their genome has a particular allele repeat, is evidence of gene-environment coaction.[33] Attachment-focused interventions for young children appear to have long-term consequences for a dyregulated stress system. There is mounting evidence for the plasticity of basic neurobiological processes[34,35] that may mitigate neuroendocrine stress.[36,37] Identifying individual differences in neurobiologically based traits,[9,38,39] including gender,[40] will allow development of specific and targeted interventions effective for a particular vulnerable group of children.

Parent-child interactions may also pose risk for specific diagnoses. Dietz and colleagues,[41] measuring affect and behavior for mothers and depressed children, observed more negativity and less positivity in their dyadic interactions than in parent-child interactions for high-risk control children. The mothers of depressed children were more disengaged than were control mothers. Bidirectional effects of low child positivity and maternal disengagement endured after recovery from the depressive episode. These may be risk factors that precede onset of major depressive disorder and predispose to recurrent depression.

Mapping Developmental Trajectories of Psychopathology

Given that biological vulnerabilities moderate effects of environment on behavior, and that environments both potentiate and mitigate biological vulnerabilities through mechanisms such as epigenetic factors and mechanisms of neuroplasticity, such as neural pruning, how do we map the trajectories of psychopathology?

More specific descriptions of biological and psychological systems allow clearer characterization of individual differences. Diverse causal processes operate differently for individuals, and can provide better explanations of risk and protective factors and resilient adaptations, and better inform treatment.[42]

Taking childhood onset bipolar disorder (BD) as an example, biological underpinnings of this condition have been explored with an MRI study using three-dimensional mapping of the hippocampus. Findings suggest a possible neural correlate for the memory deficits observed in these youngsters, and may reflect abnormal developmental mechanisms.[43] Understanding the atypical developmental mechanisms can provide a clinician with specific intervention targets to ameliorate memory deficits within the confounds of the known neurobiological constraints. Another example of a neuroanatomical marker is the size of the amygdala. Longitudinal study of amygdala volume provides preliminary evidence of decreased amygdala volume in adolescents and young adults with BD persisting over 2 years.[44] Compared with average individuals, the amygdala is smaller in bipolar children and larger in bipolar adults, suggesting that a feature of BD is abnormal patterns of growth.[45] Cortical development before and after onset of pediatric bipolar illness also reveals a distinct pattern, as shown in longitudinal mapping studies, which may reflect general affective dysregulation (lability). Mapping also demonstrated subtle, regionally specific, bilaterally asymmetrical cortical changes in children who had similar initial presentations of transient psychosis and of mood dysregulation who did not go on to develop bipolar illness.[46]

Diffusion tensor imaging methods yield findings of decreased fractional anisotropy that demonstrate abnormalities in the structural integrity of the ACC in BD, possibly contributing to altered interhemispheric connectivity in this disorder.[47] The dorsolateral prefrontal cortex (PFC), ACC, and striatum, brain regions involved with attentional circuitry, have overlapping involvement with regions affecting mood regulation. Disruption in these areas, or in the connections between them, could lead to dysfunction of mood regulation and attention.[21]

As noted, childhood trauma has long been known to lead to protean psychopathology, and recent work begins to explain why. Heim and colleagues[48] reviewed clinical studies suggesting that childhood trauma sensitizes the neuroendocrine stress response, alters glucocorticoid resistance, increases central corticotropin-releasing factor (CRF) activity, affects immune activation, and reduces hippocampal volume. This parallels neuroendocrine features of depression. The same group found that these effects of child abuse on adult depressive symptoms are moderated by genetic polymorphisms within the corticotropin-releasing hormone type-1 receptor gene,[49] supporting a gene-environment interaction.

DIAGNOSTIC FACTORS
Early Indicators/Early Recognition of Specific Conditions

Even as we gain better understanding about how neurodevelopmental processes cut across diagnoses, the heuristic of DSM diagnosis nonetheless informs subject selection for current studies. ADHD, CD, BD, schizophrenia, and anxiety disorders will be considered in turn.

An editorial review[50] of genetic and imaging studies of ADHD refers to work demonstrating subtle neuroanatomic and functional metabolic abnormalities, and the identification of several replicable candidate genes. Both these lines of inquiry provide increasing evidence of biological mediation of this most commonly diagnosed childhood disorder and show that, while the entire brain appears to be affected to some extent, the cerebellum, striatum, and prefrontal cortex seem most compromised. However, the same lines of inquiry also show that effects are not diagnosis-specific, as genetic liability for the temperamental features of ADHD and those for antisocial behavior show substantial overlap.[5]

In the emergence of conduct disorder, genetic liability is potentiated by early experience. Rutter and colleagues[5] and Caspi and colleagues[51] have demonstrated individual differences in a functional polymorphism in the promoter region of the Monoamine Oxidase A (MAOA) gene that confers lower levels of expression of MAOA, the enzyme that metabolizes norepinephrine, serotonin, and dopamine. In a study designed to show the genetic association with maltreatment, Rutter and colleagues[5] find that MAOA polymorphism is associated with the later development of conduct disorders in maltreated children.

Childhood onset of BD, as well as its observed comorbid conditions, has spurred publications at a hyperactive pace in the last decade. Recent work has clarified certain developmental factors.[52] Episodicity of mood symptoms is an important predictor:[53] episodic irritability predicts mania, while chronic, nonepisodic irritability predicts later onset of ADHD and major depressive disorder (MDD). Episodic mood lability, hypersensitivity, and anger dyscontrol and subsyndromal affective symptoms of BD occur much earlier than age 18, the average age at illness onset (for a review, see Miklowitz and Chang[21] and Liebenluft and Rich).[54] Although mania is likeliest to be preceded by early adolescent depression, childhood depression is associated with multiple clinical outcomes, an example of multifinality. Other risk factors also contribute to the development of BD. Early sexual abuse is associated with earlier age at onset of BD, with more comorbidity, suicidality, and treatment resistance, an example of an environmental potentiator.[55]

Miklowitz and Chang[21] present a model of BD development, postulating that disruptions of mood regulation and attention result if brain areas involved with mood regulation and overlapping with attentional circuitry are disrupted, or if connections between them are disrupted. Neuroimaging studies in pediatric BD support this model, showing abnormalities in subcortical-limbic brain regions, especially in the amygdala and basal ganglia. Decreased volume may mean heightened activity in the amygdala, which has been demonstrated in response to affective stress in functional imaging studies in children with BD.[56] Lacking compensatory prefrontal regulation, such heightened activation without could generate heightened experience of mood states (euphoria, sadness), which could progress to a fully syndromal mood pattern.

There is recent recognition that schizophrenia is not a neurodegenerative disorder, that pre- and perinatal adverse effects may contribute to its occurrence, and that cognitive and behavioral signs—observable during childhood—are prodromal indicators. This has led to reconceptualizing schizophrenia as a developmental disorder,[57] and has generated inquiries about the nature and the timing of factors that, in genetically susceptible individuals, increase risk. Studies seeking to identify which molecular and histogenic responses might lead to the developmental trajectory of schizophrenia have addressed stress effects on the hypothalamic-pituitary adrenal axis (HPA),[58] early disruption of white matter pathways in the hippocampal region,[59,60] progressive changes in temporal lobe structures,[61] and the possible progression from limbic system disruption seen in children and adolescents with schizophrenia to the more generalized abnormalities seen in adults.[62]

Anxiety and depressive disorders span a broad range of severity and clinical heterogeneity. Their etiology is frequently unclear, which hampers specific treatment planning beyond efforts at symptom abatement. Recent studies with genetically sensitive designs have shown environmentally mediated effects from particular risk environments for depression and anxiety (see Rutter, Moffit, and Caspi[5] for a review). Building on previous reports that the short allele of the serotonin transporter gene is associated with increased risk of depression, Caspi and colleagues[63] have presented evidence for the role of serotonin in vulnerability to depression, and that the allele variant may be dependent on gene-environment interaction.

These approaches also may illuminate the neurobiological effects of specific treatments. Commonalities in the biological mechanisms of psycho- and pharmacotherapy have been demonstrated.[64] Functional neuroimaging studies of psychotherapeutic effects of cognitive behavioral therapy in phobia and in obsessive-compulsive disorder consistently show decreased metabolism in the right caudate nucleus, similar to effects observed after successful intervention with selective serotonin reuptake inhibitors.

Other Investigative Approaches to Understanding Child Development

Recent work linking information—obtained from imaging—about activity of specific brain regions to patterns of psychopathology provides guidance to understanding symptom patterns.[65]

Efforts to link temperament and psychopathology, which have guided much psychiatric literature, are being advanced with new approaches. Caspi and Silva[66] explored the continuity between behavioral styles in 3-year-old children to their personality traits at age 18. Five temperament groups (labeled undercontrolled, inhibited, confident, reserved, and well-adjusted) were identified from behavioral ratings when children were 3 years of age. These were compared with personality styles measured with the Multidimensional Personality Questionnaire at age 18. Undercontrolled children identified at age 3 scored high at age 18 on measures of impulsivity, danger seeking, aggression, and interpersonal alienation. Children who at age 3 were inhibited, scored low at 18 on measures of impulsivity, danger seeking, aggression, and social potency; confident children at age 3 went on to develop high impulsivity scores; reserved children tend to develop low social potency scores. Children scored at age 3 as well-adjusted maintained stable normative behaviors.

An alternative approach is latent class analysis (LCA) or latent profiles analysis (LPA). The goal is to identify naturally occurring clusters of symptoms without requiring diagnostic specification by imposing cutoffs for the number of symptoms required by The Diagnostic and Statistical Manual of Mental Disorders, Fourth Edition (DSM-IV).[67] To identify children having similar underlying response profiles, temperament traits are compared with diagnostic symptomatology through individual questionnaire items, or quantitative scores for several diagnostic subscales. Applications of LCA point to categories and subtypes that differ significantly from current DSM-based conceptualizations. These clusters have been demonstrated to show higher heritability estimates than DSM-IV subtypes. For example, monozygotic co-twins are more likely to resemble one another in latent class membership than in their DSM-IV subtype classification. These finding may enable designing genetic studies that do not exclude information about what is now called "diagnostic comorbidity."

Going further, Acosta and colleagues[67] applied LCA to children with ADHD and their siblings. Their findings replicated six to eight significantly distinct clusters, which were mostly stable when comorbid diagnoses were included. They fitted data on DSM-IV symptoms of ADHD, ODD, and CD, and to seven symptoms screening for anxiety and depression, with LCA models. They found ODD symptoms in young children to be associated with either anxiety-related symptoms or conduct disorder; the combined type of ADHD to be related to externalizing disorders, especially CD; and ADHD inattentive and combined types to be strongly related to anxiety and depression.

Rettew and colleagues,[68] using the Juvenile Temperament and Character Inventory, identified four temperament traits: novelty seeking, persistence, harm avoidance, and reward dependence. LPA then identified three classes of temperament trait clusters: steady, disengaged, and moderate. Children in the moderate class had average levels of temperament traits. Children in the steady class had high persistence and low novelty seeking. Children in the disengaged class had higher harm avoidance and novelty seeking but lower persistence and reward dependence. They also had lower functioning and higher symptomatology on the Child Behavior Checklist. Yet, this variable-centered approach is limited if it is assumed that a particular temperamental trait operates independently. Other factors, including the parents' temperament and the quality of the parent-child attachment, also influence whether the child will develop symptoms consistent with a DSM diagnosis.

Rettew and colleagues[69] built on previous goodness-of-fit theories by exploring the relations between child temperament, parent temperament, and symptoms of child psychopathology. Although many child temperament dimensions were found to exert significant independent effects, they found that an association between a child temperament trait and psychopathology depends in part upon the temperament of parents. Specifically, child attentional problems were associated with high child-novelty seeking plus high maternal-novelty seeking, and increased child internalizing problems were associated with high child-harm avoidance plus high father-harm avoidance.

However, these cross-sectional data do not allow determination of the direction of causality: do temperamental traits lead to increased or decreased functioning or do children who have less involvement with family and others, fitting the disengaged class, then develop temperamental traits of high novelty seeking and low persistence?

Comorbidity

The field of child psychiatry is bedeviled methodologically by the concept of comorbidity. Comorbidities are the rule in ADHD[70,71] and conduct disorder.[72] Mood disorders are comorbid with ADHD and also CD.[73] While ODD is highly comorbid with ADHD, it also follows different developmental trajectories, ending in either anxiety or CD.

Using symptom clusters as variables for analysis rather than DSM-IV research diagnostic criteria allows a more powerful and flexible approach to exploring genetic factors and other influences on development.

PREVENTION AND INTERVENTION

Recent reframing of ideas about how psychopathology develops open the field to better strategies for prevention and early intervention. Cicchetti and Gunnar[42] suggest that liabilities in the organization of a child's biological and psychological systems, which interatively and progressively undermine adaptation to experiences, may lead to the development of patterns described as psychopathology. Their model views the emergence of clinical syndromes as the result of probabilities of development, rather than deterministic effects of either inborn or experiential factors. If attention is not paid to how constitutional, hereditable individual differences, or neurobiological bases of temperament influence the child's reaction to experience, then the conclusion will be reached that biological processes are neither malleable nor responsive to change as a result of experience. The test of this is to study environmental experience during development, specifically by evaluating, via randomized approaches, the effects of specific interventions.[74]

Early Indicators and Early Recognition

In general, the goal of prevention and early intervention is to identify periods of development when specific treatment may be more efficacious, so that intervention can be targeted to that period. Gaining insight into the mechanisms of change, the extent to which neural plasticity may be promoted and the inextricable nature of both biological and psychological processes is necessary. This will further our understanding of the developmental trajectory of psychopathology and the resilience and response indicators moderated by individual difference factors.

Advances in developmental psychopathology, neurobiology, genetics, and developmental neuroscience have contributed to new methods for early indicators and effective treatments. For example, Dawson[75] proposed a developmental model of risk, risk process, symptom emergence, and adaptation in autism spectrum disorders (ASD) that incorporates indices of genetic, environmental, and phenotypic risk that allow for early identification of vulnerability factors. For example, some studies have described that the emergence of typical social brain circuitry is contingent on the key roles of parent-child interaction. Furthermore, reciprocal interactions facilitate cortical specialization and fine tune perceptual systems.[4,76,77]

Early intervention that enhances parent-child interactions has received recent attention.[78-80] In studies of at-risk populations, behavioral interventions have been determined to be most effective when they focus on parental sensitivity and infant contingent responsiveness.[29] For example, videotaped feedback to parents, focusing on their child's risk characteristics, was most effective in facilitating early social engagement and reciprocity correlated with the child's brain circuitry.

Understanding how cumulative effects and interactions among a variety of factors contribute to biological risk is important in tailoring individual intervention approaches. For example, intervention for a child diagnosed with both an attachment disorder and a conduct disorder will need to be tailored in terms of timing, intensity, and context. A central goal of intervention is to promote resilient adaptation,[34,42,81] beginning by examining symptom clusters. Several studies have used this approach in examining ADHD and other psychiatric disorders,[82] as well as comorbidity in autism and mental retardation.[75] Understanding the complexity of diverse developmental disorders and pathways helps focus early intervention and prevention strategies. For example, for children with genetic loading for mood disorder, early psychotherapeutic interventions in conjunction with medication have been most efficacious.[83] Alternatively, for young children, where environmental or contextual factors play a predominant role in their disorder (such as attachment disorder or regulatory disorders), interventions that focus on parent-child interactions and protective factors in the social environment may be most effective in promoting positive developmental outcomes.[21]

If, as suggested by LCA studies, particular temperament profiles are common to more than one category of psychiatric disorder, then high rates of comorbidity described in child and adolescent psychiatric literature may be observed because the symptom descriptors are nonspecific. Conversely, recognition of particular temperament profiles, such as the combination of high harm avoidance and high novelty seeking with low persistence and low reward dependence will indicate that the extent to which social and family situations may buffer the child from negative reactions to ordinary experiences is relatively minimal. Obviously, identifying family factors that potentiate or mitigate child temperament profiles must inform treatment planning.

Monitoring Intervention

Monitoring the effects of treatment requires tracking change over time using clear and measurable outcomes. Standards and requirements for evidence-based interventions, requiring monitoring and accountability, have been developed for this reason.

Biological vulnerabilities are progressively potentiated by and modified by epigenesis, neural plasticity, and neural pruning, and these are influenced by the infant or child's environment, including interpersonal experience.[9] This may occur in prenatal development; examples are the association of maternal nicotine exposure to the development of externalizing behaviors in children[84] and the well-known spectrum of fetal alcohol syndrome disorders. It may occur in perinatal and infant development; developmental sequelae of infant neglect and trauma have been abundantly documented.[19] Potentiation of biological vulnerability may also occur during childhood. Genetic predisposition toward fearfulness, interacting with events in the environment, may alter neural circuits involved in the emotional experience and expression, perpetuating and amplifying anxious behavior throughout the lifespan.[85]

As noted, child maltreatment and neglect may alter biobehavioral function of children, altering their diurnal pattern of cortisol secretion even several years after adverse experiences.[86] Higher levels of externalizing behaviors have been associated with higher basal levels of cortisol; school-aged children with normal activity have lower basal levels of cortisol. A recent study examined the effects on daily cortisol of an attachment-based intervention for young children.[31] The intervention focused on skills associated with cognitive and behavioral school readiness, skills highly contingent on the development of the executive regulatory systems during the preschool years.[87,88]

Intervention may mollify or modulate the course of even the most significant genetically influenced early developmental disorders. Autism has been shown to be associated with genetic differences driving abnormalities in cerebellar development, bringing about reduced Purkinje cells in the cerebellar cortex,[89,90] altering interneuronal development and connectivity, and creating early overgrowth followed by premature arrest of growth. Yet early behavioral and pharmacological intervention may positively influence brain plasticity and prevent full expression of ASD.[75]

Clearer characterization of the genetic and experiential contributors to self-regulation may inform targeted interventions for vulnerable children. For example, genetic variation in the Catechol-0-methyltransferase (COMT) gene, which codes for the COMT enzyme that regulates dopamine levels in the prefrontal cortex, influences function in response to stress. Individuals with methionine on both genes at codon 158 have more available dopamine in the PFC and display better executive functioning than those with valine on both, but are more sensitive to stress levels that disrupt cognitive function. Therefore, promotion of self-regulation, considered as a means of preventing school failure,[88] must take into account both vertical and horizontal integration across levels of biological and social influences.

CLINICAL IMPLICATIONS

Etiological heterogeneity among high-risk groups should predict differential treatment response.[39,91] While neuroscientific principles in the theoretical formulation of

Table 1
Clinical implications of new findings in neurodevelopment

New Finding	Concept	Clinical Implication
Biological factors		
Genetic research	Gene-environment interactions	Challenges received wisdom about how psychiatric disorders develop
	Gene-environmental correlations	Child and parent factors affect environmental risk exposure
	Epigenetic effects influence environmental expression of genes	Effects of genes and environment cannot be supposed to be separate
ERP, MRI, and fMRI studies describe morphometric changes over time	Phenotypic bridge between genes and development of behaviors	Links between neurolo-developmental changes and earliest signs of disorders
Biological markers of vulnerability to specific disorders (eg, taxometric analyses)	Heritability increases over the lifespan	Better prediction of psychopathology; allostatic load differs for some disorders
Identification of core temperamental dimensions, and their correlation with volumetric measures of brain regions	Neuroanatomical correlates of temperament	Better understanding of individual (temperamental) factors allows tactical prevention and early intervention
Explication of molecular mechanisms for influence of experience	Manifestations of emerging disorders change over time	Conceptual change to categorical diagnostic schemes
Up-regulation of glucocorticoid receptors in hippocampus	Equifinality; multifinality	Failure of up-regulation → pervasive problems seen in maltreated children
Common dysfunction in mesolimbic DA system in externalizing disorders	Homotypic disorders: co-occur within a spectrum (eg, externalizing: ADHD and CD)	Be aware of different treatment approaches for different disorders
Neuroplasticity		
Blunted activation in CD and ADHD during reward tasks	Heterotypic disorders: co-occurrence of disorders in both internalizing and externalizing spectrum (eg, depression and CD)	Recognize underlying features common to both (eg, central dopamine dysfunction); Recognize that externalizing and internalizing disorder may develop sequentially because of underlying neurobiology

Separate biological traits moderate each other	For example: DA-mediated blunted reward systems interact with septohippocampal system → high anxiety → depression, and interact with serotonergic system → delinquency	Evaluate child in multiple domains (eg, anxiety, depression, impulsivity, cognition), not just "symptom checklists" to predict psychopathology
Attachment		
Heritable factors (specific allele repeat) influence child response to parenting through gene-environment co-action	Child dopamine level influences whether insensitive parenting → externalizing or internalizing behavior pattern	Identifying individual neurobiology will inform specific and targeted interventions for particular vulnerable groups of children
Mapping developmental trajectories		
3-D MRI mapping of hippocampus in bipolar disorder points to neural correlates of memory	Abnormal developmental mechanisms underlie cognitive impairment in depression	Allows specific intervention targets to ameliorate memory deficits within the confounds of the known neurobiological constraints
Decreased amygdalar volume in persistent BD (adolescents and young adults)	A feature of bipolar disorder is abnormal pattern of neural growth	Better understanding of general affective dysregulation (lability)
Diffusion tensor imaging: abnormalities in ACC → dorsolateral PFC and striatum	Possibly contributes to altered interhemispheric connectivity in bipolar disorder	Explains co-occurrence of dysfunction of mood regulation and attention
Childhood trauma sensitizes neuroendocrine stress response, increases central CRF activity, and reduces hippocampal volume	Neuroendocrine features of depression are paralleled by neuroendocrine features of trauma	Explains protean clinical features of PTSD and points to need for comprehensive clinical response
Early indicators/recognition of specific conditions		
ADHD: cerebellum, striatum, and prefrontal cortex are most compromised	Biological mediation of ADHD	Effects are not specific to the diagnosis of ADHD
CD: functional polymorphism in promoter region of MAOA gene	Genetic liability is potentiated by early experience	Children with MAOA polymorphism who are maltreated, are at greater risk of CD
BD: episodic irritability predicts mania; chronic, nonepisodic irritability predicts ADHD and MDD	Subsyndromal affective symptoms of bipolar disorder can be recognized	Because subsyndromal symptoms precede full clinical onset, prevention and early intervention can be initiated for BD

(continued on next page)

Table 1
(continued)

New Finding	Concept	Clinical Implication
Childhood schizophrenia: stress effects on HPA, disrupted hippocampal white matter, early limbic system disruption, progressive temporal lobe changes	Evidence that schizophrenia is a developmental (not neurodegenerative) disorder	Recognition of neuroanatomical and subsyndromal features allow aggressive early intervention
Anxiety and depression:short allele of serotonin transporter gene → increased risk of depression	Environmentally mediated effects potentiate gene-environment interaction	Recognition of genetic risk may influence more comprehensive preventive treatment
Other investigative approaches to understanding child development		
LCA- or LPA-identified temperament profiles show higher heritability than DSM diagnoses	Temperament categories and subtypes differ from current DSM conceptualizatons	Allows designing genetic studies that do not exclude "comorbidity"
LCA of ADHD and ADHD siblings allow recognition of risk for ODD, anxiety, or CD	LCA profiles are more stable over time than DSM diagnoses	Allows prediction of "comorbid" risk and, accordingly, informs treatment planning
LPA-identified classes temperament clusters in parents and children	Association between child and parent temperament predicts child psychopathology	Informs family-based components of treatment
Prevention and early intervention: early indicators/early recognition		
ASD: emergence of typical social brain circuitry depends on parent-child interaction	Reciprocal interactions facilitate cortical specialization	Identifying family factors that potentiate or mitigate child temperament profiles informs treatment planning
Monitoring intervention		
Autism associated with genetic differences driving abnormal cerebellar development	Early behavioral and pharmacological intervention may positively influence brain plasticity and prevent full expression of ASD	Intervention may mollify or modulate the course of even the most significant genetically influenced early developmental disorders
Genetic variation in COMT influences function in response to stress	Promotion of self-regulation, must take into account both vertical and horizontal integration across levels of biological and social influences	Characterization of genetic and experiential contributors may inform targeted interventions for vulnerable children

Taxometric analyses: description of behavioral and endophenotypic markers, such as impaired attention, saccadic intrusions in smooth pursuit, eye tracking, and spatial working memory deficits.

prevention and intervention are not yet pervasive in the literature (see Refs. 30 and 92 for exceptions), understanding vulnerability based on specific genetic and neurobiological markers is critical to designing a benign environmental impact for the specific child, namely specific treatment.[39,91] Clinical implications of new findings are summarized in **Table 1**.

Individual differences in response to early intervention may be the result of several factors, including the nature and severity of the genetic and environmental risk factors and comorbidity. It has been well documented that early intervention has positive effects on developmental trajectories.[92,93] However, to fully understand the mechanisms responsible for effective interventions, integrating biological processes into both the design and evaluation of interventions is required, which may include conducting brain imagining studies before assigning early intervention.[75] Neural areas that underlie capability for executive function include structures in dorsolateral prefrontal anterior cingulate and parietal cortex, with extensive interconnections with ventral, medial frontal, and limbic brain structures associated with emotional reactivity and regulation. Interventions that promote the development of executive function skill will enable development of other academic and social skills.[94,95]

Stress is a known common factor in the development of psychopathology. New findings on the stress system elucidate two components: the locus ceruleus/noradrenergic sympathetic system and the HPA axis.[36] Stress influences and modifies the functioning of the HPA axis, as has been amply documented.[96] This effect evolves over the course of development. As noted in preschool children, higher basal levels of cortisol (hyperactivity) are associated with higher levels of externalizing behavior, and in school-aged children externalizing behavior is associated with lower basal levels of cortisol (hypoactivity). Better understanding of links between neuroendocrine changes following trauma and specific neuroendocrine features of depression may lead to improved clinical care and prevention of adverse outcomes for traumatized children.[48]

Intervention studies that quantify and target stress will contribute to our understanding of how malleable these processes may be. Bakermans-Kranenburg and colleagues[31] targeted the relationship of the DRD4 gene, to insensitive parenting as a predictor of later externalizing behaviors. Children with the 7-repeat allele exposed to insensitive care compared with children without these combined risks have a sixfold increase in risk of developing externalizing behaviors. If assessment approaches include measures of genetic factors, it may be possible to define interventions that go beyond a "spray and pray" approach to all potentially stressed parent-infant dyads and devise interventions that will specifically target the most vulnerable infants and young children.[97]

Foster children are an obvious specific high-risk group. For example, the 7-repeat allele of the DRD4 gene has been linked to lower dopamine-reception efficiency, influencing how the dopaminergic system engages in attentional, motivational, and reward mechanisms. The dopamine system may affect the susceptibility to environmental influences, playing an important role in gene-environment interactions. Bakermans-Kranenburg and colleagues,[31] Fisher and colleagues,[30] and Gunnar and colleagues[86] have observed atypical patterns of cortisol production among infants and preschool children in foster care, pointing to possible down-regulation of the HPA system over time as the result of initially high levels of circulating cortisol.[98]

An application to treatment of childhood schizophrenia is the demonstration[99] that cognitive behavioral therapy combined with a low dose of Risperidone reduced the onset of first-episode psychosis in high-risk patients with a positive family history and incipient, subthreshold symptoms. An application to BD is the finding of Chang and colleagues[100] and Miklowitz,[101] that early intervention may delay the age of onset of the full syndrome, showing that early intervention may delay the age of onset for BD.[100,101]

Recognizing homotypic comorbidity (as among externalizing or internalizing disorders) and heterotypic comormbidity (as in the co-occurrence of both internalizing and externalizing disorders), and informed by LCA approaches to underlying temperamental or biodevelopmental factors, we see that it is important to develop prevention and early intervention programs that do not focus on single disorders.

Instead, intervention programs should be designed to anticipate homotypic continuity or heterotypic manifestations of underlying factors. Recognition of the importance of temperamental traits and the social environmental context should guide the development of empirically supported adjunctive treatment. Standardized measures for assessment and outcome should be employed for intensive, regular follow-ups not only of psychopathology symptoms but also of expression of temperamental traits and the impact of social environmental context.

REFERENCES

1. Dawson G, Munson J, Estes A, et al. Neurocognitive function and joint attention ability in young children with autism spectrum disorder versus developmental delay. Child Dev 2002;73:345–58.
2. Grelotti D, Gauthier I, Schultz R. Social interest and the development of cortical face specialization: what autism teaches us about face processing. Dev Psychobiol 2002;40:213–25.
3. Johnson M, Griffin R, Csibra G, et al. The emergence of the social brain network: evidence from typical and atypical development. Dev Psychopathol 2005;17: 599–619.
4. Kuhl P. Is speech learning "gated" by the social brain? Int J Dev Neurosci 2007; 10:110–20.
5. Rutter M, Moffitt TE, Caspi A. Gene-environment interplay and psychopathology: multiple varieties but real effects. J Child Psychol Psychiatry 2006;47(3–4): 226–61.
6. Grossman T, Johnson M. The development of the social brain in human infancy. Eur J Neurosci 2007;25:909–19.
7. Shaw P, Kabani NJ, Lerch JP, et al. Neurodevelopmental trajectories of the human cerebral cortex. J Neurosci 2008;28(14):3586–94.
8. Giedd JN, Lenroot RK, Shaw P, et al. Trajectories of anatomic brain development as a phenotype. Novartis Found Symp 2008;289:101–12.
9. Beauchaine TB, Neuhaus E, Brenner SL, et al. Ten good reasons to consider biological processes in prevention and intervention research. Dev Psychopathol 2008;20(3):745–74.
10. Beauchaine TP, Gatzke-Kopp L, Mead HK. Polyvagal theory and developmental psychopathology: emotion dysregulation and conduct problems from pre-school to adolescence. Biol Psychiatry 2007;61:720–4.
11. Strakowski SM, DelBello MP, Adler CM. The functional neuroanatomy of bipolar disorder: a review of neuroimaging findings. Mol Psychiatry 2005;10:105–16.
12. Bryant RA. Longitudinal psychophysiological studies of heart rate: mediating effects and implications for treatment. Ann N Y Acad Sci 2006;1071:19–26.
13. Sharp C, Petersen N, Goodyer I. Emotional reactivity and the emergence of conduct problems and emotional symptoms in 7–11-year olds, a 1 yr follow-up study. J Am Acad Child Adolesc Psychiatry 2008;47(5):565–73.

14. Aston-Jones F, Cohen JD. An integrative theory of locus coeruleus-norepineph-rine function adaptive gain and optimal performance. Annu Rev Neurosci 2005; 28:403–50.
15. Packard MG, Knowlton BJ. Learning and memory functions of the basal ganglia. Annu Rev Neurosci 2002;25(3):563–93.
16. Graybiel AM. Habits, rituals and the evaluative brain. Annu Rev Neurosci 2008; 31:359–87.
17. Whittle S, Yucel M, Fornito A, et al. Neuroanatomical correlates of temperament in early adolescence. J Am Acad Child Adolesc Psychiatry 2008;47(6):682–93.
18. Ogren MP, Lombroso PJ. Epigenetics: behavioral influences on gene function part II: molecular mechanisms. J Am Acad Child Adolesc Psychiatry 2008;47: 374–8.
19. Perry BD, Pollard R, Blakely T, et al. Childhood trauma, the neurobiology of adaptation and "use-dependent" development of the brain: how "states" become "traits". Infant Ment Health J 1995;16(4):271–91.
20. Cicchetti D, Toth SL. The development of depression in children and adoles-cents. Am Psychol 1998;53:221–41.
21. Miklowitz DJ, Chang KD. Prevention of bipolar disorder in at-risk children: theo-retical assumptions and empirical foundations. Dev Psychopathol 2008;20(3): 881–98.
22. Cohen P, Chen H, Crawford TN, et al. Personality disorders in early adolescence and the development of later substance use disorders in the general population. Drug Alcohol Depend 2007;88:S71–84.
23. Gatzke-Kopp LM, Beauchaine TP. Central nervous system substrates of impul-sivity: implications for the development of attention-deficit/hyperactivity disorder and conduct disorder. In: Coch D, Dawson G, Fischer K, editors. Human behav-ior and the developing brain: atypical development. New York: Guilford Press; 2007. p. 239–63.
24. Ferdinand RF, Dieleman G, Ormel J, et al. Homotypic versus heterotypic conti-nuity of anxiety symptoms in adolescents: evidence for distinction between DSM-IV subtypes. J Abnorm Child Psychol 2007;35:325–33.
25. Forbes EE, Shaw DS, Dahl RE. Alterations in reward-related decision making in boys with recent and future depression. Biol Psychiatry 2007;61:633–9.
26. Nestler EJ, Carlezon WA. The mesolimbic dopamine reward circuit in depres-sion. Biol Psychiatry 2006;59:1151–9.
27. Shankman SE, Klein DN, Tenke CE, et al. Reward sensitivity in depression: a bio-behavioral study. J Abnorm Psychol 2007;116:95–104.
28. Lyons-Ruth K. Attachment relationships among children with aggressive behav-ior problems: the role of disorganized early attachment patterns. J Consult Clin Psychol 2001;64:32–40.
29. Bakersman-Kraneburg MK, Van Ijzendoorn MH, Juffer F. Less is more: meta-analysis of sensitivity and attachment interventions in early childhood. Psychol Bull 2003;129:195–215.
30. Fisher PA, Gunnar MR, Chamberlain P, et al. Preventive intervention for maltreated preschool children: impact on children's behavior, neuroendocrine activity, and foster parent functioning. J Am Acad Child Adolesc Psychiatry 2000;39:1356–64.
31. Bakermans-Kranenburg MJ, Van Ijzendoorn MH, Mesman J, et al. Effects of an attachment-based intervention on daily cortisol moderated by dopamine recep-tor D4: a randomized control trial on 1- to 3-year-olds screened for externalizing behavior. Dev Psychopathol 2008;20(3):805–20.

32. Bakermans-Kranenburg M, Van Ijzendoorn M. Genetic vulnerability or differential susceptibility in child in child development: the case of attachment. J Child Psychol Psychiatry 2007;48:1160–73.

33. Rutter M. Gene-environment interdependence. Dev Sci 2007;10:12–8.

34. Cicchetti D, Curtis WJ. The developing brain and neural plasticity: implications for normality, psychopathology, and resilience. In: Cicchetti D, Cohen D, editors. 2nd edition, Developmental psychopathology: vol. 2. Developmental neuroscience. New York: Wiley; 2006. p. 1–64.

35. Kreppner JM, Rutter M, Beckett C, et al. Normality and impairment following profound early institutional deprivation: a longitudinal examination through childhood. Dev Psychol 2007;43:931–46.

36. Gunnar MR, Quevedo K. The neurobiology of stress and development. Annu Rev Psychol 2007;58:145–73.

37. Kaufman A, Meaney M. Role of BDNF in bipolar and unipolar disorder: clinical and theoretical implications. J Psychiatr Res 2007;41:979–90.

38. Conrod P, Stewart S, Comeau N, et al. Efficacy of cognitive-behavioral interventions targeting personality risk factors for youth alcohol misuse. J Clin Child Adolesc Psychol 2006;35:550–63.

39. Beauchaine TP, Marsh P. Taxometric methods: enhancing early detection and prevention of psychopathology by identifying latent vulnerability traits. In: Cichetti D, Cohen D, editors. Developmental pyschopathology. Hoboken (NJ): Wiley; 2006, p. 931–67.

40. Beauchaine TP, Hong J, Marsh P. Sex differences in autonomic correlates of conduct problems and aggression. J Am Acad Child Adolesc Psychiatry 2008;47:788–96.

41. Dietz L, Birmaher B, Williamson D, et al. Mother-child interactions in depressed children and children at high risk and low risk for future depression. J Am Acad Child Adolesc Psychiatry 2008;47:574–82.

42. Cicchetti D, Gunner M. Integrating biological measures into the design and evaluation of preventive interventions. Dev Psychopathol 2008;20:737–43.

43. Bearden CE, Soares JC, Klunder A, et al. Three-dimensional mapping of hippocampal anatomy in adolescents with bipolar disorder. J Am Acad Child Adolesc Psychiatry 2008;47(5):515–25.

44. Blumberg HP, Fredericks C, Wang F, et al. Preliminary evidence for persistent abnormalities in amygdala volumes in adolescents and young adults with bipolar disorder. Bipolar Disord 2005;7(6):570–6.

45. DelBello MP. The neurophysiology of childhood and adolescent bipolar disorder. CNS Spectr 2006;11:298–311.

46. Gogtay N, Ordonez A, Herman DH, et al. Dynamic mapping of cortical development before and after the onset of pediatric bipolar illness. J Child Psychol Psychiatry 2007;48(9):852–62.

47. Wang F, Kalmar JH, Edmiston E, et al. Abnormal corpus callosum integrity in bipolar disorder: a diffusion tensor imaging study. Biol Psychiatry 2008;64(8): 730–3.

48. Heim C, Newport DJ, Mletzko T, et al. The link between childhood trauma and depression: insights from HPA axis studies in humans. Psychoneuroendocrinology 2008;33(6):693–710.

49. Bradley RG, Binder EB, Epstein MP, et al. Influence of child abuse on adult depression: moderation by the corticotropin-releasing hormone receptor gene. Arch Gen Psychiatry 2008;65(2):190–200.

50. Rapoport J, Shaw P. Defining the contribution of genetic risk to structural and functional abnormalities in ADHD. J Am Acad Child Adolesc Psychiatry 2008; 47:2–3.
51. Caspi A, McClay J, Moffit T, et al. Role of genotype in the cycle of violence in maltreated children. Science 2002;297:851–4.
52. Leibenluft E, Thompson PM, Rapoport JL. Dynamic mapping of cortical development before and after the onset of pediatric bipolar illness. J Child Psychol Psychiatry 2007;48(9):852–62.
53. Liebenluft E, Cohen P, Gorrindo T, et al. Chronic vs. episodic irritability in youth: a community based, longitudinal study of clinical and diagnostic associations. J Child Adolesc Psychopharmacol 2006;16:456–66.
54. Liebenluft E, Rich BA. Pediatric bipolar disorder. Annu Rev Clin Psychol 2008;4: 163–87.
55. Leverich GS, McElroy SL, Suppes T, et al. Early physical and sexual abuse associated with an adverse course of bipolar illness. Biol Psychiatry 2002;51: 288–97.
56. Rich BA, Vinton DT, Roberson-Nay R, et al. Limbic hyperactivation during processing of neutral facial expressions in children with bipolar disorder. Proceedings of the National Academy of Sciences of the USA 2006;103: 8900–5.
57. Lewis DA, Levitt P. Schizophrenia as a disorder of neurodevelopment. Annu Rev Neurosci 2002;25:409–32.
58. Walker E, Mittal V, Tessner K. Stress and the hypothalamic pituitary adrenal axis in the developmental course of schizophrenia. Annu Rev Clin Psychol 2008;4: 189–216.
59. Nugent TF 3rd, Herman DH, Ordonez A, et al. Dynamic mapping of hippocampal development in childhood onset schizophrenia. Schizophr Res 2007; 90(1–2):62–70.
60. White T, Kendi AT, Lehéricy S, et al. Disruption of hippocampal connectivity in children and adolescents with schizophrenia—a voxel-based diffusion tensor imaging study. Schizophr Res 2007;90(1-3):3002–7.
61. Jacobsen L, Rapoport J. Research Update: Childhood-onset schizophrenia: Implications of clinical and neurobiological research. J Child Psychol Psychiatry 1998;39:101–13.
62. White T, Cullen K, Rohrer LM, et al. Limbic structures and networks in children and adolescents with schizophrenia. Schizophr Bull 2008;24(1):18–29.
63. Caspi A, Sugden K, Moffitt TE, et al. Influence of life stress on depression: moderation by a polymorphism in the 5-HTT gene. Science 2003;301(5631): 386–9.
64. Linden DEJ. How psychotherapy changes the brain—the contribution of functional imaging. Mol Psychiatry 2006;11:526–38.
65. Sugden SG, Kile SJ, Hendren RL. Neurodevelopmental pathways to aggression: a model to understand and target treatment in youth. J Neuropsychiatry Clin Neurosci 2006;18(3):302–17.
66. Caspi A, Silva PA. Temperamental qualities at age three predict personality traits in young adulthood: longitudinal evidence from a birth cohort. Child Dev 1995; 66:486–98.
67. Acosta MT, Castellanos FX, Bolton KL, et al. Latent class subtyping of attention-deficit/hyperactivity disorder and comorbid conditions. J Am Acad Child Adolesc Psychiatry 2008;47(7):797–807.

68. Rettew DC, Althoff RR, Dumenci L, et al. Latent profiles of temperament and their relations to psychopathology and wellness. J Am Acad Child Adolesc Psychiatry 2008;47(3):273–81.
69. Rettew DC, Stanger C, McKee L, et al. Interactions between child and parent temperament and child behavior problems. Compr Psychiatry 2006;47(5): 412–20 [Epub 2006 Apr 21].
70. Eiraldi RB, Power TJ, Nezu CM. Patterns of comorbidity associated with sub-types of attention-deficit/hyperactivity disorder among 6- to 12-year-old children. J Am Acad Child Adolesc Psychiatry 1997;36(4):503–14.
71. Jensen PS, Hinshaw SP, Kraemer HC, et al. ADHD co-morbidity findings from the MTA study: comparing co-morbid subgroups. J Am Acad Child Adolesc Psychiatry 2001;40:147–58.
72. Loeber R, Farrington DP, Stouthamer-Loeber M, et al. Male mental health prob-lems, psychopathy, and personality traits: key findings from the first 14 years of the Pittsburgh youth study. Clin Child Fam Psychol Rev 2001;4(4):273–97.
73. Biederman J, Mick E, Wozniak J, et al. Can a subtype of conduct disorder linked to bipolar disorder be identified? Biol Psychiatry 2003;53:952–60.
74. Cicchetti D, Curtis WJ, editors. A multilevel approach to resilience. Dev Psycho-pathol. 2007;19:627–955.
75. Dawson G. Early behavioral intervention, brain plasticity, and the prevention of autism spectrum disorder. Dev Psychopathol 2007;20(3):775–804.
76. Dawson G, Webb S, McPartland J. Understanding the nature of face processing impairment in autism: insights from behavioral and electrophysiological studies. Dev Neuropsychol 2005;27:403–24.
77. LaBar KS. Beyond fear: emotional memory mechanisms in the human brain. Curr Dir Psychol Sci 2007;16:173–7.
78. Adamson L, Bakeman R, Deckner D. The development of symbol-infused joint engagement. Child Dev 2004;75:1171–87.
79. Beckwith L. Adaptive and maladaptive parenting: implications for intervention. In: Meisels SJ, Shonkoff JP, editors. Handbook of early childhood intervention. New York: Cambridge University Press; 1990.
80. Siller M, Sigman M. The behaviors of parents of children with autism predict the subsequent development of their children's communication. J Autism Dev Disord 2002;32:77–89.
81. Luthar SS. Resilience in development: a synthesis of research across five de-cades. In: Cicchetti D, Cohen D, editors. 2nd edition, Developmental psychopa-thology: vol. 3. Risk, disorder, and adaptation. New York: Wiley; 2006. p. 739–95.
82. Kunwar A, Dewan M, Faraone S. Treating common psychiatric disorders associ-ated with attention-deficit/hyperactivity disorder. Expert Opin Pharmacother 2007;8:555–62.
83. Mikllowitz D, George E, Richards J, et al. A randomized study of family-focused psychoeducation and pharmacotherapy in the outpatient management of bipo-lar disorder. Arch Gen Psychiatry 2003;60:904–12.
84. Winzer-Serhan UH. Long-term consequences of maternal smoking and develop-mental chronic nicotine exposure. Front Biosci 2008;13:636–49.
85. Fox NA, Hane AA, Pine DS. Plasticity for affective neurocircuitry: how the envi-ronment shapes gene expression. Curr Dir Psychol Sci 2007;16:1–5.
86. Gunnar MR, Vazquez DM. Stress neurobiology and developmental psychopa-thology. In: Cicchetti D, Cohen D, editors. 2nd edition, Developmental psy-cholopathology: vol. 2. Developmental neuroscience. New York: Wiley; 2006. p. 533–77.

87. Blair C. School readiness: integrating cognition and emotion in a neurobiological conceptualization of children's functioning at school entry. Am Psychol 2002;57: 111–27.

88. Blair C, Diamond A. Biological processes in prevention and intervention: The promotion of self-regulation as a means of preventing school failure. Dev Psychopathol 2008;20:899–912.

89. Courchesne E. Brain development in autism: early overgrowth followed by premature arrest of growth. Ment Retard Dev Disabil Res Rev 2004;10:106–11.

90. Courchesne E, Pierce K. Brain overgrowth in autism during a critical time in development: implications for frontal pyramidal neuron and interneuron development and connectivity. Int J Dev Neurosci 2005;23:153–70.

91. Cicchetti D, Rogosch FA. Psychopathology as risk for adolescent substance use disorders: a developmental psychopathology perspective. J Clin Child Psychol 1999;28:355–65.

92. Dawson G, Toth K, Abbott R, et al. Early social attention impairments in autism: social orienting, joint attention, and attention to distress. Dev Psychol 2004;40: 271–83.

93. Kasari C. Assessing change in early intervention programs for children with autism. J Autism Dev Disord 2002;32:447–61.

94. Bierman K, Nix R, Greenberg M, et al. Executive functions and school readiness intervention: impact, moderation, and mediation in the head start redi program. Dev Psychopathol 2008;20:821–43.

95. Zill N, Resnick G, Kiim K, et al. Head start FACES 2000: a whole-child perspective on program performance. Retrieved from USDHHS Administration for Child and Family Web page. Available at: http://www.acf.hhs.gov/programs/opre/hs/faces/reports/faces00.

96. De Kloet ER, Joëls M, Holsboer F. Stress and the brain: from adaptation to disease. Nat Rev Neurosci 2005;6:463–75.

97. Dozier M, Peloso E, Lewis E, et al. Effects of an attachment-based intervention on the cortisol production of infants and toddlers in foster care. Dev Psychopathol 2008;20(3):854–60.

98. Davies PT, Sturge-Apple ML, Cicchetti D, et al. The role of child adrenocortial functioning in pathways between interparental conflict and child maltreatment. Dev Psychol 2007;43:918–30.

99. McGorry PD, Yung AR, Phillips LJ, et al. Randomized controlled trial of interventions designed to reduce the risk of progression to first episode psychosis in a clinical sample with sub-threshold symptoms. Arch Gen Psychiatry 2007;59: 921–8.

100. Chang K, Gallelli K, Howe M. Early identification and prevention of early-onset bipolar disorder. In: Romer D, Walker EF, editors. Adolescent psychopathology and the developing brain. Oxford: Oxford University Press; 2007. p. 315–46.

101. Miklowitz DJ. The role of the family in the course and treatment of bipolar disorder. Curr Dir Psychol Sci 2007;16:192–6.

Towards a Neurodevelopmental Model of Clinical Case Formulation

Marjorie Solomon, PhD[a,b,c,]*, David Hessl, PhD[a,b], Sufen Chiu, MD, PhD[b], Emily Olsen, BS[c], Robert L. Hendren, DO[a,b]

KEYWORDS

- Neurodevelopment • Case formulation
- Fragile X Syndrome
- Pervasive developmental disorder • Endophenotypes

Rapid advances in molecular genetics and neuroimaging over the last 10 to 15 years have been a catalyst for research in neurobiology, developmental psychopathology, and translational neuroscience.[1] Methods of study in psychiatry are becoming sufficiently sophisticated to effectively investigate the biology of higher mental processes and complex forms of psychopathology.[2] These advances have the potential to add depth to our understanding of psychiatric symptoms and to facilitate more targeted interventions.

Rett syndrome and Down syndrome are examples of conditions thought of as being neurodevelopmental disorders:[3] disorders where the interaction of genes and the environment lead to the biochemical processes involved in pathologic development of the brain and central nervous system. However, aspects of almost all psychiatric disorders likely involve the interaction of multiple genes with environmental factors. Thus, schizophrenia, autism spectrum disorders, attention-deficit hyperactivity disorder (ADHD), Tourette's disorder, and bipolar disorder also can be approached from a perspective emphasizing the importance of neurodevelopment.

Historically, mental health professionals have used heuristic case-formulation models to help organize complex information about psychologic, interpersonal, and

During the preparation of this manuscript, Dr. Solomon was supported by NIH Grant K-08 MH-074967; Dr. Hessl was supported by NIH Grant MH-77554.

[a] Department of Psychiatry and Behavioral Sciences, University of California, Davis, Sacramento, CA, USA

[b] The M.I.N.D. Institute, University of California, Davis, Sacramento, CA, USA

[c] Imaging Research Center, University of California, Davis, Sacramento, CA, USA

* Corresponding author.

E-mail address: majorie.solomon@ucdmc.ucdavis.edu (M. Solomon).

behavioral problems, and to guide the development of treatment plans.[4] A biopsycho-social formulation, particularly when applied through a developmental lens for children, can bring a rich perspective to the case. However, some cases lend themselves to an even more specific focus, that of the neurodevelopmental formulation, which also brings to bear genetic and neurologic information, which is becoming more readily available to the clinician because of rapidly advancing research in these areas.

A neurodevelopmental model of case formulation has not yet been clearly articulated. This is probably because of the enormous complexity inherent in explaining the relationship between genes and behaviors and our often nascent knowledge base, and skepticism about whether this type of formulation model could improve clinical practice in terms of accuracy, treatment, or cost. The goal of this article, which is written as a clinical case conference, is to begin to articulate a neurodevelopmental model of case formulation, to illustrate its value, and to explore the evolution of clinical psychiatry if this type of case formulation became standard practice.

TOWARDS A NEURODEVELOPMENTAL MODEL OF CASE FORMULATION: BRIDGING THE GAP BETWEEN GENES AND BEHAVIORS

Pennington[5] articulated a model of developmental psychopathology that offers an organizing framework for examining critical elements in neurodevelopment. This framework traces four levels between genes and behavior. Level 1, Etiology, is concerned with the genetic and environmental influences and the role they play in the development of symptoms and disorders. Level 2, the Brain and Central Nervous System, includes development of the neuroarchitecture of the brain. In this model, Level 3, Neuropsychology, performs a "bridging" function between the internal and external manifestations of psychopathology through the use of noninvasive assays of brain functioning, such as neuropsychologic tests. Level 4, Symptoms, consists of observable behaviors. During development, interactions between these four levels are continuous, bi-directional, and interactive.[6] In considering schizophrenia research, Tandon and colleagues[7] suggest that pathophysiology, including neurochemical alterations in brain regions, should be considered as part of Level 2, and that the Symptoms level should be expanded to include treatment. See **Fig. 1** for a schematic diagram of this model. The authors propose that the practice of clinical psychiatry can

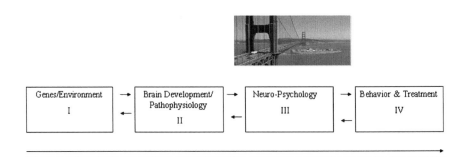

Fig. 1. Four levels in a neurodevelopmental model. (*Adapted from* Pennington BF. The development of psychopathology. New York: Guilford; 2002; and Tandon R, Keshavan, MS, Nasrallah, HA. Schizophrenia, "just the facts," what we know in 2008. 2. Epidemiology and etiology. Schizophr Res 2008;102:1–18; with permission.)

be advanced and enhanced by using diagnostic formulations that consider and orga-nize information using these levels of analysis.

Below, a case is presented in a Grand Rounds Format to illustrate the application of a neurodevelopmental model of case formulation and the clinical issues it raises. In this case, a neurodevelopmental formulation reveals that a complex constellation of psychiatric and learning problems has arisen from a "single-gene" disorder with a well-described phenotypic presentation. Case materials are presented using the Levels, starting with the presenting Symptoms. This case was chosen because it illus-trates how case formulation would be affected when a genetic "cause" can be iden-tified, although there also are many aspects of the case that conform to the more common situation of disorders related to multiple genes or environmental factors or those with no known genetic origin. Similar case materials with a different emphasis have been presented previously.[8]

CASE PRESENTATION: "SARAH," A GIRL WITH MILD INTELLECTUAL DISABILITY, ANXIETY, BEHAVIORAL DYSREGULATION, AND SYMPTOMS OF AUTISM
Dr. Hendren

At level 4, the Symptom level, we evaluate Sarah's presenting problems, her medical and developmental history, and her medical examination. At age 8, Sarah was referred for a multidisciplinary evaluation because of longstanding difficulties with social skills, learning, aggression, and anxiety. She is described as an extroverted and pleasant girl. However, she becomes severely emotionally dysregulated and engages in tan-trums, aggression, and self-injury when she becomes frustrated in academic or social situations. Academic performance is a relative strength, although she has trouble with mathematics.

Sarah was born weighing 7 pounds, 2 ounces following an uncomplicated delivery. Motor milestones and language development were within normal limits. Hand flap-ping, poor eye contact, and tactile defensiveness began during the first year of life. Her preschool years were unremarkable.

She was referred for evaluation at age 6 when kindergarten teachers observed that her play and social skills were delayed. She also demonstrated echolalia, obsessive-ness, and intolerance for changes in her routine. In first grade, issues related to inat-tention, following instructions, and reading comprehension became apparent, and her academic performance was well below average. She began to display behavioral problems including talking out, provoking other children, difficulty transitioning be-tween activities, and having tantrums or sulking when upset. She did not have any friends and exhibited autistic-like symptoms, including poor eye contact, solitary play, sensory hypo- and hyper-responsiveness, and hand flapping.

It was hypothesized that Sarah's emergent behavioral problems were directly re-lated to her frustration and desperation that her academic and social skills were failing to keep pace with environmental demands. Sarah's behavioral difficulties destabilized the institutional and family systems that supported her, as teachers and parents strug-gled to respond. Likely, at least initially, Sarah's problems led to increased anger on the part of her teachers and feelings of guilt and loss in her parents.

Sarah was initially tried on atomoxetine at 18 mg and then later at 40 mg for distract-ible inattention, impulsivity, hyperactivity, and anxiety. She became more irritable and this was discontinued. She was subsequently started on sertraline at 50 mg, at which dose she displayed decreased anxiety, fewer emotional outbursts and aggression, and improved behavior at school. Her attention problems and impulsivity persisted, however, and an additional 36-mg of once-daily methylphenidate was added. This resulted in improved attention and concentration, and further reduction in aggressive behavior.

During her medical examination, Sarah presented as an attractive overweight girl. She was appropriately dressed and well groomed. Ear pinna were prominent, with significant cupping. Hyperextensible joints and macrocephaly were noted. Her features were mildly dysmorphic: she had a long face and prominent ears. She made poor eye contact and had difficulty sitting still during the interview. Her speech was of normal rate, but volume was loud and prosody was monotone and slightly robotic. Her mother reported no evidence of auditory, visual, or tactile hallucinations. However, Sarah was reportedly often "in her own world," where she engaged in self-talk and recited lines from favorite television shows and videos. Thought content was generally appropriate for the interview. She displayed no suicidal ideation.

DISCUSSION
Dr. Hessl

In consideration of Level 1, Etiology, we were impressed by similarities between Sarah's symptom presentation and the neuropsychiatric phenotype of Fragile X Syndrome (FXS), and referred her for hi-resolution cytogenetic and Fragile X DNA testing. Fragile X DNA testing was positive for the full mutation, with 486 to 845 CGG repeats, and fragile X mental retardation 1 (FMR1) protein studies demonstrated 48% of normal protein expression. These results documented a full mutation of the fragile X mental retardation 1 (*FMR1*) gene and Sarah was subsequently diagnosed with FXS.

FXS is a "single gene" disorder caused by a trinucleotide repeat expansion $(CGG)_n$ in the 5′ untranslated region of the *FMR1* gene located on the X chromosome. It is the most common form of inherited mental retardation. The full mutation, as in Sarah's case, occurs when individuals have more than 200 CGG repeats, leading to methylation, subsequent transcriptional silencing of the *FMR1* gene, and absence or deficiency of the FMR1 protein, FMRP.[9]

Individuals with FXS demonstrate a behavioral phenotype characterized by hyperarousal, social anxiety and withdrawal, social deficits, abnormalities in communication, unusual responses to sensory stimuli, stereotypic behavior, gaze aversion, inattention, impulsivity, and hyperactivity.[10–16] Autistic disorder is present in 15% to 33% of individuals with FXS.[17–20] Studies of females with FXS have shown that reduced FMRP expression is associated with internalizing behaviors, such as anxiety and social withdrawal,[16] and reduction of task-specific areas of brain activation during fMRI studies of math calculation.[21] Sophisticated neurogenetic studies have even documented that functional brain activation during arithmetic processing and executive-function tasks involving response inhibition in females with FXS are linearly related to FMR1 protein expression.[21,22] Consistent with these research studies, this patient's most prominent referral concerns were anxiety and social withdrawal, artithmetic-learning problems, and impulsivity.

Our clinical research program has begun to examine secondary genetic factors that might explain why some boys with FXS develop more severe aggression or anxiety symptoms than others.[23] As part of a study protocol approved by the Univeristy of California Davis Institutional Review Board, Sarah's DNA sample also was analyzed for polymorphisms known to be associated with anxiety and aggression in the general population, including the serotonin transporter gene and the monoamine oxidase A (MAOA) polymorphism. The functional polymorphism in the promoter region of the serotonin transporter gene (*SLC6A4*) has been associated with reduced glucocorticoid-regulated human serotonin transporter (5-HTT) expression and function, increased fear and anxiety-related behaviors, and greater amygdala neuronal activity in response to fearful stimuli.[24] In the our study, it was found that boys with FXS who were homozygous for the short genotype (S/S) had the least aggression. Those with the long (L/L) genotype had the highest levels of stereotyped behaviors. It was also surprising to observe that individuals in the study taking selective serotonin reuptake inhibitor or selective serotonin and norepinephrine reuptake inhibitor medication were more likely to have the high-activity MAOA-variable number of tandem repeats 4-repeat genotype. Writing about a sample of boys with autism, Brun and colleagues[25] found that the short S/S and S/L genotypes were associated with the failure to use nonverbal communication to regulate social interaction, whereas the L/L phenotype was associated with more severe stereotyped motor mannerisms and aggression. The probe of Sarah's serotonin transporter gene revealed two copies of the short allele (S/S). Additional empirical studies, and studies specifically about girls, clearly will be needed to confirm that these polymorphisms are associated with psychiatric symptoms in individuals with FXS. Preliminarily, however, Sarah's aggression symptoms do not conform to the our research findings about individuals with the short allele (S/S); however, she does have difficulty using nonverbal communication to regulate social interactions, as discussed by Brun and colleagues.

MAOA is a mitochondrial enzyme active in degrading all of the monoamines: namely serotonin, dopamine, and norepinephrine. Although the present study did not demonstrate a relationship between MAOA levels and aggression, self-injurious behavior, or stereotypy in boys with FXS, the 3-repeat allele has been implicated in the pathogenesis of aggression and impulse-control disorders,[26,27] autism symptom severity,[28] conduct/aggression disorders co-morbid with ADHD,[29] and unmanageable aggressive behaviors in schizophrenia[30] and Alzheimer's disease.[27] Examination of Sarah's MAOA status showed that she carries one allele with 3.5 repeats and one allele with 3 repeats. Although findings regarding the significance of this are contradictory at the present time, the relationship between Sarah's MAOA status and her behavior may become clearer with future research, and such information may help to better delineate the relative responsibility of genes and environment in Sarah's presentation.

In sum, for this case, knowledge of genetic information about the fragile X phenotype, combined with knowledge about the serotonin transporter gene and MAOA polymorphisms provides the clinician with a richer understanding of factors mediating symptom expression.

Dr. Chiu

At the Brain Level, one can consider what is known about neuronal growth and development in individuals with FXS. Greenough and colleagues[31] have provided strong evidence that FMRP is required for the refinement of dendritic spine morphology, an important neural correlate of brain changes linked to development and learning. FMRP is expressed in all brain regions of typically developing individuals. Therefore, FXS is characterized by effects on all of brain development and all cognitive domains are likely to have developed at least somewhat atypically.[11] However, fMRI, neurohistologic, and neuropsychologic studies show that particular brain regions may demonstrate higher FMRP expression and therefore some brain functions, such as those subserving sequential information processing,[21] visual tracking,[24] and inhibitory processes[22] may be especially affected in patients with FXS. Again, knowledge about neurodevelopment associated with the fragile X phenotype provides a more complete appreciation of the patient and her symptoms, given that it enables one to anticipate problem areas of cognitive and adaptive functioning, and vulnerability to psychopathology.

Dr. Solomon

At Level 3, Neuropsychology, it is known that the cognitive profile of individuals with FXS, is characterized by relative strengths in language, long-term memory, holistic information processing[32] and, as mentioned above, relative weaknesses in attention, visuospatial cognition, short-term memory, sequential information processing, and inhibition. Most individuals with FXS exhibit symptoms of ADHD,[15,33]and up to one-third meet criteria for autism.[19]

On the Kaufman Assessment Battery for Children,[34] Sarah obtained a Mental Processing Component of 72 (borderline range of intellectual functioning), and scales on nonverbal items were significantly depressed to others. Consistent with this pattern, Sarah's academic achievement scores (Woodcock-Johnson Psychoeducational Battery III)[35] ranged from a high of 105 in reading to 78 in mathematics. Scores on a developmental examination of visual motor integration revealed that Sarah's scores were below average.

To see whether the atypical language, reciprocal social deficits, and restricted and repetitive behavior symptoms associated with autism were present, an Autism Diagnostic Observation Schedule (ADOS)[36] – Module 3 was completed. Sarah showed a wide range of affect on the ADOS. She was able to engage in imaginary play with the examiner. Her speech was odd in its sing-song prosody and repetitive use of catch phrases. She did not comment on others' emotions, demonstrate true empathy, or engage in perspective-taking during the testing. Her score on the ADOS was in the autism-spectrum disorder range, but below the cut-off for full autism. Her score on the Social Communication Questionnaire,[37] a parent-report inventory of items related to the *Diagnostic and Statistical Manual of Mental Disorders* diagnosis of autism, was consistent with this.

Dr. Hendren

For most children presenting in our clinics with a constellation of cognitive, learning, emotional, and social difficulties, the etiology is unknown and somewhat mysterious. In Sarah's case, however, we are fortunate because the neurodevelopmental formulation rests on the foundation of a wealth of genetic, biologic, and behavioral knowledge about FXS. At levels 3 and 4, there are a wide range of seemingly disparate symptoms and cognitive strengths and weaknesses, including social deficits, anxiety, and mathematics learning difficulties. Studies have documented that each of these are features of the phenotype of FXS. At levels 1 and 2, the etiological/genetic and brain/pathophysiologic levels, it is recognized that many of Sarah's difficulties have been directly linked to the dysfunction of the fragile X gene, *FMR1*, through neuropsychologic and neuroimaging studies. Although many of these phenotypic features may be modified by environmental factors,[26] Sarah's experience starts from a point of significantly increased genetic susceptibility. In addition to her fragile X status, Sarah carries two additional genetic risk factors: a less efficient serotonin transporter gene and a MAOA polymorphism predisposing her to aggressive behavior.

Dr. Solomon

We sought to reduce Sarah's anxiety by accentuating her strengths and by bolstering her functioning in problem areas. Psychopharmacologic interventions were used to target her anxiety and attentional problems, as previously noted. Sarah's presentation includes aspects of a nonverbal learning disorder profile (NLD)[38] commonly seen in girls with FXS. Hence, her teachers and parents were encouraged to recognize and help her use her excellent rote memory for facts and other information delivered verbally, and to use her relatively strong fund of knowledge to compensate for areas such as abstract reasoning, which are more difficult for her. It was recommended that teaching methods be tailored to Sarah's sequential information-processing problems and that Sarah receive more assistance in mathematics, as this is a relative weakness for her as it is with other individuals with NLD. She has been able to use assistive technology during math class. To help desensitize her to social challenges and to provide extra scaffolding and practice, Sarah attends a social skills group, which includes lessons on stress and anger management.

Hopefully, advances in our understanding of the phenotype of FXS will lead to improved pharmacologic and psychosocial interventions targeted to these individuals.

Dr. Hendren

Environmental and psychodynamic factors, including those involving adoption and family dynamics, play a role in Sarah's experience, as does learned behavior. Explanations for her behavioral dysregulation, however, should not over-emphasize the role of her parents or other caregivers. Sarah's emotional dysregulation may be at least in part because of deficits and immaturities in inhibitory neural circuits, which permit self-soothing, diminution of negative affect, and enhanced emotion regulation.[39,40] It is important to note that Sarah's academic achievement exceeds what would be expected given her cognitive level, speaking to the ability of her parents to provide a supportive learning environment for her.

Dr. Chiu

This diagnosis has direct genetic counseling implications for Sarah's extended family. The identification of FXS has implications for *FMR1* screening in her siblings and other extended family members. In addition, the recent discovery of fragile X-associated tremor ataxia syndrome,[41] a neurodegenerative disorder occurring in elderly carriers of the *FMR1* premutation, indicates that Sarah's grandfather is at risk for a late-onset disease that arises from an abnormality of the same gene but with completely different phenotypic expression.

FUTURE IMPLICATIONS
Dr. Hendren

One can imagine a time in the future when it will be the standard of care to draw blood and order several genetic tests to ascertain a patient's vulnerabilities and even make diagnoses. More will be known about the genes involved in schizophrenia, ADHD, autism, and bipolar disorder. Single nucleotide polymorphism profiles that are characteristic of different disorders will be established. Gene-expression profiling with DNA microarrays, which assess the expression of thousands of mRNA transcripts simultaneously using tissue samples, also will come into more widespread use because of the ability to use whole blood.[42,43] Unique gene-expression profiles will have been identified for many disorders. For example, a pilot study at the Medical Investigation of Neurodevelopmental Disorders Institute has recently demonstrated that there are different gene-expression profiles for children with autism with and without symptoms of regression.[44] These genetic information profiles will help clinicians by providing comparative contexts within which to evaluate symptoms, prognoses, and potential efficacy of intervention strategies.

Dr.Hessl

The tremendous challenge of understanding what happens between Levels 1 and 4 can be facilitated by the use of the intermediate "endophenotypes."

Phenotypes represent the full expression of an individual's genes in the environment. They are heterogeneous and potentially include multiple symptoms in the diagnostic category. Endophenotypes are partial "internal phenotypes" or collections of traits.[45,46] Conceptually, they are closer to the site of genes or primary causative agents than symptoms, and are therefore considered to be more homogeneous. They distinguish individuals with the disorder from a control population; are stable over time; are more prevalent in family members of the affected individual; precede the development of clinical manifestations of the disorder; and are more accurately measured than clinical features. Schizophrenia researchers were the first to suggest this approach 30 years ago.[45] Endophenotypes have received renewed attention, and are being used to study ADHD[47,48] and, to a lesser extent, autism[49] and bipolar disorder.[50]

Dr. Chiu

While it is too early to attempt to interpret this information, some research programs have begun to collect age- and gender-normed developmental data sets about the size and volume of brain structures for typical and atypical populations.[51] One day it may be possible to chart the growth trajectory of an individual's brain structures relative to established developmental norms. At that point, we may also know more about the pathophysiology resulting in these size patterns and their relationship to behavioral symptoms. For example, researchers have demonstrated that children and adolescents with autism demonstrate a different trajectory of amygdala growth than typically developing control subjects,[52] and efforts currently are underway to understanding the etiology of these differences and their functional significance.

"Pharmaco fMRI" also is now being used in ADHD research. This work has begun to clarify which forms of the disorder are most responsive to medication[53] and mechanisms of stimulant action on the neural circuitry of individuals with the disorder.[54] Similarly, diffusion tensor imaging, which is used to measure white-matter tracts, and computational modeling will help further our understanding of neural circuits and patterns of regional connectivity.

Dr. Solomon

If cost barriers can be overcome, fMRI may be used more routinely to provide a window into brain activation associated with cognitive and affective processes. This would lead to a merger between the Brain and Neuropsychology Levels as it becomes feasible to study brain function during cognitive testing. Measures of key neural processes will evolve as the result of imaging technology, and developmental norms for these new cognitive science-based measures will be established. Given that these new assays will derive from cognitive neuroscience and fMRI-based investigation, they will relate more closely to endophenotypes than currently available neuropsychologic tasks. For example, as mentioned above, measures of context processing have developed this way in schizophrenia research.[55,56] Neuroimaging will also serve as a source of converging evidence in understanding the effects of genes on neural circuitry, as genetic testing is more routinely incorporated in fMRI studies, and relationships between genes and neural circuitry-activation patterns are investigated.

Dr. Hessl

Some of the biggest potential benefits of a neurodevelopmental model that enhances our understanding of pathophysiology occur at the levels of treatment-development and treatment-matching. Advances in the field of proteomics are likely to serve as a catalyst for the development of new pharmaceutics, which may help with cognitive, social, and adaptive functioning. In this case, as a single-gene disorder, Fragile X, provides a relatively simple model for studying the effects of secondary or tertiary modifying genes because the primary genetic deficit and phenotype are known.[23] It is known that the lack of a fragile X mental retardation 1 gene protein in fragile X leads to dramatic up regulation of the metabotrophic glutamate 5 pathway, which affects synaptic plasticity, leading to long-term depression and subsequent development of weak and immature synaptic connections.[57] The use of metabotrobic glutatmate 5 antagonists has been helpful in improving cognition and in decreasing seizures in animal models of FXS. Initial Phase I clinical trials in human beings are now underway; it is hoped that they may be further developed to play an important clinical role in human beings. Neural retraining programs are already used to remediate reading,[58] attention,[59,60] and face-processing[61] problems, as well as general cognition and working memory in schizophrenia.[62] Based on our understanding of the endophenotype of FXS, it is reasonable to expect that these interventions can also be usefully applied to patients with FXS. Once we can reliably augment an individual's phenotypically derived diagnosis with a neurodevelopmental formulation, we can better establish a well-targeted treatment plan.

Dr. Hendren

Some readers may wonder if the authors believe there is room for environmental factors, including early childhood experience, in this neurodevelopmental model. The answer to this question is clearly "yes." Better understanding the origin of Sarah's symptoms enabled those around her to be more helpful and responsive. Sarah's parents were able to stop blaming themselves or their parenting for many of her problems. They were empowered by knowing more of what to expect in her development, by having a more elaborated treatment armamentarium to draw upon, and by having a new-found supportive community of other families and clinicians dealing with FXS. They were able to better educate teachers, service providers, and relatives about how to help Sarah. Sarah was of course a beneficiary of this attuned and responsive environment, which has enabled her to achieve her full potential.

The authors hope, however, that this neuordevelopmentally focused discussion will encourage more systematic thought about the role of biologic factors, which are highly complex as well. Interestingly, basic science research using animal models clearly demonstrates the profound impact of early caregiving on an offspring's gene expression related to stress responses, which are critical for survival.[63] In this instance, a neurodevelopmental approach to formulation is consistent with psychodynamic models' emphasis on the critical role of early experience, even if the underlying theory is quite different.

Dr. Chiu

Finally, it should be evident that a neurodevelopmental case-formulation model may serve as a catalyst for the development of a taxonomy of mental disorders informed by pathophysiology. Once a better understanding of the genes, endophenotypes, and prodromal symptoms underlying psychiatric disorders is possessed, it is likely that unappreciated relationships between symptom clusters will be discovered. It is expected that this will lead to the revision of our conceptualization of many psychiatric disorders.

ACKNOWLEDGMENT

The authors acknowledge Flora Tassone, PhD for providing genetic data information, and Dr. Randi Hagerman for providing helpful comments on prior drafts.

REFERENCES

1. Jensen PS. Developmental psychopathology courts developmental neurobiology: current issues and future challenges. Semin Clin Neuropsychiatry 1998;3:333–7.
2. Skuse DH. Behavioural neuroscience and child psychopathology: insights from model systems. J Child Psychol Psychiatry 2000;41:3–31.
3. Hagerman RJ. Neurodevelopmental disorders: diagnosis and treatment. New York: Oxford University Press; 1999.
4. Eells TD, editor. Psychotherapy Case Formulation. New York: The Guilford Press; 1997.
5. Pennington BF. The development of psychopathology. New York: Guilford; 2002.
6. Cannon TD, Rosso IM. Levels of analysis in etiological research on schizophrenia. Dev Psychopathol 2002;14:653–66.
7. Tandon R, Keshavan MS, Nasrallah HA. Schizophrenia, "just the facts," what we know in 2008. 2. Epidemiology and etiology. Schizophr Res 2008;102:1–18.
8. Solomon M, Hessl D, Chiu S, et al. A genetic etiology of pervasive developmental disorder guides treatment. Am J Psychiatry 2007;164(4):575–80.
9. Tassone F, Hagerman RJ, Ikle DN, et al. FMRP expression as a potential prognostic indicator in Fragile X Syndrome. Am J Med Genet 1999;84(3):250–61.
10. Reiss AL, Freund L. Behavioral phenotype of Fragile X Syndrome: DSM-III-R autistic behavior in male children. Am J Med Genet 1992;43:35–46.
11. Bregman JD, Leckman JF, Ort SI. Fragile X Syndrome: genetic predisposition to psychopathology. J Autism Dev Disord 1988;18:343–54.
12. Cohen IL, Fisch GS, Sudhalter V, et al. Social gaze, social avoidance, and repetitive behavior in fragile X males: a controlled study. Am J Ment Retard 1988;92(5):436–46.
13. Cohen IL, Brown WT, Jenkins EC, et al. Fragile X syndrome in females with autism. Am J Med Genet 1989;34(2):302–3.
14. Cohen IL, Sudhalter V, Pfadt A, et al. Why are autism and the Fragile-X Syndrome associated? Conceptual and methodological issues. Am J Hum Genet 1991;48(2):195–202.
15. Hagerman RJ, Amiri K, Cronister A. Fragile X checklist. Am J Med Genet 1991;38: 283–7.
16. Hessl D, Dyer-Friedman J, Glaser B, et al. The influence of environmental and genetic factors on behavior problems and autistic symptoms in boys and girls with Fragile X Syndrome. Pediatrics 2001 Nov;108(5):E88.
17. Bailey DB Jr, Mesibov GB, Hatton DD, et al. Autistic behavior in young boys with Fragile X Syndrome. J Autism Dev Disord 1998;28(6):499–508.
18. Hagerman RJ, Jackson AW 3rd, Levitas A, et al. An analysis of autism in fifty males with the Fragile X Syndrome. Am J Med Genet 1986;23(1–2):359–74.
19. Rogers SJ, Wehner DE, Hagerman R. The behavioral phenotype in fragile X: symptoms of autism in very young children with Fragile X Syndrome, idiopathic autism, and other developmental disorders. J Dev Behav Pediatr 2001;22: 409–17.
20. Sudhalter V, Cohen IL, Silverman W. Wolf-Schein EG: conversational analyses of males with Fragile X, Down syndrome, and autism: comparison of the emergence of deviant language. Am J Ment Retard 1990;94(4):431–41.
21. Rivera SM, Menon V, White CD, et al. Functional brain activation during arithmetic processing in females with Fragile X Syndrome is related to FMR1 protein expression. Hum Brain Mapp 2002;16(4):206–18.
22. Rivera SM, Reiss AL, Eckert MA, et al. Developmental changes in mental arithmetic: evidence for increased functional specialization in the left inferior parietal cortex. Cereb Cortex 2005;15(11):1779–90.

23. Hessl D, Tassone F, Cordeiro L, et al. Aggression and stereotypic behavior in males with Fragile X Syndrome: moderating secondary genes in a "single gene" disorder. J Autism Dev Disord 2008;38(1):184–9.
24. Hariri AR, Mattay VS, Tessitore A, et al. Dextroamphetamine modulates the respone of the human amygdala. Neuropsychopharmacology 2002;27(6): 1035–40.
25. Brune CW, Kim SJ, Salt J, et al. 5-HTTLPR Genotype-specific phenotype in children and adolescents with autism. Am J Psychiatry 2006;163(12):2148–56.
26. Manuck SB, Flory JD, Ferrel RE, et al. A regulatory polymorphism of the monoamine oxidase-A gene may be associated with variability in aggression, impulsivity, and central nervous system serotonergic responsivity. Psychiatry Res 2000; 95(1):9–23.
27. Swann AC. Neuroreceptor mechanisms of aggression and its treatment. J Clin Psychiatry 2003;64:26–35.
28. Cohen IL, Liu X, Schutz C, et al. Association of autism severity with a monoamine oxidase A functional polymorphism. Clin Genet 2003;63(3):190–7.
29. Lawson DC, Turic D, Langley K, et al. Association analysis of monoamine oxidase A and attention deficit hyperactivity disorder. Am J Med Genet B Neuropsychiatr Genet 2003;116(1):84–9.
30. Jonsson EG, Norton N, Forslund K, et al. Association between a promoter variant in the monoamine oxidase A gene and schizophrenia. Schizophr Res 2003;61: 31–7.
31. Greenough WT, Klintsova AY, Irwin SA, et al. Synaptic regulation of protein synthesis and the fragile X protein. Proc Natl Acad Sci USA 2001;98(13):7101–6.
32. Freund LS, Reiss AL. Cognitive profiles associated with the fra (X) syndrome in males and females. Am J Med Genet 1991;38:542–7.
33. Cornish K, Munir F, Wilding J. A neuropsychological and behavioural profile of attention deficits in fragile X syndrome. Rev Neurol 2001;33:S24–9.
34. Kaufman AS, Kaufman NL. Kaufman Assessment Battery for Children. Circle Pines (MN): American Guidance Services; 1983.
35. Woodcock RW, Mather N. Woodcock-Johnson III Tests of Achievement. Itasca (IL): Riverside Publishing; 2001.
36. Lord C, Risi S, Lambrecht L. The autism diagnostic observation schedule generic: a standard measure of social and communication deficits associated with the spectrum of autism. J Autism Dev Disord 2000;30:205–23.
37. Berument SK, Rutter M, Lord C, et al. Autism screening questionnaire: diagnostic validity. Br J Psychiatry 1999;175:444–51.
38. Rourke BP. Nonverbal learning disabilities: syndrome and the model. New York: Guilford; 1989.
39. Rothbart M, Bates J. Temperament, in Handbook of Child Psychology. New York: John Wiley & Sons, Inc.; 1998. p.105–76.
40. Bhangoo RK, Leibenluft E. Affective neuroscience and the study of normal and abnormal emotion regulation. Child Adolesc Psychiatr Clin N Am 2002;11: 519–32.
41. Jacquemont S, Hagerman R, Leehey J, et al. Fragile X premutation tremor/ataxia syndrome: molecular, clinical, and neuroimaging correlates. Am J Hum Genet 2003;72:869–78.
42. Yang SZ, Dong JH, Li K, et al. Detection of AFPmRNA and melanoma antigen gene-1mRNA as markers of disseminated hepatocellular carcinoma cells in blood. Hepatobiliary Pancreat Dis Int 2005;4(2):227–33.

43. Yang SZ, Dong JH, Zhu K, et al. Detection of alpha-fetoproteins mRNA and melanoma agen-1 mRNA in peripheral blood of patients with hepatocellular carcinoma and its clinical significance. Zhonghua Wai Ke Za Zhi 2004; 42(17):1060–3.

44. Sharp F. Gene expression profiles for children with and without symptoms of regression in autism. Davis (CA): M.I.N.D. Institute Research Meeting, Sacramento, CA; March 2005.

45. Gottesman II, Gould TD. The endophenotype concept in psychiatry; etymology and strategic intentions. Am J Psychiatry 2003;160:636–45.

46. Gottesman I, Shields J. Schizophrenia and Genetics: a twin study vantage point. New York: Academic Press; 1972.

47. Heiser P, Friedel S, Dempfle A, et al. Molecular genetic aspects of attention-deficit/hyperactivity disorder. Neurosci Biobehav Rev 2004;28(6):625–41.

48. Nigg JT, Blaskey LG, Stawicki JA, et al. Evaluating the endophenotype model of ADHD combined and inattentive subtypes. J Abnorm Psychol 2004;113:614–25.

49. Dawson G, Webb S, Schellenberg GD, et al. Defining the broader phenotype of autism: genetic, brain, and behavioral perspectives. Dev Psychopathol 2002;14: 581–611.

50. Leibenluft E, Charney DS, Towbin KE, et al. Defining clinical phenotypes of juvenile mania. Am J Psychiatry 2003;160:430–7.

51. Gogtay N, Giedd JN, Lusk L, et al. Dynamic mapping of human cortical development during childhood through early adulthood. Proc Natl Acad Sci USA 2004; 101(21):8174–9.

52. Schumann CM, Hamstra J, Goodlin-Jones BL, et al. The amygdala is enlarged in children but not adolescents with autism; the hippocampus is enlarged at all ages. J Neurosci 2004;24:6392–401.

53. Durston S, Fossella JA, Casey BJ, et al. Differential effects of DRD4 and DAT1 genotype on fronto-striatal gray matter volumes in a sample of subjects with attention deficit hyperactivity disorder, their unaffected siblings, and controls. Mol Psychiatry 2005;10:678–85.

54. Vaidya CJ, Austin G, Kirkorian G, et al. Selective effects of methylphenidate in attention deficit hyperactivity disorder: a functional magnetic resonance study. Proc Natl Acad Sci USA 1998;95:14494–9.

55. Lewis DA, Volk DW, Hashimoto T. Selective alterations in prefrontal cortical GABA neurotransmission in schizophrenia: a novel target for the treatment of working memory dysfunction. Psychopharmacology (Berl) 2004;174:143–50.

56. Barch DM, Mitropoulon V, Harvey PD, et al. Context-processing deficits in schizotypal personality disorder. J Abnorm Psychol 2004;113(4):556–68.

57. Dölen G, Bear MF. Role for metabotropic glutamate receptor 5 (mGluR5) in the pathogenesis of Fragile X Syndrome. J Physiol 2008;586(6):1503–8 .Epub 2008.

58. Temple E, Deutsch GK, Poldrack RA, et al. Neural deficits in children with dyslexia ameliorated by behavioral remediation: evidence from functional MRI. Proc Natl Acad Sci USA 2003;100:2860–5.

59. Rueda MR. Training children's executive attention. Sacramento (CA): UC Davis M.I.N.D. Institute; 2005.

60. Rueda MR, Rothbart MK, McCandliss BD, et al. Training, maturation, and genetic influences on the development of executive attention. Proc Natl Acad Sci USA 2005;102(41):14931–6.

61. J. Tanaka C. Klaiman K. Koenig Plasticity of the neural mechanisms underlying face processing in children with ASD: behavioral improvements following

perceptual training with faces. International Meeting for Autism Research, Boston, MA: May 2005.

62. Hogarty GE, Flesher S, Ulrich R, et al. Cognitive enhancement therapy for schizophrenia: effects of a 2-year randomized trial on cognition and behavior. Arch Gen Psychiatry 2004;61:866–76.

63. Erikson K, Gabry KE, Schulkin J, et al. Social withdrawal behaviors in nonhuman primates and changes in neuroendocrine and monoamine concentrations during a separation paradigm. Dev Psychobiol 2005;46:331–3.

Child and Adolescent Psychiatry for the Future: Challenges and Opportunities

Malia McCarthy, MD*, Jimmark Abenojar, MD, Thomas F. Anders, MD

KEYWORDS

- Opportunities • Challenges • Future • Child psychiatry
- Consultation • Workforce

"Change is the law of life. And those who look only to the past or present are certain to miss the future."

—John F. Kennedy

Psychiatry is perhaps the most fascinating and challenging field of medicine. Child and adolescent psychiatry (CAP) shares in these rewards and challenges; yet, there are relatively few child and adolescent psychiatrists despite the fact that the need for children's mental health services remains enormous. Can recruitment to child and adolescent psychiatry be enhanced? Should new roles for child and adolescent psychiatrists be promulgated to enlarge their scope of professional activity? Can the interests and skills of general psychiatrists, who are currently treating more and more adolescents and even younger school-aged children, be expanded? In this article, the authors focus on three particularly salient sets of issues that face the field of CAP as a subspecialty of general psychiatry today: those related to workforce, public perception, and professional identity. In an article directed at the general psychiatrist, the authors present possibilities for expanding the activities of the child and adolescent psychiatrist to include more consultative and collaborative roles with general psychiatrists, pediatricians, family physicians and other allied health providers. The authors embrace working in systems of care with communities and families as partners. Finally, they discuss the training implications of such shifts in professional identity, and the need to maintain the centrality of a scientifically-based, developmental, biopsychosocial formulation in all of our work.

Department of Psychiatry and Behavioral Sciences, University of California, Davis, School of Medicine, Medical Investigation of Neurodevelopmental Disorders (M.I.N.D.) Institute, 2825 50th Street, Sacramento, CA 95817, USA
* Corresponding author.
E-mail address: mmccarthy@ucdavis.edu (M. McCarthy).

Psychiatr Clin N Am 32 (2009) 213–226
doi:10.1016/j.psc.2008.11.008
0193-953X/08/$ – see front matter © 2009 Elsevier Inc. All rights reserved.
psych.theclinics.com

REWARDS OF CHILD AND ADOLESCENT PSYCHIATRY

What is it that draws us to child psychiatry? The satisfaction of working directly with children and families; developing effective and collaborative relationships with other skilled and committed professionals including physicians, teachers, therapists, and social workers; entering complex matrices of maladaptation and identifying creative ways to catalyze change; and the joy of observing a return to a healthier developmental trajectory for a child and family, are enormous. In fact, child psychiatrists as a group, when surveyed early in their careers, have reported feeling very satisfied with their career choice.[1]

As with general psychiatry, there has never been a better time to be a child psychiatrist. The ability to understand our patients' mental illness and to offer effective treatments is being fed by explosive advances in molecular medicine, proteinomics, neuroimaging, gene mapping, brain mapping, pharmacogenetics, and the identification of genetic polymorphisms and endophenotypes.[2–6] (See the article by Solomon and colleagues elsewhere in this issue for further discussion of this topic.) The contributions of cultural, spiritual, and resilience factors in our understanding of mental health are also increasingly being understood and appreciated.[7–11] We have embarked on an era of innovative, individualized, evidence-based interventions. At the same time that we improve individual treatments, epidemiologic approaches to children's mental health is gaining greater salience as the public health priorities of children become apparent.[12,13] These advances have greatly expanded the elegant, original, and descriptive work of some of our profession's founders—Anna Freud, Margaret Mahler, John Bowlby and Eric Erikson—to mention just a few whose seminal observations and theories preceded the current biologic era. Today, we have begun to better understand the interconnections between inner life, brain, behavior, and development. Our exponentially expanding knowledge base offers unprecedented opportunities.

SOME CHALLENGES FACING CHILD AND ADOLESCENT PSYCHIATRY

However, despite rapid advances, there are equally compelling challenges that face our profession. The authors review some of these challenges in three broad categories: workforce issues, public perception, and scope of practice and professional identity. As portrayed in **Fig. 1**, the three areas are inter-related, yet each is complex and deserving of significant discussion and multiple solutions. The ways in which the field of child and adolescent psychiatry meets these challenges may well determine the future of our practice activities and professional identity with repercussions for general psychiatry and related disciplines.

Workforce Issues

The U.S. Dept of Health and Human Services estimates that 20% of youth develop a mental illness over the course of a year.[14,15] Prevalence estimates of serious emotional disturbance (SED) in youth range from 6% to 17%.[16] It is estimated that 30,000 child and adolescent psychiatrists are needed to meet our nation's needs. Currently, in the United States, child and adolescent psychiatrists number fewer than 7000.[16] However, in terms of full-time equivalents, the number of child and adolescent psychiatrists who treat children is inflated because most child and adolescent psychiatrists do not spend 100% of their time with children. Some also treat adult patients and others are engaged in nondirect professional service activities. Thus, if child and adolescent psychiatrists restricted their practice to only those children with SED, and if there were 7000 of us practicing full time with children, each of us would need to carry

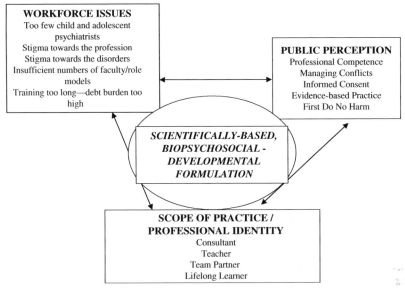

Fig. 1. Challenges to child and adolescent psychiatry.

a minimum caseload of 750.[16,17] And since inner city and rural areas are particularly underserved, many of us would need to move to meet this need.[18]

Why are there so few child and adolescent psychiatrists? A number of reasons account for the low recruitment rates into the field. Stigma against psychiatry and child psychiatry persists in both the general public and within medicine.[8,19–21] This stigma is manifest when teachers and mentors discourage students and residents from pursuing our specialty and subspecialty, suggesting that it lacks sufficient rigor. Related to this stigma are our relatively small faculties in academic settings. Most medical students have little, if any, exposure to child and adolescent psychiatrists during their schooling, and especially not early on when role models and career trajectories are first considered.[22] Later, residents who begin general psychiatry training with an expressed interest in children often lack sufficient opportunities (clinical or mentoring) at the outset of their training to sustain their initial interest in child psychiatry. During their years of general psychiatry training, they become exposed to other exciting aspects of psychiatric practice.[23] These interests often diminish their resolve to pursue the longer course of training leading to certification in CAP, especially when the choice entails a delay in entering the workforce and adding to an already large debt burden.[16,24]

In response to concerted efforts and innovative programs, recruitment has recently increased and will likely continue to increase. A grant program from the Klingenstein Third Generation Foundation has stimulated efforts that: (1) support medical student CAP- interest groups, (2) provide medical students with opportunities to find CAP faculty mentors, (3) engage students in early clinical experiences, and in some instances, the opportunity to participate in research or outreach programs during their first two years of medical school.[22] The American Academy of Child and Adolescent Psychiatry (AACAP) has developed an online mentoring program and has mentoring at its annual meeting for interested medical students. AACAP additionally supports a medical student-friendly Web site and offers free membership and journal subscriptions to interested students.

In addition to a focus on medical students early in training, expanded options and new portals of entry to CAP postgraduate training have emerged. The psychiatry Residency Review Committee (RRC) has provided more flexibility in the sequences for training in general psychiatry and CAP, permitting greater opportunity for concurrent and integrated child and general psychiatry clinical experiences starting in the first postgraduate year. With earlier and sustained exposure to children and adolescents, and to child and adolescent faculty role models throughout the 5 years of training, it is hoped that residents entering general psychiatry training with an interest in children will persist in their interest.[25]

The triple board program, begun in the 1980s with 10 programs currently in existence, is an integrated 5-year program of pediatrics and psychiatry training from which residents graduate as board-eligible pediatricians, psychiatrists, and child and adolescent psychiatrists. Many graduates of these programs enter academic CAP using their skills in providing consultation-liaison services to departments of pediatrics.[26]

The Post Pediatrics Portal Project (PPPP), recently approved by the American Council on Graduate Medical Education, is another new portal of entry into CAP training. The PPPP recruits physicians who are board eligible or certified in pediatrics for 3 years of integrated general and CAP training leading to board-eligibility in both.[26–28] Finally, a research training track begun at the Yale Child Study Center provides medical students motivated for academic careers in CAP the opportunity for a 6-year program that integrates research and clinical training in both general and child psychiatry. Several other university programs have also begun to offer integrated academic research training tracks.[22,29]

Even if these new avenues to CAP training are highly successful, however, it is unlikely that the workforce will be able to keep pace with the mental health needs of the children and families in our country. The field has therefore begun to consider other potential options for expanding the workforce to meet the needs of children with mental and developmental disorders and their families. Future options that are currently being debated include certificate programs for general psychiatrists, pediatricians, and family physicians, that document an expertise in the diagnosis and treatment of childhood mental disorders; increased partnering with psychiatric nurse practitioners or physician assistants as front-line providers; and limited prescription authority for psychologists.[30–32] Although controversial and not without potential pitfalls, some variation of these initiatives is likely to occur.

Finally, and most pertinent to this discussion, many general psychiatrists in the community are beginning to treat young adolescents and school-aged children with mental and behavioral disorders.[33] Expanded training within the general psychiatry training sequence might incorporate the developmental models with which we work and the knowledge base from which we draw. Such an expanded curriculum, or track, within general psychiatry training would seem to be a natural way to support general psychiatrists in developing discrete niches in which they might effectively treat youth, while at the same time, extending child and adolescent psychiatric services.

Public Perception

Psychiatry, including CAP, has been party to the recent vigorous public scrutiny of the U.S. health care system. All of medicine is suffering from a crisis of confidence resulting, in part, from the high cost of care, issues involving the efficiency and quality of care, and real and perceived conflicts of interest between industry and the medical profession.[34–36] Serious concerns around these issues have been raised by editors of medicine's major scientific journals, by our academic centers, and by our professional organizations.[34]

How have we come to find ourselves in this position? In many ways, psychiatry is a natural focus for media attention, easily inciting passions. We deal not only with the brain and behavior but we also deal with the mind and the meaning of human experience, emotionally loaded subjects. Society and families attribute different and often powerful meanings to the diagnostic labels that we use, often with implications of moral judgments in reference to our patients. In CAP, our practice involves working with children, the most vulnerable members of our society, and their families; our treatments focus on their developing brains. The vulnerability of children appropriately unleashes highly protective instincts at the social level. The use of pharmacotherapy and polypharmacy with children, especially young children, has been increasing in recent years,[37–39] concurrent with increasing societal and economic pressures on families, including increased public interest in parenting practices. And while research funding for new psychopharmacologic treatments in general psychiatry has advanced the field exponentially, research progress has not been as rapid with children. Psychopharmacologic clinical trials, for the most part, have largely been performed with adult patients; thus, efficacy and safety data are often not available, or are not as comprehensive or convincing for children.[40–43] In addition, the rapid advances in pharmacotherapy have dwarfed the advances in new and validated psychosocial therapies, often the first line of treatment in CAP because children's dependency and developmental immaturity renders them so sensitive to relational and environmental stressors.[44] There is concern that our fields, both general and child and adolescent psychiatry, have developed a diagnostic system that is primarily phenomenological, yet we rely principally on a set of treatments that are largely biological. Too often, the biological underpinnings of our treatments for children have not been adequately validated. It is not difficult to understand why the public might be confused and concerned.

An overly biologic approach directed primarily at symptom management is fraught with risk to our patients and to our field. Our future must include a return to our roots of formulating cases from a biopsychosocial-developmental perspective, with judicious use of targeted interventions focused on the obstacles to typical development. At some level, implicit in its scrutiny, the public seems to be urging us not to lose sight of the complexity of the disorders that we treat, and the individuals who suffer from them, and to focus on the most appropriate and least restrictive treatments.

The public's confidence is required for CAPs to function effectively. Conflicts of interest, real or perceived, arise when research is predominantly funded by the same industry that profits from the product being tested; when "thought leaders" in the field take on marketing roles for industry rather than educational roles; and when practitioners accept gifts and enticements from industry. We should embrace absolute transparency, high quality validated treatments, and strict adherence to our ethical principles, especially *primum non nocere*. By maintaining the establishment of individualized, balanced, comprehensive, and developmentally informed treatment plans, guided by evidence-based medicine whenever possible, the public's trust in us can be restored.

Scope of Practice and Professional Identity

The balance of this article will focus on the third issue that is closely intertwined with the workforce challenges and our public perception–ie, the challenges involving scope of practice, and consequently, our identity as a profession. The term "scope of practice" is not used here in the technical sense, as referring to the clinical activities permitted by state licensure boards; it is used in the broader sense, as encompassing the following questions. What is the nature of the work that child and adolescent psychiatrists are doing? How can this focus be shifted to better serve mentally ill children and their families?

Child and adolescent psychiatrists working in private practice, universities, and community-based settings are clearly struggling to meet the needs of an ever-expanding and increasingly ill populace. As a result, many, in recent years, have been thrust into the position of providing primarily medication management to mentally ill youth while clinical social workers, master's-level therapists, psychologists, and others provide psychosocial therapies and case management services. Although child and adolescent psychiatrists are the ones best able to provide essential medical prescriptions, this fragmentation of care is often less than optimal for patients and their families.[45] More lucrative reimbursement rates for medication support set by third-party payers combined with more stringent prior authorization requirements for psychosocial treatments provided by psychiatrists have clearly fed this current.[46,47] Yet, many child and adolescent psychiatrists, particularly those with strong neurobiological orientations who practice in communities saturated with clinicians with strong psychosocial treatment skills, find this practice effective and fulfilling. But such a limited scope of practice for our field as a whole is not in the best interests of the children that we treat.

Child and adolescent psychiatrists are the only medical professionals working with mentally ill children who are in a position to bring together the medical, neurological, developmental, psychological, dyadic, familial, social, and behavioral factors that together affect a developing child's functioning. However, under pressure to narrow our focus to the identification and treatment of target symptoms, trusting that others will tend to other aspects of treatment, we may be adversely affecting our future professional identity. When we fail to understand the predisposing, precipitating, and perpetuating factors and the meaning and impact of symptoms in developing a treatment plan, we increase the likelihood that medications will be used prematurely or inappropriately, and that other modalities will be underutilized. Our interventions become less comprehensive and our work becomes less challenging and satisfying.

But how can we simultaneously adhere to a biopsychosocial-developmental approach, which may be more time-consuming than a pharmacologic assessment, while meeting clinical demand for psychopharmacologic management of symptoms? Certainly, psychopharmacologic interventions often remain a critical component of treatment.

CHILD AND ADOLESCENT PSYCHIATRY IN THE FUTURE
Collaboration and Consultation

One solution to maintaining a broad perspective in addressing service needs and concerns regarding quality of care involves shifting the focus and identity of the field from one in which individual child and adolescent psychiatrists provide direct services to patients, to one in which they extend themselves by primarily working in consultative and collaborative capacities.

This shift is synchronous with an emerging climate in children's mental health. As family centered care models ascend in dominance and parents become more visible and effective advocates for their children's needs, the medical model, wherein the physician dictates the treatment or leads the team, is giving way to models in which physicians work collaboratively with informed families and allied providers. The particular expertise of each member of the team, patients and families included, is considered. Consensus about diagnosis and treatment is achieved and treatment proceeds in a concerted manner. The more complex families and systems problems that characterize multiple diagnoses or gravely disorganized families, are also often better treated in collaborative care settings.

A variant of the child and adolescent psychiatrist as team member is the child and adolescent psychiatrist as consultant. (See the article by Milam-Miller elsewhere in this issue for further exploration of this topic.) Development of a consultative role would allow us to influence the treatment of a greater number of children; to teach our colleagues, including general psychiatrists, skills, perspectives, and knowledge which they can then use to treat a large segment of children who present early in the course of their illness or who present with a minimal amount of complexity.

The field of child psychiatry has a long history of consultation to pediatric services, schools, juvenile justice systems, and social services that can form the basis for this paradigm shift toward more extensive consultative work. Those drawn to child psychiatry often enjoy working within systems (family and otherwise) and bringing together disparate perspectives. These are skills that are fundamental to working as collaborators and consultants. Many child psychiatrists are natural teachers. Finally, unlike other physicians, psychiatrists' psychotherapeutic skills may augment our ability to work effectively with others.

Several programs have capitalized upon this movement. The Massachusetts Child Psychiatry Access Project is an example of an innovative program in which primary care physicians are provided timely access to child psychiatric consultation, with 96% of all primary care physicians in the state reportedly enrolled (http://mcpap. com/).[48,49] In Illinois, a new program called "DocAssist" provides child psychiatric consultation and other resource support to primary care physicians (www.illinois. gov/news/HealthHuman.cfm).[50] Other programs are being implemented on smaller scales.[51,52] For example, AACAP supports regional meetings between primary care providers and local child psychiatrists. These group events often occur over lunch or dinner and focus on consultations around challenging cases, discussions about psychopharmacologic management, or indications and best practices for referral. Finally, child and adolescent psychiatrists in many areas of the country have extended themselves using telepsychiatry.[53–56]

Training and Education

In many ways, the system-of-care and consultation movements are well underway. But is our field ready to embrace a major paradigm shift from individual practitioner to consultant or team member? And how do we train the next generation of child psychiatrists to assume these roles?

We must embrace technological advances. Interactive, online learning has assumed great salience with the ever increasing popularity of the Internet and the technological sophistication of our patients, their families, and our trainees. The American Academy of Child and Adolescent Psychiatry (AACAP) is providing leadership in this area by its eAACAP initiative, an electronic source of information with three portals: one for child and adolescent psychiatrists, one for professionals who are not child and adolescent psychiatrists, and one for parents and teens.[57] The interactive nature of eAACAP has begun to provide users with different levels of knowledge and experience an opportunity to ask questions about children's mental health and be directed to reliable and scientifically sound answers. Technological and communication advances will provide opportunity for further development of formal collaborative consultative networks. Using the Internet to educate families and communities about prevention strategies and wellness is a high priority opportunity. To capitalize upon this role of technology, we need to ensure that our residents are provided the resources and training to access clinical and research data electronically, and the support to use technology in innovative ways to expand and improve care (Joel Yager, "Challenges for Psychiatric Education in the 21st Century" UC Davis Grand Rounds presentation, 4/8/2004).[58,59]

Consultative experiences are frequently provided in CAP training, often to inpatient pediatrics services and schools, and occasionally to social services, and the courts as well. Continued inclusion and even expansion of these experiences, including opportunities to reflect thoughtfully upon them, is important.

However, we need to ensure that our training programs specifically focus on teaching residents how to function effectively within systems. Our current generation of trainees must move beyond the goal of an acceptance and comfort in working with systems, to becoming expert at working between and within them, and to becoming confident in their ability to create and partner in innovative, strong, and effective systems. Support from AACAP for the pilot Systems of Care teaching module is an excellent start. Our trainees must be comfortable speaking the languages of related disciplines. They must be able to understand and respect the perspectives (as well as the strengths and limitations) of our various partners in education, social work, pediatrics, nursing, public health, and our patients' families.

Conjoint training and seminar experiences, and provision of training in effective multidisciplinary settings under thoughtful guidance, will further enhance respect, experience, and skill. Supervision and seminars might specifically focus upon issues of conflict resolution, problem solving, advocacy, management, and leadership. Leadership experiences during training should be provided. At least one program has already begun to explicitly teach leadership skills to their child and adolescent psychiatry fellows (Dorothy Stubbe, MD, Yale Child Study Center, personal communication, 2008). Service delivery might become a specific focus of training.

To become effective as a consultant, child psychiatrists must possess effective teaching skills. At the clinical level, child and adolescent psychiatrists frequently teach patients, as well as their families. As consultants, we must also be able to learn from, listen to, and teach our various colleagues. To become an effective teacher, we must have effective teachers. The recent AACAP initiative for the development of master child psychiatric educators through the AACAP-Harvard Macy Teaching Scholars Program, is advancing this goal.[60] These educators' ability to teach and inspire other child and adolescent psychiatrists as educators, particularly regarding the scholarship of education including the principles of adult and small-group learning, will pay dividends through generations of trainees. Providing trainees with supervised and progressive opportunities to teach patients, parents, colleagues, and clinical partners is a rich and useful learning experience that should be welcomed at a range of levels. The AACAP medical educator initiative also addresses the workforce shortage by ensuring that master teachers serving as role models participate early in a medical student's education.

As clinicians and teachers, we must feel comfortable and confident in our ability to speak the scientific language of various related disciplines—both basic science and clinical. We must develop our own skills for life-long learning to assimilate the rapidly expanding base of new knowledge.[61,62] This is a priority supported by the AACAP Maintenance of Certification Modules for Lifelong Learning and the American Board of Psychiatry and Neurology recertification process. As our science develops new risk markers and endophenotypes for mental illness, we will be able to focus more effectively on prevention and early intervention. We will be the team member counted upon to bring this science to the table to interpret for the team.

Finally, we must recruit CAP trainees who possess the motivation and interpersonal skills to thrive in consultative and community-based settings. It will be interesting to see whether a focus on consultative practice may increase our pool of prospective child and adolescent psychiatrists. Our workforce needs compel us to actively seek trainees interested in community-based work, and then to nurture this interest.

However, despite these modifications to training, we must continue to emphasize the importance of maintaining our core. Perhaps the most important skill that a child and adolescent psychiatrist consultant must possess is the time-honored ability to formulate a case from a biopsychosocial-developmental perspective. As we consider a future that possibly involves the establishment of certificate programs for other physicians, greater partnering with nurse practitioners, and collaboration with psychologists with limited prescription authority, adherence to the biopsychosocial-developmental perspective assumes increased importance. If the profession is to embrace a major professional identity shift to child and adolescent psychiatrists as consultants and collaborative team members, our training programs need to be modified to ensure that the knowledge base and skill sets required for professional teaching, consultation, and systems analysis are adequately learned. However, CAP training curricula must remain comprehensive. Theories and the science of development and an understanding of the inner life of the child and of family dynamics must be prioritized,[63] and skills in formulation must be explicitly taught.[64] Only in this way will the child and adolescent psychiatric consultant and collaborator be able to teach and support the consultees in their understanding of the child, and in the development and implementation of an effective and comprehensive treatment plan.

The Role of the General Psychiatrist

So how does the general psychiatrist fit into this future? As noted earlier in this discussion, many general psychiatrists in clinical practice are already treating children; many others might be willing to do so with appropriate support and guidance. This is a legitimate way in which to expand our provision of services.

The roles in which general psychiatrists currently seem best suited to working with children and adolescents include the treatment of late adolescents, whose issues and presenting diagnoses are more similar to those of early adulthood; the psychopharmacologic management of adolescents with heavily neurobiologically driven disorders; and, perhaps, monitoring the medications of adolescents with more complex clinical presentations, in consultation with a child and adolescent psychiatrist. The issues facing latency and preschool-aged children are sufficiently unique that their treatment may be better "turfed" to a child and adolescent psychiatrist, or, if none are available, treated in consultation with one. However, expanded training during the general psychiatry sequence, followed by further continuing education programs, perhaps leading to certificates of special competence, might expand the scope of practice for general psychiatrists.

Supports currently available to general psychiatrists include annual AACAP meetings; regional continuing education institutes sponsored by AACAP such as the Mid-Year Psychopharmacology Institute; Practice Parameters published in the *Journal of the American Academy of Child and Adolescent Psychiatry* and available free online through the AACAP Web site (www.aacap.org); *Facts for Families*, informational handouts about a range of child psychiatric issues and conditions, available free at the AACAP Web site (translated into eight languages); and *eAACAP*, the online resource for practitioners and families, described earlier in this discussion. It is hoped that there will soon be much more.

General psychiatrists are encouraged to become familiar with the systems of care for children and adolescents in their community, as well as the systems of care movement.[65] (See the article by Winters and Metz elsewhere in this issue.) It is recommended that consultative relationships be developed with one or more child and adolescent psychiatrists in a community; and that general psychiatrists consider developing or joining other consultative networks if available.

OTHER CONSIDERATIONS

The consultative/collaborative model is not without its difficulties in implementation. Who will pay for the consultations and what is the liability of the consultant? Will consultations be reimbursed by insurance companies? How will this be paid for in systems of care such as county mental health systems or managed care networks? Another important consideration is the liability of the consulting child and adolescent psychiatrist. If a child is cared for by a pediatrician, or other physician extender who prescribes psychiatric medication and recommends treatments based on consultation with the child and adolescent psychiatrist, who is liable when there is a negative outcome to treatment? Although one child and adolescent psychiatrist could possibly inform the care of a large number of children as a consultant to an entire school district, pediatric medical group, or several general psychiatrists, a role change to consultant will require a change in the reimbursement structure. New models of reimbursement for consultation and collaboration are now being tested–a change that has only become feasible because of the tremendous unmet need and the resulting societal pressure for economic restructuring.

The role of the child and adolescent psychiatrist in providing direct clinical care will never become obsolete. In fact, the ability to provide high quality consultation and to engage in effective team collaboration is dependent upon the highly honed skills of clinical practice leading to the ability to develop comprehensive and complex formulations. Perhaps the future holds that child and adolescent psychiatrists will devote a portion of their practice to collaborative and consultative services; or, some will continue predominantly as front-line clinicians, and others will become more specialized in consultation and collaboration. Triple board graduates, for example, are ideally suited to consult or collaborate with pediatric practitioners.

How might these changes impact our identity within medicine? Does increased consultation and collaboration make CAP more central to medicine as a whole, or more peripheral? By taking a broader role, we will ensure that psychiatry continues to be connected with medicine. For if we, as a profession, do not take the lead in shaping the future of mental health care for children, others will–others who may not have the breadth of knowledge and skills that we have gained over the many years of providing care to mentally ill children and youth.

SUMMARY

As with general psychiatry, our work as child and adolescent psychiatrists is robust and rewarding. Expanding resources, increased public awareness of children's mental health needs, and an exploding scientific knowledge base offers tremendous opportunity. Yet, challenges face our field, some of which are unique to CAP, others of which are shared by general psychiatry and the larger field of medicine. Our workforce shortage is improving; however, it is not improving fast enough. This has clearly affected the nature of our practice and of our professional identity. As we take stock of the nature of our work and the forces shaping our practice, it becomes clear: We must step away from the medical model and the medication management role and learn to work collaboratively and in consultative roles with a broader array of partners. To best serve the millions of children who suffer from untreated and under-treated mental illness in this country and their families, we must fundamentally change some key aspects of the way we practice. Ironically, by stepping outside of our current role and by strengthening our relationships with others in related disciplines (ie, by broadening our role) we will strengthen our niche. As child and adolescent psychiatrists, our thinking must become even more integrative as we assimilate knowledge from a broad and burgeoning range of bases, and as we learn to appreciate and integrate the perspectives of others. Fortunately, we already have a framework with which to do so effectively: the scientifically based biopsychosocial-developmental approach which must remain central to our work. General psychiatrists can play a critical role in extending services to children and adolescents by taking advantage of increasingly available consultative networks and resources, familiarizing themselves with principles of systems-based work and the system of care available in their community, and by working collaboratively with child and adolescent psychiatrists. Finally, enriched opportunities for postgraduate and continuing medical education can enhance skill sets for working with children and adolescents.

REFERENCES

1. Stubbe DE, Thomas WJ. A survey of early-career child and adolescent psychiatrists: professional activities and perceptions. J Am Acad Child Adolesc Psychiatry 2002;41(2):123–30.
2. Ladouceur CD, Almeida JR, Birmaher B, et al. Subcortical gray matter volume abnormalities in healthy bipolar offspring: potential neuroanatomical risk marker for bipolar disorder? J Am Acad Child Adolesc Psychiatry 2008;47(5):532–9.
3. Pauly K, Seiferth NY, Kellermann T, et al. Cerebral dysfunctions of emotion-cognition interactions in adolescent-onset schizophrenia. J Am Acad Child Adolesc Psychiatry 2008;47(11):1299–310.
4. Laucht M, Becker K, Frank J, et al. Genetic variation in dopamine pathways differentially associated with smoking progression in adolescence. J Am Acad Child Adolesc Psychiatry 2008;47(6):673–81.
5. Lombroso PJ, Ogren MP. Fragile X syndrome: keys to the molecular genetics of synaptic plasticity. J Am Acad Child Adolesc Psychiatry 2008;47(7):736–9.
6. Whittle S, Yucel M, Fornito A, et al. Neuroanatomical correlates of temperament in early adolescents. J Am Acad Child Adolesc Psychiatry 2008;47(6):682–93.
7. Josephson AM, Dell ML. Religion and spirituality in child and adolescent psychiatry: a new frontier. Child Adolesc Psychiatr Clin N Am 2004;13(1):1–15.
8. Pescosolido BA. Culture, children, and mental health treatment: special section on the national stigma study-children. Psychiatr Serv 2007;58(5):611–2.
9. Lim RF, Lu FG. Culture and psychiatric education. Acad Psychiatry 2008;32(4): 269–71.
10. Greenberg MT. Promoting resilience in children and youth: preventive interventions and their interface with neuroscience. Ann N Y Acad Sci 2006;1094:139–50.
11. Riley AW, Valdez CR, Barrueco S, et al. Development of a family-based program to reduce risk and promote resilience among families affected by maternal depression: theoretical basis and program description. Clin Child Fam Psychol Rev 2008;11(1–2):12–29.
12. Demyttenaere K, Bruffaerts R, Posada-Villa J, et al. Prevalence, severity, and unmet need for treatment of mental disorders in the World Health Organization World Mental Health Surveys. JAMA 2004;291(21):2581–90.

13. Patel V, Flisher AJ, Hetrick S, et al. Mental health of young people: a global public-health challenge. Lancet 2007;369(9569):1302–13.

14. Satcher DS. Executive summary: a report of the Surgeon General on mental health. Public Health Rep 2000;115(1):89–101.

15. USDeptHHS. Mental health: a report of the surgeon general-executive summary. U.S. Department of Health and Human Services, Substance Abuse and Mental Health Services Administration, Center for Mental Health Services, National Institutes of Health. Rockville (MD): National Institute of Mental Health; 1999.

16. Kim WJ. Child and adolescent psychiatry workforce: a critical shortage and national challenge. Acad Psychiatry 2003;27(4):277–82.

17. Kim W. Recruitment. Child Adolesc Psychiatr Clin N Am 2007;16(1):45–54, viii.

18. Thomas CR, Holzer CE 3rd. The continuing shortage of child and adolescent psychiatrists. J Am Acad Child Adolesc Psychiatry 2006;45(9):1023–31.

19. Pescosolido BA, Jensen PS, Martin JK, et al. Public knowledge and assessment of child mental health problems: findings from the National Stigma Study-Children. J Am Acad Child Adolesc Psychiatry 2008;47(3):339–49.

20. Pescosolido BA, Perry BL, Martin JK, et al. Stigmatizing attitudes and beliefs about treatment and psychiatric medications for children with mental illness. Psychiatr Serv 2007;58(5):613–8.

21. Cutler JL, Harding KJ, Mozian SA, et al. Discrediting the notion "working with 'crazies' will make you 'crazy'": addressing stigma and enhancing empathy in medical student education. Adv Health Sci Educ Theory Pract. 2008 Sep 3. [Epub ahead of print].

22. Martin A, Bloch M, Pruett K, et al. From too little too late to early and often: child psychiatry education during medical school (and before and after). Child Adolesc Psychiatr Clin N Am 2007;16(1):17–43.

23. Cadinouche A, Gainza F. Choosing a career in child and adolescent psychiatry. Psychiatr Bull 2006;30(5):194.

24. Rodriguez C, Stowell K. Want your voice to count? Join us at the AMA. Psychiatr News 2008;43(19):17.

25. Moran M. Residency program combines child, general psychiatry. Psychiatr News 2006;41(5):9.

26. Gray DD, Bilder DA, Leonard HL, et al. Triple board training and new "portals" into child psychiatry training. Child Adolesc Psychiatr Clin N Am 2007;16(1):55–66, viii.

27. Training program in pediatrics, child psychiatry developed. AAP News 1985;1(6):3.

28. Schneider ME. Pilot project aims to address shortage in child psychiatry. Clinical Psychiatry News 2007;35(8):11.

29. Gilbert AR, Tew JD Jr, Reynolds CF III, et al. A developmental model for enhancing research training during psychiatry residency. Acad Psychiatry 2006;30(1):55–62.

30. Harpaz-Rotem I, Rosenheck RA. Prescribing practices of psychiatrists and primary care physicians caring for children with mental illness. Child Care Health Dev 2006;32(2):225–38.

31. Staller JA. Service delivery in child psychiatry: provider shortage isn't the only problem. Clin Child Psychol Psychiatry 2008;13(1):171–8.

32. Staller JA. Psychiatric nurse practitioners in rural pediatric telepsychiatry. Psychiatr Serv 2006;57(1):138.

33. Douglas Mossman M, Christina G, Weston M. Going outside your area of expertise: How far is too far? Current Psychiatry 2008;7(10):53–6. Available at:

http://www.currentpsychiatry.com/pdf/0710/0710CP_Malpractice.pdf. Accessed October 28, 2008.

34. Martin A, Faraone SV, Henderson SW, et al. Conflict of interest. J Am Acad Child Adolesc Psychiatry 2008;47(2):119–20.

35. Anders TF. Child and adolescent psychiatry: the next 10 Years. Psychiatric Times 2008;25(6):1–4.

36. Anders TF. The pharmaceutical industry, academic medicine, and the FDA. J Child Adolesc Psychopharmacol 2007;17(5):727–30.

37. Zito JM, Tobi H, de Jong-van den Berg LT, et al. Antidepressant prevalence for youths: a multi-national comparison. Pharmacoepidemiol Drug Saf 2006;15(11): 793–8.

38. Zito JM, Safer DJ, dosReis S, et al. Psychotropic practice patterns for youth: a 10-year perspective. Arch Pediatr Adolesc Med 2003;157(1):17–25.

39. Zito JM, Safer DJ, dosReis S, et al. Rising prevalence of antidepressants among US youths. Pediatrics 2002;109(5):721–7.

40. Sonuga-Barke Edmund. Editorial: building therapeutic innovation on scientific foundations in child psychology and psychiatry. J Child Psychol Psychiatry 2007;48(7):629–30.

41. March JS, Szatmari P, Bukstein O, et al. AACAP 2005 Research Forum: speeding the adoption of evidence-based practice in pediatric psychiatry. J Am Acad Child Adolesc Psychiatry 2007;46(9):1098–110.

42. Cohen JD, Insel TR. Cognitive neuroscience and schizophrenia: translational research in need of a translator. Biol Psychiatry 2008;64(1):2–3.

43. Wang PS, Heinssen R, Oliveri M, et al. Bridging bench and practice: translational research for schizophrenia and other psychotic disorders. Neuropsychopharmacology 2009;34(1):204–12.

44. Graeff-Martins AS, Flament MF, Fayyad J, et al. Diffusion of efficacious interventions for children and adolescents with mental health problems. J Child Psychol Psychiatry 2008;49(3):335–52.

45. Gabbard GO, Kay J. The fate of integrated treatment: whatever happened to the biopsychosocial psychiatrist? Am J Psychiatry 2001;158(12):1956–63.

46. Glever J. Talk therapy loses popularity with psychiatrists. MedPage Today 2008. Available at: http://www.medpagetoday.com/Psychiatry/GeneralPsychiatry/10418. Accessed October 30, 2008.

47. Mojtabai R, Olfson M. National trends in psychotherapy by office-based psychiatrists. Arch Gen Psychiatry 2008;65(8):962–70.

48. Connor DF, McLaughlin TJ, Jeffers-Terry M, et al. Targeted Child Psychiatric Services: a new model of pediatric primary clinician–child psychiatry collaborative care. Clin Pediatr 2006;45(5):423–34.

49. Cheung A. Review: 3 of 4 RCTs on the treatment of adolescent depression in primary care have positive results. Evid Based Med 2007;12(1):27.

50. Governor Blagojevich announces program to help doctors address children's mental health needs. Illinois DocAssist will improve diagnosis and treatment of mental illness, substance abuse in children. Office of the Governor NEWS. 2008. Available at: http://www.illinois.gov/PressReleases/ShowPressRelease. cfm?SubjectID=3&RecNum=7153. Accessed January 7, 2009.

51. Levin A. Pediatricians gain 'Safety Net' through psychiatric consults. Psychiatr News 2008;43(18):14–27.

52. Thinking Outside the Box to Stretch Resources. Psychiatr News 2008;43(18): 14–27.

53. Hilty DM, Marks SL, Urness D, et al. Clinical and educational telepsychiatry applications: a review. Can J Psychiatry 2004;49(1):12–23.

54. Urness D, Wass M, Gordon A, et al. Client acceptability and quality of life - telepsychiatry compared to in-person consultation. J Telemed Telecare 2006; 12(5):251–4.

55. Hakak R, Szeftel R. Clinical use of telemedicine in child psychiatry. Focus 2008; 6(3):293–6.

56. Myers KM, Valentine JM, Melzer SM. Child and adolescent telepsychiatry: utilization and satisfaction. Telemed J E Health 2008;14(2):131–7.

57. Hendren RL. Casting a wide net to nurture mentally healthy children. J Am Acad Child Adolesc Psychiatry 2008;47(2):123–8.

58. Hilty DM, Hales DJ, Briscoe G, et al. APA Summit on Medical Student Education Task Force on Informatics and Technology: learning about computers and applying computer technology to education and practice. Acad Psychiatry 2006;30(1):29–35.

59. Srinivasan M, Keenan CR, Yager J. Visualizing the future: technology competency development in clinical medicine, and implications for medical education. Acad Psychiatry 2006;30(6):480–90.

60. Hunt J, Stubbe DE, Hanson M, et al. A 2-year Progress Report of the AACAP-Harvard Macy Teaching Scholars Program. Acad Psychiatry 2008;32(5):414–9.

61. March JS, Chrisman A, Breland-Noble A, et al. Using and teaching evidence-based medicine: the Duke University child and adolescent psychiatry model. Child Adolesc Psychiatr Clin N Am 2005;14(2):273–96.

62. Lim RF, Hsiung BC, Hales DJ. Lifelong learning: skills and online resources. Acad Psychiatry 2006;30(6):540–7.

63. Fox G, Katz DA, Eddins-Folensbee FF, et al. Teaching development in undergraduate and graduate medical education. Child Adolesc Psychiatr Clin N Am 2007; 16(1):67–94.

64. Winters NC, Hanson G, Stoyanova V. The case formulation in child and adolescent psychiatry. Child Adolesc Psychiatr Clin N Am 2007;16(1):111–32.

65. Pumariega AJ, Winters NC, Huffine C. The evolution of systems of care for children's mental health: forty years of community child and adolescent psychiatry. Community Ment Health J 2003;39(5):399–425.

Index

Note: Page numbers of article titles are in **boldface** type.

A

ADHD (Attention deficit/hyperactivity disorder), atomoxetine for, 46, 49
    ethnicity and response to, 156–157
  bipolar disorder vs., 75
  causes of, 40
  diagnosis of, DSM-IV-TR criteria for, 41–42
    practice parameters for, 42
    rating scales for, 41–43
  differential diagnosis of, 44
  early indicators/recognition of, 183, 189
  epidemiological studies of, 40
  importance of early treatment of, 40
  investigative approaches to, symptom clusters vs. DSM-IV diagnostic criteria, 185, 190
  latent class analysis of, diagnostic comorbidity and, 184–185, 190
    of temperament clusters, 185, 190
  methylphenidate for, ethnicity and response to, 156
  off label medications for, 46, 49
  pharmaco fMRI research in, 206
  pharmacotherapies for, cardiovascular concerns, 51
    growth effects of, 50
    monitoring of, 51
  presentation in pediatric population, 40–41
  prevalence of, 39–40
  psychiatric disorder comorbidity, 44
  psychopharmacologic treatment of, 112–113
  review for general psychiatrist, **39–56**
  sex and, 40
  treatments for, behavioral, 44–45
    family education and support, 44–45
    in adolescents, 52–53
    in preschool children, 51–52
    pharmacotherapy, 45, 50–51
  with bipolar disorder, 76
Adjustment disorder with depressed mood, bipolar disorder vs., 76
Adolescent psychiatry. See *Child and adolescent psychiatry (CAP).*
Adolescents, ADHD in, treatment of, 52–53
  cognitive-behavioral therapy for, for anxiety disorders, 96–99
    for depression, 99–102
  suicidal, dialectical behavior therapy for, 102–105
Affective disorders, with psychotic features, in Prader-Willi syndrome, 25

Psychiatr Clin N Am 32 (2009) 227–241
doi:10.1016/S0193-953X(09)00009-4
0193-953X/09/$ – see front matter © 2009 Elsevier Inc. All rights reserved.

psych.theclinics.com

Aggression, in bipolar disorder, 73–74
    in disruptive behavior disorders, psychopharmacologic treatment of, 114–115
Alpha2-adrenergic medications, for ADHD, 46, 49
Alpha-adrenoceptor agonists, for ADHD, 113
    for autism, 122
Alzheimer's disease, early-onset in Downs syndrome, 23
Amphetamines, for ADHD, 46, 48, 112–113
    for autism, 7
    in autistic spectrum disorders, 122
Amygdala, in bipolar disorder, 183
Anticonvulsants, for bipolar disorder, 117–119
Antidepressants. See also *Selective serotonin reuptake inhibitors (SSRIs).*
    monitoring of, 115–116
    tricyclic, for pediatric depression, 115
Antipsychotics, atypical. See *Atypical antipsychotics.*
    first generation, 124
Anxiety disorder(s)
    autoimmune neuropsychiatric disorders, streptococcal infection-associated, 62–64
    childhood onset, early indicators/recognition of, 184, 190
    cognitive-behavioral therapy for, alliance with adolescent in, 98
        case example of, 97
        developmental differences and, 97–98
        homework in, 98
        parent/caregiver role in, 98
        treatment excerpt, 99
    DSM-IV-TR criteria differences for, 57–59
    for adolescents, cognitive-behavioral therapy for, 96–97
        implementation of, 97–99
    generalized anxiety disorder, 59–60
    obsessive-compulsive disorder, 61–62
    prevalence of, 57–58
    psychopharmacologic treatment of, 118, 120–121
    separation anxiety disorder, 57–59
    social phobia, 60–61
    update on, **57–64**
    with bipolar disorder, 76
Anxiety/mood disorders, in ADHD, 44
Applied behavior analysis (ABA), for autism, 6–7
Aripiprazole (Abilify), for aggression in disruptive behavior disorders, 115–116
    for autism, 7
    for autism and pervasive developmental disorders, 122
    for bipolar disorder, 117–119
    for psychotic disorders, 123
Asperger's disorder, 3
Atomoxetine (Strattera), ethnicity and response to, 156–157
    for ADHD, 46, 49, 113
        adverse effects of, 50–51
    growth effects of, 50
    in adolescents, 52
Attachment system, and neurodevelopment, heritable factors in, 181, 189
        nuturing experience and adaptation to stress, 181

        parent-child interactions and diagnostic risk, 181–182
Attention deficit/hyperactivity disorder (ADHD), in fragile X syndrome (FXS), 21
Atypical antipsychotics, for autism, 7, 122
    for bipolar disorder, 118–119
        in childhood, 77
    for disruptive behavior disorders, 114–115
    for psychotic disorders, 124
    side effects of, 123
Autism, behaviors in, 3, 6
    characterization of, 1
    comorbities with, 6
    diagnosis of, 2–4
        characteristic features of, 2–3
        demographic findings on, 2
        differentiation from other pervasive disorders, 3
        tools for, 3
    early identification of, 4
    families and, working with, 9–10
    forms of, 6
    genetics in, 4–5
    in Down syndrome, 23–24
    new developments in, **1–14**
    pathophysiology of, genetic susceptibility to environmental trigger in, 4–6
    prevalence of, 1–2
    psychomarmacologic treatment of, 121–122
    psychostimulants in, for inattention and hyperactivity, 121
    symptoms in, 7
    treatment of, 6–9
        behavioral interventions for, 6–7
        biomedical, 8–9
        implementation of, 9
        pharmacologic, 7–8
Autism Diagnostic Interview, Revised (ADI-R), 3
Autism Diagnostic Observation Schedule (ADOS), 3
Autism spectrum disorders (ASDs), 2
    early intervention in parent-child interactions for, 186
    in fragile X syndrome (FXS), 21
    intervention and prevention in, behavioral and pharmacological, 187, 190
    in velocardiofacial syndrome, 18
    risk for, developmental model of, 186

B

Basal ganglia, in bipolar disorder, 183
Behavioral disorders, with bipolar disorder, 76
Behavioral interventions, for autism, 6–7
Behavioral therapy, for ADHD, 44–45
Behaviors, in autism, 2–3, 7
    in Prader-Willi syndrome, 25
Biomedical treatments, for autism, 8–9

Bipolar disorder, **71–80**
  broad spectrum of, Jack's case, 73
  childhood onset, early indicators/recognition of, 183, 189
  classic presentation in childhood, Jill's case, 72
  comorbidity in, 76
  criteria in, for depressive episode, 74
    for mania, 74–75
  cycling in, 74
  diagnostic issues in, **71–80**
  differential diagnosis of, 75–76
  early intervention and prevention in, 191–192
  epidemiology of, 76–77
  in children vs. adults, 77
  in youths vs. adults, 74
  irritability and aggression in, 73–74
  prevalence of, 76
  prognosis for, before age 12, 78
    in adolescents, 77–78
  psychopharmacologic treatment of, 117–118
  symptoms in, context of, 75
    episodic vs. continuous, 74
    hallmark, 74–75
  treatment of, 77
  vs. ADHD, 75
Bipolar disorder (BD), childhood onset, biological underpinning of, 182
    diffusion tensor imaging in, 182, 189
    trauma in, 182, 189
Brain, in autism, 5–6
  in bipolar disorder development, 183
  in Kleinfelter's syndrome, 28
  in Turner's syndrome, 26–27
Bupropion (Wellbutrin, Zyban), for ADHD, 49

C

Cannabis use, as risk factor, for early-age onset schizophrenia, 86
    for psychosis, 86
Carbamazepine, for bipolar disorder, 117–118
Center for Mental Health Services (CMHS), children's mental health and, 136
  definition of serious emotional disturbance by, 136–137
  outcome evaluation of, 136
Child and adolescent psychiatrists, recruitment strategies for, expanded training within
  general psychiatry training, 216
    focus on medical students, 215–216
    postgraduate training, 216
    triple board program, 216
Child and adolescent psychiatry (CAP)
  biologic symptom management in, 217–218
  biopsychosocial-developmental perspective in, need for return to, 217
  challenges and opportunities in, **213–226**
  consultative/collaborative model of, implementation of, 222

front-line clinicians in, 222
general psychiatrist in, in consultation with child and adolescent psychiatrist, 221
    supports for, 221
    systems of care knowledge of, 222
in future, collaboration and consultation in, 218–219
    training and education for, 219–221
public perception of, 216–217
rewards of, 214
scope of practice and, as nature of practice, 218
    limitations on, 217–218
    professional identity in, 217–218
training and education for, as consultant, 220
    as teachers, 220
    for collaboration in system of care, 220
    life-long learning in, 220
    recruitment of trainees and, 221
workforce issues in, 214–216
    recruitment rates and, 215–216
    shortage of psychiatrists, 214–215
Childhood disintegrative disorder, 3
Childhood trauma, effects of, 182
Child psychiatry. See *Child and adolescent psychiatry (CAP)*.
Cholinesterase inhibitors, for Down syndrome, 24
Citalopram, for posttraumatic stress disorder, 120
    in autism, 121
Clomipramine, in autism, 121
Clonidine (Catapres), for ADHD, 46, 48–49, 113
    for autism, 122
    for posttraumatic stress disorder, 120
Clozapine, for treatment-resistant schizophrenia, 123–124
Cognitive-behavioral therapy (CBT), culturally adapted forms of, 160
    developmental approach to, 95
    for adolescents, parent/caregiver role in, 98, 102
    for anxiety disorders, in adolescents, 96–99
    for depression, in adolescence, 99–100
        in adolescents, models of, 101
    for eating disorders, 105–106
    for pediatric autoimmune neuropsychiatric disorders associated with streptococcal
        infections, 64
    for somatoform disorders, 105
    implementation of, for anxiety disorders in adolescents, 96–99
        for depressive disorders in adolescents, 100–102
    research on, for anxiety disorders in adolescents, 96–97
        implementation of, 99–100
    with medication, for anxiety disorders, 120
    with sertraline, for obsessive-compulsive disorder, 96
    with SSRI therapy, for refractory depression, 116–117
Communication, in autism, 2
Comorbidity, genetic factors and development of, 185–186
    homotypic and heterotypic, 180–181, 188, 190
Complementary and alternative medical (CAM) treatments. See *Biomedical treatments*.

Comprehensive Community Services for Children and Youth and Their Families, establishment of, 136
Compulsions, in Prader-Willi syndrome, 25
Conduct disorder, early indicators/recognition of, 183, 189
    in ADHD, 44
Confidentiality, evaluation of youth in custody and, 172
    in juvenile justice system, 166
Consent, in treatment of minors, 166
Cortisol production of, 191
Cultural diversity, and under-utilization of psychiatric services, by racial and ethnic minorities, 154–155
        cultural factors in, 157
    cultural beliefs about causes and treatments, 157
    culturally competent physician and, 160–161
    culturally competent psychotherapy research and, cognitive-behavioral therapy, 160
        family therapy, 159–160
        storytelling therapy adaptation, 159
    culture and, 154
    ethnicity and, 154
    evolution in the United States, 153–154
        increase in Asian and Hispanic immigrants, 154
        race-based practices in, 154
    of racial and ethnic minorities, and under-utilization of psychiatric services, 154–155, 157
        disparities in psychotropic medication treatment, 155–156
        disparities in treatment of ADHD, 156
        pediatric ethnopsychopharmacology and, 156–157
    race and, 154
Culturally competent physician, ethnocentrisim of physicians and, 161
    functional qualities of, 160
    learning curve for cultual competence, 160
Culturally diverse children and adolescents. See also Cultural diversity.
    treatment disparities in, **153–163**
Culture, defined, 154

    D

D-cycloserine, for autism, 122
Depression. See also Bipolar disorder; Major depressive disorder (MDD).
    childhood onset, early indicators/recognition of, 184, 190
    in adolescence, cognitive-behavioral therapy therapy for, 100–102
    in generalized anxiety disorder, 60
    social phobia and, 61
    unipolar, bipolar disorder vs., 76
Depression not otherwise specified, bipolar disorder vs., 76
Dialectical behavior therapy (DBT), 95
    for suicidal adolescents, 102–103
        caregiver involvement in skills training in, 103
        duration of, 103
        family sessions in, 104–105
        implementation of, 103–105

middle path in, 104
   research on, 102–103
Disruptive behavior disorders (DBDs), psychopharmacologic treatment of, 114–115
Divalproex sodium, for autism, 8
Divalproic acid (DVPX), for bipolar disorder, 117–118
   for disruptive behavior disorders, 114
Donepezil, for Down syndrome, 24
Down syndrome, anatomic and medical features of, 22
   autism in, 23–24
   behavioral problems in, 22
   chromosome 21 and trisomy 21 in, 22
   depression in, 23
   detection of, 22
   mental retardation in, 23
   microencephaly in, 23
   pharmacotherapy for, 24

E

Early Detection and Intervention for the Prevention of Psychosis Program (EDIPPP), 90–91
Eating disorders, cognitive-behavioral therapy for, 105–106
Endotypes, description of, 206
   vs. phenotype use, in neurodevelopmental model for case-formulation, 206
Environment, as trigger in pathophysiology of autism, 4–6
   factors associated with autism, 5
   in neurodevelopment, case presentation, 205, 207
      correlation and interaction with genes, 177–178, 181, 188
Epileptiform abnormalities, autism and, 5
Escitalopram, in autism, 121
Ethical issues, in psychiatric consultation, 166, 170–171
Ethnicity, defined, 154

F

Family, in dialectical behavior therapy for suicidal adolescents, 104–105
   of autistic persons, education of, 9
      working with, 9–10
Family therapy, culturally adapted forms of, 159–160
Fluoxetine, for major depressive disorder, 115
   for obsessive-compulsive disorder, 120
Fluvoxamine, for obsessive-compulsive disorder, 120
Fragile X gene *(FMR1)*, 202, 204–205
Fragile X mental retardation protein (FMRP), in Sarah case, 202–203
Fragile X syndrome (FXS), as model for study of modifying genes, 207
   carriers of, medical issues in, 21–22
      permutation condition (55–200 CGG repeats), 21
   FMR1 gene permutation in, 19
   phenotypes in, 19–22
     cognitive, 20
     physical, 20
     psychiatric and behavioral, 20–21
   sex differences in, 19–21
   vs. autism, 6

G

Generalized anxiety disorder (GAD), course and outcome of, 60
    DSM-IV-TR criteria for youth, 59
    prevalence of, 59
    psychiatric comorbidity in, 60
Growth hormone therapy, for Prader-Willi syndrome, 25
Guanfacine (Tenex), for ADHD, 46, 48–49, 113

H

Hepatic toxicity, atomoxetin and, 51
Hypothalamic/pituitary/adrenergic axis (HPA), stress and, 191

I

Immune abnormalities, autism and, 5
Irritability, in bipolar disorder, 73–74

K

Kleinfelter's syndrome (KS), as sex chromosome disorder, 27
    brain deficiency in, 28
    cognitive deficits in, 17–18
    hormone replacement therapy for, 27
    psychiatric symptoms in, 27

L

Latent class analysis (LCA), of ADHD, 184–185, 190
Lisdexamphetamine (Vyvanse), for ADHD, 113
Lithium, for bipolar disorder, 117
    for disruptive behavior disorders, 114
Locus ceruleus/noradrenergic sympathetic system, stress and, 191

M

Major depressive disorder (MDD). See also *Bipolar disorder; Depression.*
    and posttraumatic stress disorder, prodromal period in, 82
    antidepressants for, differences in pediatric and adult populations, 115
        risk for bipolar disorder and, 117
    bipolar disorder vs., 76
    generalized anxiety disorder and, 60
    psychopharmacologic treatment of, 115–117
    psychotherapeutic treatment of, 116
Methylphenidate, ethnicity and response to, 156
    for ADHD, 46–47, 112
    for autism, 7
    for inattention and hyperactivity, in pervasive developmental disorders, 121–122
    in adolescents, 52–53
    in preschool children, 52

new formulations of, 112–113
transdermal system, 112
Monoamine oxidase A (MAOA) polymorphism, defined, 203
    in boys with fragile X syndrome, 202–203
    in case presentation of Sarah, 202–203
Mood disorders, bipolar disorder vs., 75–76
    in ADHD, 44
Mood stabilizers, for aggression, 114
    for autism, 8, 122
    for bipolar disorder, in childhood, 77
    for disruptive behavior disorders, 114

N

Neurodevelopment, attachment system and, heritable factors in, 181, 189
        nuturing experience and adaptation to stress, 181
        parent-child interactions and diagnostic risk, 181–182
    biological factors in, 187
        event-related potenial study in, 178–179, 188
        gene-environment correlations, 177–178, 188
        gene-environment interactions, 177, 188
        imaging studies of, 177, 179
        markers of vulnerability and, 179, 188
        neuroanatomical correlates of temperament and, 179–180, 188
    clinical implications of, 187–191
        foster children and, 191
        stress and, 191
    clinical implications of current findings in, **177–197**
    current findings in, 177–189
        clinical implications of, 188–190
    diagnostic factors in, early indicators/early recognition of specific conditions, 182–184,
        189–190
    early intervention, individual responses to, 191
    investigative approaches to, 184–185, 190
        latent class analysis, 184–185, 190
    monitoring intervention in, 187, 190
    neurobiological effects of specific treatments and, 184
    neuroplasticity in, 180–181, 188
    prevention and intervention, 185–186
        early indicators and recognition in, 186–187, 190
    psychopathology and,, mapping developmental trajectories of, 182, 189
    temperament and neuropsychology in, 184
Neurodevelopmental model for case-formulation, **199–211**
    biologic factors in, 207
    case presentation of Sarah, 201
        anxiety in, presentation and treatment of, 204–205
        at brain level, 203, 205
        at neuropsychology level, 204
        environmental and psychodynamic factors in, 205
        etiology in, fragile X syndrome and, 202–203
        fragile X mental retardation protein in, 202–203

Neurodevelopmental model (*continued*)
    genetic counseling for family and, 205
    monoamine oxidase A polymorphism in, 202–203
    serotonin transporter gene in, 202–203
    symptom level evaluation, 201
    treatment of, 202
  diagram of, 200
  environmental factors in, 207
  future implications, endotypes vs. phenotype use in, 206
  future implications of, merger of brain and neuropsychology levels of, 206
    pathophysiology in development of taxonomy of mental disorders, 207
    treat development and treatment matching, 206
  levels in, brain and central nervous system, 200
    etiology, 200
    neuropsychology, 200
    symptoms, 200
Neurogenetic disorder(s), Down syndrome, 22–24
  fragile X-associated tremor/ataxia syndrome, 19, 22
  fragile X syndrome, 19–22
  Kleinfelter's syndrome, 27–28
  Prader-Willi syndrome, 24–25
  psychiatric phenotypes associated with, **15–37**
  Turner's syndrome, 25–27
  velocardiofacial syndrome (VCFS), 16–19
  48,XXYY karyotype, 28
  47,XYY karyotype, 28
Neuroplasticity, comorbidity and, 180
  defined, 180
  heterotypic disorders and, 181, 188
  homotypic disorders and, 180–181
Neuropsychiatric disorders, autoimmune streptococal infection-associated, 62–63
  case example of, 63–64
    diagnosis and treatment of, 64
    symptoms in, 63–64
Neurotransmitter abnormalities, autism and, 5
Norepinephrine reuptake inhibitor (Strattera), for autism, 7

O

Obsessive-compulsive disorder (OCD), age of onset, bimodal pattern to, 62
  clinical presentation of, 61–62
  cognitive-behavioral therapy for, 99
  DSM-IV-TR criteria for, 58, 61–62
  prevalence of, 62
Occupational therapy, for autism, 7
Olanzapine, for aggression in disruptive behavior disorders, 115–116
  for autism and pervasive developmental disorders, 122
  for psychotic disorders, 123
Oppositional defiant disorder, in ADHD, 44
Oxcarbazepine, for bipolar disorder, 117–118
Oxidative stress, autism and, 5

P

Panic disorder, 121
Pediatric autoimmune neuropsychiatric disorders associated with streptococcal infections
(PANDAS), 62
    case example of, 63–64
    diagnostic criteria for, 62
    obsessive compulsive disorder in, 64
    treatment of, 64
Pervasive developmental disorder not otherwise specified (PDD-NOS), 3
Pervasive developmental disorders, 3
    autism, 2
    in velocardiofacial syndrome, 18
    methylphenidate for, 121–122
    psychopharmacologic treatment of, 121–122
Phenotypes, description of, 206
Portland Identification and Early Referral (PIER) program, for early detection of psychosis,
90–91
Posttraumatic stress disorder (PTSD), 64–69
    cognitive-behavioral therapy for, 99
    course and outcome of, 65
    in infants and young children, 64–65
    in older children and adults, 64
    prevalence of, 65
    risk factors associated with, 65
    update on, **64–69**
Prader-Willi syndrome (PWS), characteristic phenotype in, 24
    treatment of, 24–25
Propranolol, for panic disorder, 121
    for posttraumatic stress disorder, 121
Psychiatric consultant, as clinician, in direct evaluation/treatment of children, 172
    as collaborator with school, 173
    as systems expert and collaborator in program development, 173
    as teacher, 171–172
    entry into system, 167–168
        answers to series of questions in, 168
        assessment of consultee and, 167
    professional liability insurance for, 170
    role as consultant vs. as psychiatrist, 167
    to schools, courts, and primary care, current trends in, 171–173
    training for, 173
Psychiatric consultation, case-based, 168–169
    confidentiality in, 166, 170–171
    conflict of interest in, 171
    consent in, 166, 170
    consultant roles in, 167, 171–173
    consultee-based, 168–169
    outcome measurement of, in schools, 170
        self-report data from administrators, teachers, students, 170
        through consultee feedback, 169
    professional and ethical issues in, 170

Psychiatrist as consultant, **165–176**
    in juvenile justice system, 166
    in primary care, 169–170
    in schools, 165–168, 170
Psychopharmacology update, child and adolescent, **111–133**
    for anxiety disorders, 118, 120–121
    for attention deficit hyperactivity disorder, 112–113
    for autism, 121–122
    for bipolar disorder, 117–119
    for disruptive behavior disorders, 114–115
    for major depressive disorder, 115–117
    for pervasive developmental disorders, 121–122
    for psychotic disorders, 122–124
Psychosocial therapies, by nonmedical professionals vs. psychiatrists, 218
Psychotic disorders, at-risk groups for, 84
    development over time, 87
    duration of untreated and outcome, 87–88
    early intervention in, **81–94**
        as prevention, 88
        benefits of, 86–89
        cognitive-behavioral therapy in, 89
        future directions of, 90–91
        identification of target population for, 89
        medications in, 90
        prospective MRI studies in, 90
        rate of conversion from ultra-high risk to psychosis with, 89
        risk factors for conversion to psychosis and, 90
    early intervention studies, of assertive care vs. standard care, 88–89
        reduction in duration of untreated psychosis, 88
    in velocardiofacial syndrome, 18
    Kelly case: first-break schizophrenia, 84–85
    Max case: marijuana and cocaine use as risk factors, 85–86
    Nick case, depression and anxiety at presentation, 82
        diagnosis of major depression and posttraumatic stress disorder, 82
    predictive symptoms of, 84
    prodromal period in, phases of, 83
        retrospective of, 83
        shift to prospective studies of at-risk patients, 83–85
    psychopharmacologic treatment of, 122–124
    risk factors for, trait (genetic) and state (functional decline), 84
    schizoaffective disorder. See *Schizoaffective disorder.*
    schizophrenia. See *Schizophrenia.*
    treatment/management of, of ultra-high risk population, 89

Q

Quetiapine (Seroquel), for aggression in disruptive behavior disorders, 115–116
    for autism, 7, 122
    for pervasive developmental disorders, 122
    for posttraumatic stress disorder, 120–121

R

Race, defined, 154
Rett's sydrome, 3
Risperidone, for aggression in disruptive behavior disorders, 115
    for autism, 7, 122
    for bipolar disorder, 117–119
    for pervasive developmental disorders, 122
    for psychotic disorders, 123
Rivastigmine, for Down syndrome, 24

S

Schizoaffective disorder, early-onset, 122
    in velocardiofacial syndrome, 18–19
    psychopharmacotherapy for, 123–124
Schizophrenia, cannabis use and, 86
    childhood onset, as neurodevelopmental vs. neurodegenerative disorder, 183–184, 190–191
    early intervention and prevention in, 191
    early-onset, 86, 122
    first-break, Kelly case, 84–85
        mood and anxiety symptoms in ultrahigh risk populations, 85
        prodromal symptoms in, 85
    in velocardiofacial syndrome, 18–19
    psychopharmacotherapy for, 123–124
    treatment-resistant, clozapine for, 123–124
        haloperidol and, 124
Selective serotonin reuptake inhibitors (SSRIs). See also *Antidepressants.*
    for anxiety disorders, 120
    for autism, 7, 121
    for obsessive-compulsive disorder, 120
    for pediatric autoimmune neuropsychiatric disorders associated with streptococcal infections, 64
    safety issues with, 116
Separation anxiety disorder (SAD), as risk factor for anxiety and depression in adulthood, 59
    clinical presentation of, 57–58
    course and outcome of, 58–59
    DSM-IV-TR criteria for youth, 58
    prevalence of, 58
Serious emotional disturbance (SED), definition of, 136–137
    prevalence of, 214
Serotonin transporter gene, as depression risk factor, 183
    in case presentation of Sarah, 202–203
Sertraline, in autism, 121
Sex chromosome aneuploidy, in men, 47,XYY karyotype, 28
        48,XYY karyotype, 28
Sleep disturbance, in bipolar disorder, 75
Social deficits, in fragile X syndrome (FXS), 21

Social phobia, comobidity in, 61
   course and outcome, 61
   DSM-IV-TR criteria for youth, 58, 60–61
Somatoform disorders, cognitive-behavioral therapy for, 105
Stimulant medication, for ADHD, 45–46
     adverse effects of, 49–50
     cardiac events and, 113
     in adolescents, 52
   for autism, 7
   selection of, 46
Storytelling therapy, culturally adapted forms of, 159
Stress, HPA axis and, 191
   locus ceruleus/noradrenergic sympathetic system and, 191
   neurodevelopment and, 191
Substance dependence, social phobia and, 61
Suicidal adolescent, dialectical behavior therapy for, 102–105
Suicidality, atomoxetin and, 51
   with SSRIs, 116
System of care programs, community-based services in, 137–138
   family-driven care in, 138
   wraparound approach in, historical context of, 135–138
   youth-guided care in, 138

T

Topiramate, for bipolar disorder, 117–118
Tricyclic antidepressants, for pediatric depression, 115
Turner's syndrome (TS), behavioral phenotype in, 26
   brain neuroimaging findings in, 26–27
   in girls, 25–26
   neurocognitive phenotype in, 26
   physical characteristics of, 25

V

Velocardiofacial syndrome (VCFS) (22q11.2 deletion syndrome), 16
   as risk factor for schizophrenia, 16, 17
   cognitive disabilities in, 17
   congenital medical defects in, 16–17
   laboratory diagnosis of, 17
   psychiatric symptoms in, 17–18
Venlafaxine, for anxiety disorders, 120

W

Wraparound approach, applications of, 145–145
   as team process, 139–140
   case examples of, ADHD, 141–142
     behavior and mood problems, 142–143
   Center for Mental Health Services and, 136
   Child and Adolescent Service System Program and, 135–136

child in, 139
comparison with intensive community-based interventions, intensive case
    management, 145–146
    multidimensional treatment foster care, 145
    multisystemic therapy, 143–145
Comprehensive Community Services for Children and Youth and Their Families and,
    136
defined, 138
essential elements of, 138–139
evidence base in, 143
family partner in, 139–140
future research and implentation of, 147
historical context of, 135–138
in systems of care, **135–151**
intensive community-based interventions, evidence supporting, 145
limitations of, 146
    access to, 146
    administrative issues, 146
    lack of manuals for, 146
    natural or informal community-based supports in, 141
    network of supportive relationships in, 141
    phases in, 140
    population selection for, 145–146
    studies of, 143

Z

Ziprasidone, for autism and pervasive developmental disorders, 122

Related Interest:

Child and Adolescent Psychiatry Clinics of North America
Eating Disorders and Obesity, January 2009
Beate Herpertz-Dahlmann, MD and Johannes Hebebrand, MD, Guest Editors

Section I: Diagnostic Concerns

1. Diagnostic Issues in Eating Disorders and Obesity, Johannes Hebebrand, MD

2. Eating Disorders of Infancy and Childhood: Definition, symptomatology, epidemiology and comorbidity, Dasha Nicholls and Rachel Bryant-Waugh

3. Adolescent Eating Disorders: Definitions, Symptomatology, Epidemiology and Comorbidity, Beate Herpertz-Dahlmann

4. Psychological and Psychiatric Aspects of Pediatric Obesity, Johannes Hebebrand and Beate Herpertz-Dahlmann

Section II: Etiologic and Neurobiologic Findings

5. Environmental and genetic risk factors for eating disorders: What the clinician needs to know, Suzanne E. Mazzeo, PhD and Cynthia M. Bulik, PhD

6. Environmental and genetic risk factors in obesity, Johannes Hebebrand and Anke Hinney

7. Neuroimaging in eating disorders and obesity: Implications for research, Dr Frederique Van den Eynde & Professor Janet Treasure

8. Leptin mediated neuroendocrine alterations in anorexia nervosa: somatic and behavioural implications, Timo D. Müller, Manuel Föcker, Kristian Holtkamp, Beate Herpertz-Dahlmann, Johannes Hebebrand

Section III: Treatment Modalities

9. Overview of Treatment Modalities in Adolescent Anorexia Nervosa, Beate Herpertz-Dahlmann and Harriet Salbach-Andrae

10. Cognitive Behavioral Approaches in Adolescent Anorexia and Bulimia Nervosa, U. Schmidt

11. Family Interventions in Adolescent Anorexia Nervosa, Daniel le Grange, PhD, and Ivan Eisler, PhD

12. Pharmacotherapy for Eating Disorders and Obesity, Pauline S. Powers

13. Evidence-based behavioral treatment of obesity in children and adolescents, Dr Laura Stewart and Professor John J Reilly

14. Preventing Eating Disorders, Heather Shaw, Eric Stice, and Carolyn Black Becker

15. Obesity prevention in children and adolescents, Boyd Swinburn

16. Outcome of eating disorders, Hans-Christoph Steinhausen

Moving?

Make sure your subscription moves with you!

To notify us of your new address, find your **Clinics Account Number** (located on your mailing label above your name), and contact customer service at:

E-mail: elspcs@elsevier.com

800-654-2452 (subscribers in the U.S. & Canada)
314-453-7041 (subscribers outside of the U.S. & Canada)

Fax number: 314-523-5170

Elsevier Periodicals Customer Service
11830 Westline Industrial Drive
St. Louis, MO 63146

*To ensure uninterrupted delivery of your subscription, please notify us at least 4 weeks in advance of move.